Surgery for Crohn's Disease

Second Edition

nova
Medicine & Health
New York

Digestive Diseases - Research and Clinical Developments

More information about this series can be found at
https://novapublishers.com/product-category/series/digestive-diseases-research-and-clinical-developments/

Surgery - Procedures, Complications, and Results

More information about this series can be found at
https://novapublishers.com/product-category/series/surgery-procedures-complications-and-results/

Stephen M. Kavic
Rebecca Brown
Kerri Lopez
Editors

Surgery for Crohn's Disease

Second Edition

nova
Medicine & Health
New York

DOI: https://doi.org/10.52305/NYLW2724

Library of Congress Cataloging-in-Publication Data

ISBN: 979-8-89530-676-5 (Hardcover)
ISBN: 979-8-89530-739-7 (eBook)

Published by Nova Science Publishers, Inc. † New York

To my loving wife, Jennifer, and my lovely daughter, Emily.
Stephen M. Kavic

To my patients, who trust me at their most vulnerable moments,
my mentors, who still "talk" to me in the OR, and my family,
who continue to support this ongoing journey.
Rebecca Brown

To my wonderful husband and our spectacular little sons.
Kerri Lopez

Contents

Preface

Welcome to the second edition of *Surgery for Crohn's Disease.*

Crohn's Disease can be a devastating disorder. It afflicts people in their prime, often crossing the border of adolescence into adulthood. Crucially, it interferes with eating, which is supposed to be one of the great joys in life.

Surgery for Crohn's disease is challenging. Ideally, those operating on patients with this problem have a deep understanding of the process, as well as good relationships with the gastroenterologists and primary care physicians who diagnose and initiate therapy for these patients.

The initial edition of this book was borne out of frustration for not having one reference to help guide the surgeon. In the ten years since its initial publication, there have been significant advances in the medical management of patients with Crohn's disease. However, there have also been novel surgical approaches, some of which may supplant the current standard of care. This new edition has been thoroughly revised and updated to reflect these changes.

The format of the book has also changed. We have divided the book into three sections, based on a surgical perspective. The first section is on medical management, including diagnosis, nutritional support, medical therapy, and endoscopy. The second section concentrates on surgery, from preoperative optimization to dealing with Crohn's disease in all portions of the gastrointestinal tract. The third and final section discusses postoperative care, including complications, short bowel syndrome, and surveillance.

This book includes chapters written by gastroenterologists and surgeons, residents, fellows, and attendings, because it takes all of us to counter such a wily foe. It has been said that "we are all preop for something." If that something happens to be Crohn's disease, we hope this book prepares you for it.

Editors' Note

There is a movement in medicine to eliminate the possessive from eponyms. In this case, the preferred term may be Crohn disease, rather than Crohn's disease.

However, there has been markedly uneven acceptance of this. Literature searches curiously show more "hits" for "Crohn's" instead of "Crohn." As such, we have retained the possessive form in the title and the text.

Given how common the term is referred to in this text, we have consistently used the abbreviation "CD."

Section I. Medical Therapy

Chapter 1

Crohn's Disease: History, Epidemiology, and Etiology

Leyla J. Ghazi*, MD
Concord Hospital Gastroenterology, Concord, New Hampshire, USA

Abstract

Crohn's disease is a chronic, inflammatory bowel disease characterized by periods of relapsing symptoms. The disease received its eponym in 1932, but its existence probably dates back hundreds of years. Millions of people suffer from Crohn's disease, and its incidence is on the rise. Crohn's disease is an immune-mediated phenomenon, and its true etiology remains obscure. However, there has been increasing research that demonstrates the importance of genetic factors such as *NOD2/CARD15*, environmental factors, and alterations in the immune system itself.

History

Crohn's disease is a chronic inflammatory bowel disease (IBD) characterized by periods of relapsing symptoms caused by immune-mediated inflammation. The eponym "Crohn's disease" (CD) was adopted after a landmark *JAMA* publication by Crohn, Ginzberg, and Oppenheimer in 1932, which documented 'terminal ileitis' as an objective finding [1] (see Figure 1.1). However, clinicopathologic descriptions of similar processes date back to 1761 when Morgagni described chronic intestinal inflammation [2]. Subsequently, there were published case reports of intestinal inflammatory processes in the medical and surgical literature by Fenwick (1889), Dalziel (1913), Weiner (1914), and Muschowitz and Wilensky (1923) [2, 3]. After the identification of tuberculosis by Koch in 1882, the similarities between CD and intestinal tuberculosis became clear; nonetheless, the lack of tubercle bacillus distinguished these diagnoses.

Lockhart-Mummery and Morson ultimately described granulomatous colitis, and the disease process was understood to affect the large bowel and have distinguishing features compared to ulcerative colitis (UC) [4, 5]. Fistulization was also reported as a common manifestation. In 1938, Penner noted eight of fifty patients (16%) had perianal fistula as an early manifestation of ileal disease, some without preexisting luminal symptoms [6]. Thus, by the end of the 1930's, CD was recognized to present over almost all of the lower GI tract, and with major manifestations of stricture, perforation, and fistula.

* Corresponding Author's Email: ljghazi@crhc.org

In: Surgery for Crohn's Disease. Second Edition
Editors: Stephen M. Kavic, Rebecca Brown and Kerri Lopez
ISBN: 979-8-89530-676-5

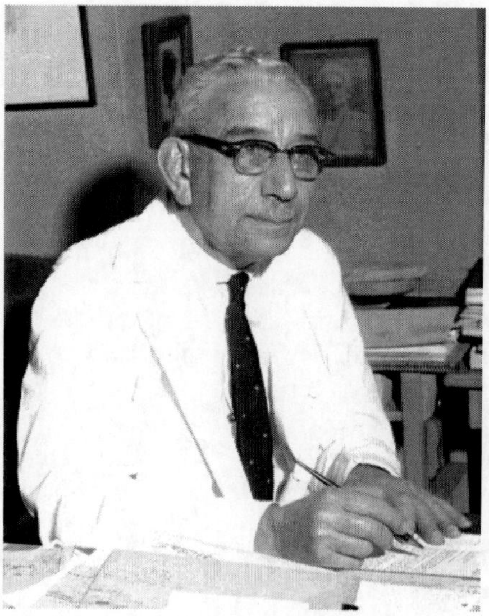

Figure 1.1. Burrill B. Crohn (Courtesy of Mt. Sinai archives).

Early on, the treatment algorithm involved primarily operative intervention. The most common procedures were fecal diversion, ileal resection, and closure of perianal and rectovaginal fistulas. Since that time, the development of targeted anti-inflammatory medications has allowed surgery for CD to become more refined, employing a variety of surgical techniques. For instance, surgical bypass was replaced by resection for stricturing and inflammatory phenotypes. The principle of bowel preservation to avoid short bowel syndrome became an important consideration, and led to the adoption of small bowel strictureplasty when feasible [7]. Most recently, the incorporation of laparoscopy and other minimally invasive approaches has reduced length of hospital study and accelerated recovery time.

However, early case reports documented patients with anastomotic recurrence and stricture formation after surgery [4]. With the recognition and further support of the chronic and recurrent nature of the disease, there were attempts to treat the disease by both medical and surgical methods. Initial medical therapies included antibacterial and anti-tuberculous drugs, Dakin's solution, anti-dysentery serum, *Escherichia coli* vaccine, and anti-amoebic drugs [2]. Given the lack of success, the use of these drugs was mostly abandoned.

Sulfasalazine was deemed the first effective agent in IBD when it was discovered that it resolved both diarrhea and arthralgias in patients with UC and joint inflammation. In the 1970's, further experimentation revealed that the active moiety of sulfasalazine was 5-aminosalicylate (5-ASA) [8]. Additionally, therapeutic agents that targeted immune-mediated activation of inflammation were subsequently developed. Corticosteroids were proven to be highly effective in treating IBD [9]. Nevertheless, later studies have shown that they are associated with a worse overall prognosis, including increased risk of surgery and risk of disability [10].

As a result, immunomodulatory agents such as 6-mercaptopurine (6MP)/azathioprine and methotrexate were deemed effective for the maintenance of remission for steroid-refractory or steroid-dependent CD [11-13]. Highly effective biologic therapies, such as anti-tumor necrosis factor-α (anti-TNF-α), anti-α4B7 integrin antibody, interleukin (IL)-12/23 blockers, JAK inhibitors, and S1PR modulators have been studied in multicenter trials and FDA approved for the treatment of IBD.

Epidemiology

Epidemiologic data of the incidence and prevalence of CD is impacted by a lack of a diagnostic gold standard. For instance, for those patients suffering with colitis, there is broad overlap between ulcerative colitis and CD. In some cases, there is no conclusive decision even after pathologic analysis of a colectomy specimen, leading to the diagnosis of "indeterminate colitis." Indeterminate colitis may be the final diagnosis in up to 15% of patients, which highlights our difficulty in defining treatment for CD specifically.

In addition, there is a reliance on data from large referral centers. Population-based studies of disease are made possible by centers worldwide that utilize a universal health care system. In the United States, centers that have a medical healthcare linkage system often publish the largest series, but this may represent a skewed fraction of the Crohn's population as a whole.

The prevalence of CD in the United States was previously estimated to be about 200 per 100,000 adults, and 40 per 100,000 children and adolescents [14]. Based on this study, approximately 1 to 1.5 million Americans live with IBD in the United States. However, the burden of IBD and CD has increased. A recent Lancet population-based study in 2020 reported the highest prevalence values are in Europe and North America (UC: 286 per 100,000 in the USA; CD: 319 per 100,000 in Canada) [15]. CD affects women and men nearly equally (1.3:1 female:male ratio). CD is most often diagnosed in persons between 15 and 30 years of age, with a second peak in those in the sixth and seventh decade of life. Population-based studies have shown the median age of diagnosis to be approximately 30 years. Differences in clinical presentation among younger and older patients suggest that risk factors for the development of disease are different in each age group.

There are also racial differences that have been observed in IBD. Early on, it was assumed that CD was a disease of Caucasians. In the 1930s, terminal ileitis was recognized as a non-specific granulomatous infection in younger, Jewish patients. Since 2005, increasing numbers of published studies have demonstrated that between 10 – 40% of CD patients are African-American. These studies tend to focus on another important aspect, that of racial disparities. For example, one large multicenter analysis found a lower rate of surgery among African-Americans compared to Caucasians; this racial difference persisted after adjustment for disease behavior and location [16]. Other studies, however, have identified similar [17, 18], or even increased rates of surgery when comparing races [19].

Numerous epidemiological studies have been done worldwide to elucidate the incidence and prevalence of IBD. It has been hoped that a better understanding of the epidemiology may help researchers to identify the causal mechanisms of CD. For instance, geographical and temporal trends in incidence of CD have been observed [20]. IBD centers in the northern latitudes of Europe have described an increase in the rate of CD compared to those in the south [21-24]. A north-south gradient has also been reported in the United States [25]. Although this trend is clear, its significance remains obscure.

Incidence rates of CD have stabilized in some regions [25, 26], but the incidence has continued to rise in others, such as Denmark, Scotland, and Spain [25, 27, 28]. Sometimes, this rise is dramatic. For example, in Olmstead County, Minnesota, the incidence of CD steadily increased from 3 per 100,000 (1954-63) to 8 per 100,000 (1964-1973). However, from 2000 to 2005, this region had over a 22% increase in the prevalence of CD [29].

In Asia, the incidence of CD is low, ranging from 0.5 to 1.3 per 100,000 persons in China and Japan. However, the incidence may be rising in parallel with socioeconomic development [30, 31]. Conversely, in Australia, the incidence is 14 per 100,000 [31]. Although CD is a rare diagnosis in South America, Asia and Africa, the incidence has been rising in these newly industrialized countries since the 1990's [15, 20].

Etiology

The exact cause of CD remains unknown. In 1937, Jackman described four possible causal factors including anatomical peculiarities, accidental, neuromuscular or inflammatory causes (4). Today, we group the mechanisms for the development of chronic inflammation process into three broad categories: environmental, genetic, and immunological causes (see Figure 1.2).

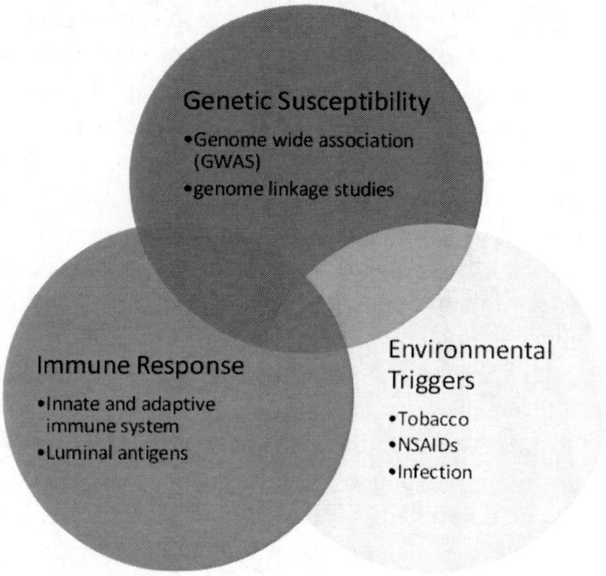

Figure 1.2. Model for pathogenesis of inflammatory bowel disease.

Genetic Factors

Genetics are known to play a role in the susceptibility to IBD. The major identified risk factor for IBD is a family history. Although IBD susceptibility genes involve all populations and ethnicities, the risk is higher in individuals of Ashkenazi Jewish background [32]. Further evidence of a genetic basis comes from twin studies, where a high concordance for CD among monozygotic twins have been observed. Monozygotic twin concordance rates range from 20 to 50% for CD [33]. Siblings of patients with Crohn's have a 30-fold increased risk of developing the disease compared to the general population.

The strong familial clustering stimulated researchers to search for IBD susceptibility genes in the late 1990s. Several mechanisms for gene mapping have been utilized, including candidate and whole genome linkage studies, as well as genome-wide association studies (GWAS) which investigates the entire human genome by testing upwards of 1,000,000 single nucleotide polymorphisms (SNPs) [34].

The first IBD gene linked to CD was the *NOD2/CARD15* gene on chromosome 16, associated with the IBD1 locus [34-37]. *NOD2* mediates signals of innate immunity from bacteria [38]. Specific gene mutations have been associated with distinct Crohn's characteristics. To date, *NOD2* has been associated with ileal disease location and stricturing phenotype [34]. The National Institutes of Health (NIH) National Institute of Diabetes and Digestive and Kidney Diseases (NIDDK) IBD Genetics Consortium has identified several other susceptibility genes including but not limited to *ATG16L1*, *CARD9*, *IRGM*, *ITLN1* and *IL23R* for CD [34]. *NOD2/CARD15* and *CARD9* are genes associated with molecular pattern recognition of pathogens, *ATG161* and *IRGM* are associated with autophagy (i.e., cellular recycling), and *IL23R* is associated with lymphocyte differentiation. However, the implications of molecular genetics for predicting disease course, genetic counseling, and therapeutic targeting is still under investigation.

Environmental Factors

Environmental influences have long been suspected of playing a role in the pathogenesis of IBD. The human gut microbiota is a complex ecosystem that is composed of mainly bacteria and other microbes such as fungi, parasites, and viruses responsible for maintaining homeostasis. Previously accepted theories for the development of IBD include the notion that mucosal inflammation was a response to pathogenic organisms [39]. There continues to be interest in the hypothesis that gut dysbiosis can result in the immune dysregulation associated with IBD. Potential pathogenic candidates have included *Escherichia coli* (*E. Coli*), *Bacteroides, Enterobacteriaceae family, Fusobacterium varium*, and *Mycobacterium paratuberculosis* (MAP) among many others [40, 41]. Although unproven, even normal flora may also contribute to the pathogenesis of IBD.

The causal role of Mycobacteria, especially MAP, in CD remains controversial. Studies have recovered the DNA of the organism in inflamed and non-inflamed intestinal samples. In Manitoba, Canada, where there is high prevalence of MAP, MAP was not serologically associated with CD [42]. Furthermore, anti-mycobacterial therapy does not appear to be effective in the treatment of CD [43]. Despite lack of strong evidence for a causal link between MAP and CD, the possibility of an association has not been definitively excluded, and further therapeutic studies are ongoing [44].

An additional element to the microbiome theories is that of timing. It has been postulated that the exposure to an organism may occur in childhood. The autoimmune response, on the other hand, begins its macroscopic destructive effects only after puberty. The delayed presentation of the response may explain why it has been so difficult to establish a definitive link between pathogen and the disease process.

The hygiene hypothesis has also been proposed to explain the rise in IBD in the 20th century. The hypothesis is that early exposure to certain antigens and infections may be ultimately protective. In the current climate, children may be subject to overly hygienic environments, which may negatively impact immune development, and in turn lead to autoimmune diseases such as IBD. Population-based studies from Canada have been supportive of this theory [34].

In a similar vein, lack of exposure to intestinal helminths has been associated with the development of IBD. The prevalence of IBD in Africa where helminth infections are common is low. Furthermore, there is evidence that luminal exposure to ova from the porcine whipworm, *Trichuris suis*, was effective in improving symptoms of active CD [45]. The response rates are relatively high nearing 80% without significant adverse events. Helminths may offer patients a novel therapy and supports the notion of the hygiene hypothesis.

Antibiotics have long been accepted to have short term efficacy for the treatment of luminal and perianal disease [46-47]. Studies have also shown the beneficial effect of antibiotics when used to prevent anastomotic recurrence [48]. Experiments in the 1980s done in surgically diverted Crohn's patients suggested that luminal bacteria were a cause of anastomotic recurrence, based on observations that diverted patients had quiescent disease [49]. The efficacy of antimicrobials and diversion provides strong but indirect evidence of the importance of gut organisms in the development and subsequent course of CD.

Other environmental factors have been noted to affect the expression and/or progression of IBD. For example, a prior history of appendectomy has also been recognized as a risk factor for the development of CD [50]. An additional important factor is tobacco use [51]. The mechanism of the effect of smoking on mucosal inflammation is unclear. Nicotine may have negative effects on cell-mediated immunity or alter mucosal secretory functions [52]. Smoking has been consistently associated with increased risk of CD [52], but is curiously protective for UC. Women smokers appear to have a greater risk of developing severe course compared to their male counterparts [45]. The effect is not permanent, as individuals who stop smoking reduce their risk [52].

Nonsteroidal anti-inflammatory drugs (NSAIDs) also play a role in the progression of CD [53]. The exact mechanism of NSAID-induced exacerbations of IBD is not clear. These agents block prostaglandin production, alter immune reactivity, and increase intestinal permeability [54], which may factor in to the clinical Crohn's flare.

Immune Response and Inflammation

The normal state of intestinal immunity requires immune tolerance. Immunologic tolerance is made possible by a wide variety of cell types that regulate the immune response. Further, the luminal milieu is important. Luminal antigens and genetic factors can predispose individuals to an abnormal immune response to the flora. Normal individuals can appropriately regulate insults to the intestinal lumen and downregulate inflammation. In individuals susceptible to IBD, these same insults can lead to a state of uncontrolled and chronic inflammation.

Host-microbial interactions may be mediated by the innate immune system, that which is essential for host defense. Pathogens can activate host defenses and trigger a cascade of events that can also initiate the adaptive immune system. Current advances in the recognition of Toll-like receptors (TLRs) and NOD-like receptors (NLRs) have clarified the mechanism by which innate immune system of normal intestine recognizes microbes. TLRs are known to play a protective role in intestinal homeostasis. Research has shown that certain TLRs are downregulated while others are activated in active CD [34]. Such observations may prove useful in drug development and therapeutic targeting.

In CD patients, T-cell activation appears to occur as a result of luminal antigens (the adaptive immune system). Differentiated T-cells produce Th1-type cytokines, interferon-γ (IFN), and tumor necrosis factor-α (TNF). Production of Th1 mediated cytokines such as interleukin (IL)-12 and 23 appear to play a role in IBD pathogenesis based upon experiments in murine models. Other animal models of IBD pathogenesis have included those with disturbed immune regulation involving interleukin (IL)-2, T-cell receptor α and IL-10 knockouts, as well as epithelial barrier dysfunction such as the G2αi knockout mouse [55]. The identification of immunologic pathways of the adaptive immune responses in CD has led to new and specific therapeutic agents that target different inflammatory pathways.

Conclusion

We have come a long way in our understanding of CD since Crohn first described terminal ileitis in 1932. We have increased our understanding that environmental, genetic, and immunological responses are responsible in varying degrees for the development of IBD. Unfortunately, much remains speculative, but powerful advances have allowed us to identify CD susceptibility genes. Understanding the complex mechanism of IBD pathogenesis including the interplay of innate and adaptive immunity, host-microbial interactions, and environmental triggers in a genetically susceptible host are important to help in the continued development of new therapeutic targets.

References

[1] Crohn BB, Ginzberg L, Oppenheimer GD. Regional ileitis, a pathological and clinical entity. *JAMA* 1932;99:1323-9.

[2] Kirsner, JB. Historical origins of current IBD concepts. *World J Gastroenterol* 2001;7:175-84.

[3] Dalziel TK. Chronic interstitial enteritis. *The British Medical Journal* 1913;2(2756):1069.

[4] Jackman WA. Terminal ileitis. *Proc R Soc Med* 1937; 30(6): 691–692.

[5] Lockhart-Mummery, HE, Morson, BC. Crohn's disease (regional enteritis) of the large intestine and its distinction from ulcerative colitis. *Gut* 1960;1:87-105.

[6] Penner A, and Crohn B. Perianal fistulae as complication of regional enteritis. *Ann Surg* 1938; 108(5): 867–873.

[7] Deutsch AA, Stern HS. Stapler stricturoplasty for Crohn's disease. *Surg Gynecol Obstet* 1989;169:458-60.

[8] Azad Khan AK, Piris J, Truelove SC. An experiment to determine the active therapeutic moiety of sulfasalazine. *Lancet* 1977;2:8925.

[9] Truelove SC, Jewell DP. Intensive intravenous regimen for severe attacks of ulcerative colitis. *Lancet* 1974;1:1067-70.

[10] Munkholm P, Langholz E, Davidsen M, Binder, V. Frequency of glucocorticoid resistance and dependency in Crohn's disease. *Gut* 1994;35:360-2.

[11] Present DH, Korelitz BI, Wisch N, et al. Treatment of Crohn's disease with 6-mercaptopurine. A long-term, randomized, double-blind study. *N Engl J Med* 1980;302:981-7.

[12] Feagan BG, Rochon J, Fedorak RN, et al. Methotrexate for the treatment of Crohn's disease. The North American Crohn's Study Group Investigators. *N Engl J Med* 1995;332:292-7.

[13] Feagan BG, Fedorak RN, Irvine EJ, et al. A comparison of methotrexate with placebo for the maintenance of remission in Crohn's disease. North American Crohn's Study Group Investigators. *N Engl J Med* 2000;342:1627-32.

[14] Kappelman MD, Rifas-Shiman L, Kleinman K. The prevalence and geographic distribution of Crohn's disease and ulcerative colitis in the United States. *Clinical Gastroenterol Hepatol* 2007;5:1424-29.

[15] Ng SC, Yun Shi H, Hamidi N et al. Worldwide incidence and prevalence of inflammatory bowel disease in the 21st century: a systematic review of population-based studies. *Lancet* 2020; 23;390(10114):2769-2778.

[16] Nguyen GC, Torres EA, Regueiro M, et al. Inflammatory bowel disease characteristics among African Americans, Hispanics, and Non-Hispanic Whites: characterization of a large North American cohort. *Am J Gastroenterol* 2006;101:1012-1023.

[17] Cross RK, Jung C, Wasan S, et al. Racial differences in disease phenotype in patients with Crohn's disease. *Inflamm Bowel Dis* 2006;12(3):192-198.

[18] Straus WL, Eisen GM, Sandler RS et al. Crohn's disease: does race matter? *Am J Gastroenterol* 2000;95(2):479-483.

[19] Goldman CD, Kodner IJ, Fry RD et al. Clinical and operative experience with non-Caucasian patients with Crohn's disease. *Dis Colon Rectum* 1986;29(5):317-21.

[20] Ng SC, Bernstein CN, Vatn MH. Geographical variability and environmental risk factors in inflammatory bowel disease. *Gut* 2013;62:630-649.

[21] Brahme F, Lindstrom C, Wenckert A. Crohn's disease in a defined population: an epidemiological study of incidence, prevalence, mortality, and secular trends in the city of Malmo, Sweden. *Gastroenterol* 1975;69:342–351.

[22] Munkholm P, Langholz E, Nielsen OH, et al. Incidence and prevalence of Crohn's disease in the county of Copenhagen, 1962–87: a sixfold increase in incidence. *Scand J Gastroenterol* 1992;27:609–614.

[23] Pinchbeck BR, Kirdeikis J, Thomson ABR. Inflammatory bowel disease in northern Alberta: an epidemiologic study. *J Clin Gastroenterol* 1988;10:505–515.

[24] Stowe SP, Redmonds SR, Stormont JM, et al. An epidemiologic study of inflammatory bowel disease in Rochester, New York: hospital incidence. *Gastroenterol* 1990;98:104–110.

[25] Loftus, EV, Silverstein MD, Sandborn WJ, et al. Crohn's Disease in Olmsted County, Minnesota, 1940–1993: Incidence, Prevalence, and Survival. *Gastroentol* 1998;114:1161–1168.

[26] Stowe SP, Redmonds SR, Stormont JM, et al. An epidemiologic study of inflammatory bowel disease in Rochester, New York: hospital incidence. *Gastroenterol* 1990;98:104–110.

[27] Barton JR, Gillon S, Ferguson A. Incidence of inflammatory bowel disease in Scottish children between 1968 and 1983; marginal fall in ulcerative colitis, three-fold rise in Crohn's disease. *Gut* 1989;30:618–622.

[28] Trallori G, Palli D, Saieva C, et al. A population-based study of inflammatory bowel disease in Florence over 15 years (1978– 92). *Scand J Gastroenterol* 1996;31:892–899.

[29] Loftus EV. Editorial: The burden of inflammatory bowel disease in the United States: A moving target? *Clinical Gastro Hepatol* 2007;5:1383-84. 22.

[30] Ng SC. Epidemiology of inflammatory bowel disease: Focus on Asia. *Best Practice & Res Clinical Gastroenterol* 2014;28:363–372.

[31] Ng SC, Tang W, Ching JY. Incidence and phenotype of inflammatory bowel disease based on results from the Asia-pacific Crohn's and colitis epidemiology study. *Gastroenterol.* 2013;145(1):158-165.

[32] Yang H, McElree C, Roth MP. Familial empirical risks for inflammatory bowel disease: differences between Jews and non-Jews. *Gut* 1993;34:517-24.

[33] Tysk C, Lindberg E, Jarnerot G. Ulcerative colitis and Crohn's disease in an unselected population of monozygotic and dizygotic twins. A study of heritability and the influence of smoking. *Gut* 1988;29:990-6.

[34] Bayless TM and Hanauer SB. Advances in Therapy in Inflammatory Bowel Disease: Volume 1, Chapter 10 and 11: IBD Pathogenesis and Genetics. Pg 63-76.

[35] Hugot JP, Laurent-Puig P, Gower-Rousseau C, et al. Mapping of a susceptibility locus for Crohn's disease on chromosome 16. *Nature*1996; 379: 821–23.

[36] Hugot JP, Chamaillard M, Zouali H, et al. Association of NOD2 leucine-rich repeat variants with susceptibility to Crohn's disease. *Nature* 2001;411: 599–603.

[37] Ogura Y, Bonen DK, Inohara N, et al. A frameshift mutation in *Nod2* associated with susceptibility to Crohn's disease. *Nature* 2001;411: 603–06.

[38] Girardin SE, Hugot JP, Sansonetti PJ. Lessons from Nod2 studies: towards a link between Crohn's disease and bacterial sensing. *Trends Immunol.* 2003;24:652–8.

[39] Podolsky DK. Inflammatory bowel disease. *N Engl J Med.* 2002;347:417–29.

[40] Cammarota G, Ianiro G, Rossella C et al. The involvement of gut microbiota in inflammatory bowel disease pathogenesis: Potential for therapy. *Pharmacology and Thera* 2015.

[41] Hermon-Taylor J, Bull T. Crohn's disease caused by *Mycobacterium avium* subspecies *paratuberculosis*: a public health tragedy whose resolution is long overdue. *J Med Microbiol.* 2002;51:3–6.

[42] Bernstein CN, Blanchard JF, Rawsthorne P et al. Population-based case control study of seroprevalence of Mycobacterium paratuberculosis in patients with Crohn's disease and ulcerative colitis. *J Clin Microbiol* 2004;42(3):1129-1135.

[43] Selby W, Pavli P, Crotty B et al. Antibiotics in Crohn's disease Study Group. Two-year combination antibiotic therapy with clarithromycin, rifabutin, and clofazimine for Crohn's disease. *Gastroenterol* 2007;132(7):2313-2319.

[44] Sartor B. Does Mycobacterium avium subspecies paratuberculosis cause Crohn's disease? *Gut* 2005;54:896-898.

[45] Summers RW, Eilliott DE, Urban JF Jr. Trichuris suis therapy in Crohn's disease. *Gut* 2008;57(1):87-90.

[46] Sutherland L, Singleton J, Sessions J, et al. Double blind, placebo controlled trial of metronidazole in Crohn's disease. *Gut* 1991;32:1071-1075.

[47] Thia KT, Mahadevan U, Feagan BG. Ciprofloxacin or metronidazole for the treatment of perianal fistulas in patients with Crohn's disease: a randomized, double-blind, placebo-controlled pilot study. *Inflamm Bowel Dis.* 2009;15(1):17-24.

[48] Swoger J, Regueiro M. Preventive therapy in postoperative Crohn's disease. *Current Opinion in Gastroenterol* 2010;26(4):337–343.

[49] Rutgeerts P, Goboes K, Peeters M et al. Effect of fecal stream diversion on recurrence of Crohn's disease in the neoterminal ileum. *Lancet* 1991;338:771–4.

[50] Andersson RE, Olaison G, Tysk C. Appendectomy is followed by increased risk of Crohn's disease. l F., Beaugerie L. Effects of cigarette smoking on the long-term course of Crohn's disease. *Gastroenterol* 1996;110(2):424–431.

[51] Odes HS, Fich A, Reif S, et al. Effects of current cigarette smoking on clinical course of Crohn's disease and ulcerative colitis. *Dig Dis Sci.* 2001;46:1717–21.

[52] Cosnes J, Beaugerie L, Carbonnel F, et al. Smoking cessation and the course of Crohn's disease: an intervention study. *Gastroenterol* 2001;120:1093–9.

[53] Bjarnason I, Zanelli G, Smith T, et al. Nonsteroidal anti-inflammatory drug-induced intestinal inflammation in humans. *Gastroenterol* 1987;93:480–9.

[54] Cipolla G, Crema F, Sacco S. Nonsteroidal anti-inflammatory drugs and inflammatory bowel disease: current perspectives. *Pharmacol Res* 2002;46(1):1-6.

[55] Sands BE. Inflammatory bowel disease: past, present, and future. *J Gastroenterol* 2007;42:16-25.

Chapter 2

Diagnosis of Crohn's Disease

Joseph Clinton[1], MD
and Lauren George[2,*], MD
[1]University of Maryland Medical Center, Baltimore, Maryland, USA
[2]University of Maryland School of Medicine, Baltimore, Maryland, USA

Abstract

Crohn's disease (CD) has the potential to involve any part of the gastrointestinal tract and may have variable symptoms and timing of the disease process. These factors combine to make Crohn's one of the more difficult diagnoses for physicians to make on initial presentation. Before arriving at a diagnosis, many patients will visit multiple physicians, and undergo a variety of cross-sectional imaging and other tests.
Clinical signs and symptoms are non-specific, and typically involve abdominal pain and altered bowel habits. Laboratory markers have also been non-specific, with elevations in erythrocyte sedimentation rate, C-reactive protein, antibodies, and serologic testing all available as options. Genetic testing remains in its infancy. Imaging modalities are evolving as a useful tool in diagnosis and disease activity assessment. However, endoscopy remains the core tool for diagnosis, as it also permits biopsy. We present here the consensus diagnostic criteria for Crohn's disease, as well as the relative value of each testing modality in establishing the diagnosis.

Presentation and Symptoms

Crohn's disease (CD) is inflammatory bowel disease that is characterized by the potential to cause transmural inflammation of any part of the gastrointestinal (GI) tract. Generally, a patient's symptoms are related to the location of inflammation within the GI tract, the severity of inflammatory burden, the presence and degree of fibrosis and the depth of bowel wall involvement of the inflammatory process. Given these variables, it is not surprising that the clinical presentation of CD can be protean.

The disease onset can also be rather insidious, with wide between-patient variations in the time-points of onset of pathology, clinical symptoms and eventual disease diagnosis. Because of the wide range of symptoms, and timing of symptoms, there are no universally accepted

---

* Corresponding Author's Email: Lauren.george@som.umaryland.edu

In: Surgery for Crohn's Disease. Second Edition
Editors: Stephen M. Kavic, Rebecca Brown and Kerri Lopez
ISBN: 979-8-89530-676-5

objective diagnostic criteria for Crohn's disease. As a result, patients with milder and less-specific symptoms may go un-diagnosed or mis-diagnosed for some time.

The classically described CD patient is a young adult Caucasian smoker who presents with diarrhea, abdominal pain and weight loss. However, as epidemiologic studies have included more representative population samples, it has become clear that the incidence and prevalence of CD cuts across racial, age, and ethnic delineations [1]. Nonetheless, classic referral and population-based studies of patients with CD note that diarrhea and abdominal pain are the most common symptoms at presentation. Other common symptoms may be unintentional weight loss and objective fever [2-4]. The most common symptoms at presentation, then, are non-specific.

The presentation and specific nature of diarrhea may be protracted and reflect several overlapping pathophysiologic mechanisms. A given patient may present with subtle changes in bowel movement frequency, consistency or urgency. The spectrum can range from large volume diarrhea with malabsorption, to incontinence, or occasional nocturnal defecation.

Due to the capability of CD to be transmural, fibrosis with strictures in the bowel can occur with resultant barodynamic changes across the stenosed segments, more commonly in the small bowel than the colon. While such strictures can be clinically silent, they often lead to symptoms of bowel obstruction. The presentations can be varied, with acute partial, acute complete, chronic intermittent or chronic partial presentations. Nausea, vomiting, and bloating are often present, depending on severity of the fibrotic lesion. Given the relative frequency of distal ileal involvement, patients most often report right lower quadrant abdominal pain [5].

Abdominal pain often occurs regardless of disease location and is usually described as crampy. Interestingly, colonic involvement is less often associated with classic abdominal pain. When a patient with Crohn's colitis has pain, it is typically described as a dull ache.

If the colon is not involved, overt bleeding is less common that in ulcerative colitis (UC) [6]. However occult blood loss manifesting as iron-deficiency anemia is commonly seen. Weight loss is usually multifactorial with malabsorption, maldigestion, decreased oral intake due to post prandial symptoms and catabolic inflammatory state all playing a role. Growth failure noted at the time of diagnosis is common, reportedly seen in 10-51% of children [7].

More specific signs and symptoms of CD (abdominal abscess, perianal or internal fistula, extra-intestinal manifestations) are seen far less frequently, and as such are far less sensitive (Figure 2.1). In addition, their frequency is less consistent between population and referral-based analyses owing to biases inherent in referral populations. Individual patients, however, present with signs and symptoms that can be quite variable. Patients often have symptoms for many years before diagnosis, especially if older in age at onset, or those carrying a pre-existing diagnosis of irritable bowel syndrome [6, 8, 9]. When present, gastroduodenal CD presents with upper abdominal pain and symptoms of gastric-outlet obstruction or rarely with fistula [10, 11].

Oral presentations of Crohn's disease are rare but have a defined constellation of symptoms. Oral Crohn's usually manifests as symptoms of sitopobia (food aversion) and/or mouth pain with erosions and/or ulcers of the gums. Patients are universally symptomatic with complaints of dysphagia, odynophagia, heartburn and/or chest pain [12].

It is relatively unusual for CD to have an initial presentation requiring surgery, though such patients certainly have been described. While appendiceal Crohn's has been described in as many as 0.55% of appendectomy specimens, it remains quite rare clinically [13]. Far more common is the 'appendicitis-like' presentation. In these cases, the patient with an acute abdomen is felt to have appendicitis based on clinical presentation. However, the intraoperative finding is significant terminal ileal inflammation from previously undiagnosed CD, and the adjacent appendix is involved only secondarily. This scenario was reported by the Lahey Clinic in 2.5% of 1,421 of their patients undergoing surgery for acute appendicitis [14].

Symptom	Frequency (%)			
	NCCDS*[2] N = 1084	ECCDS*[3] N = 452	Munkholm, et al.‡[4] N = 373	Vavricka, et al.‡[16] N = 950
Diarrhea	92	79	73	
Abdominal Pain	95	70	82	
Weight loss	85	32	56	
Fever	56	16	40	
Bleeding	61		36	
Perianal disease	36	22	4	
Extra-perianal fistula	21	7	14	
Arthritis	19		11	33 (5.7 AS)
Oral Aphthae				10
Abdominal mass		22		
Intra-abdominal abscess			12	
Any EIM		24		
Iritis/uveitis	4		4	6% uveitis
Hepatobiliary	4			0.7% PSC
Skin	5		3	1.5 PG 6 EN

* referral-based cohort.
‡ population-based cohort.
NCCDS- National Cooperative Crohn's Disease Study.
ECCDS- European Cooperative Crohn's Disease Study.
AS- Ankylosing spondylitis.
EIM- Extra-intestinal manifestation.
PG- Pyoderma gangrenosum.
EN- Erythema nodosum.

Figure 2.1. Clinical presenting signs and symptoms in patients with Crohn's disease.

Intra-abdominal or psoas abscess presentations are unusual, though CD accounts for nearly half of all psoas abscess presentations. One report noted 11 of 46 presenting CD cases had psoas abscesses, though most did not require emergent surgery. Patients with Crohn's can present already with a surgically diagnosed and managed perforating complication at the time of diagnosis. One case series review reported that 25 of the 84 free perforations in the literature to-date was the presenting disease manifestation [15]. Most specialists, however, feel that this statistic is an overestimation of complication frequency.

All of the features of Crohn's disease can be seen in other diseases (i.e., granulomas on biopsy, regional bowel inflammation, etc.,) which creates a broad clinical differential (Figure 2.2). Unfortunately, as there is no single diagnostic test adequately sensitive or specific for CD, the diagnosis of Crohn's disease is made via the constellation of supporting clinical, radiologic, endoscopic and pathologic features [16, 17].

The classic Lennard-Jones criteria (Figure 2.3) attempted to set objective diagnostic parameters, though this has evolved to a less stringent set of diagnostic criteria commonly used today. These 'diagnostic criteria' are an amalgam of clinical, endoscopic, radiologic and histologic results supporting CD and refuting alternative diagnoses serve as the current benchmark in clinical studies and practice guidelines in supporting a diagnosis of CD (Figure 2.4) [16, 18-20].

Etiology	Specific entity
Bacterial infection	Actinomyces spp. Aeromonas spp. Campylobacter spp. Clostridium difficile Salmonella spp. Shigella spp. Escheria coli (EHEC, EAEC). Yersinia spp. Mycobacterium spp.
Fungal infection	Cryptococcus neoformans Histoplasma capsulatum
Parasitic infection	Giardia lamblia Schistosomiasis Amebiasis
Viral colitis	HSV CMV
Viral gastroenteritis	Adenovirus, enterovirus, astrovirus
Parasitic infection	Giardia lamblia Schistosomiasis Amebiasis
Functional GI/ psychiatric disorder	Irritable bowel syndrome Anorexia nervosa Laxative abuse Cyclic vomiting syndrome
Carbohydrate malabsorption	Lactose intolerance
IBD	Ulcerative colitis Microscopic colitis collagenous, lymphocytic Celiac disease Gastrointestinal sarcoid Acute self-limited colitis
Vascular	Ischemic colitis Portal hypertensive colopathy Arteriovenous malformations
Immunodeficiencies	Chronic granulomatous disease
Toxins	NSAIDs Chemotherapeutics Mycophenolate Radiation-induced colitis Oral sodium phosphate solutions
Etiology	Specific entity
Malignancies	Lymphoma Adenocarcinoma Metastatic disease Neuroendocrine tumors (i.e. carcinoid) Leiomyosarcoma Neutropenic enterocolitis (typhlitis)
Anatomic	Diverticulitis Diverticular-associated colitis appendicitis Rectal prolapse Solitary rectal ulcer syndrome
Nutritional/metabolic	Diversion colitis Acute intermittent porphyria

Etiology	Specific entity
Autoimmune	Vasculitis (polyarteritis nodosa, Churg- Strauss, Wegener's granulomatosis, Behcet's syndrome, Henoch-Schöenlein purpura Hereditary angioedema
Infiltrative	Amyloidosis Eosinophilic gastroenteritis Systemic mastocytosis

*Representative but not all-inclusive.

Figure 2.2. Differential diagnosis of Crohn's disease.

Macroscopic discontinuity
Transmural inflammation
Fibrosis
Lymphoid aggregates
Discontinuous inflammation on histology
Non-caseating granulomas
Diagnosis of Crohn's favored if Granuloma + any 1 additional criteria or any 3 criteria without granuloma.

Figure 2.3. Lennard-Jones criteria for diagnosis of Crohn's disease.

Historical features	Diarrhea +/- blood, +/- mucus Nocturnal stools Abdominal pain Rectal bleeding Weight loss Fatigue Growth retardation (children) Family history of IBD Other autoimmune disease History of anemia Current or former smoker Extra-intestinal manifestations Prior perianal abscess or fistula
Physical exam findings	Abdominal tenderness RLQ Abdominal mass Malnourishment Growth retardation Perianal findings (abscess, fistula, stenosis, anal ulcer, numerous or large skin tags, non-midline fissure Aphthous stomatitis Oral ulcers Extra-intestinal manifestations Pyoderma gangrenosum, Erythema nodosum, arthritis, uveitis, episcleritis, Active smoking history Minimal NSAID use

Figure 2.4. (Continued).

Serum Labs	Elevated Erythrocyte sedimentation rate Anemia Iron-deficiency, macrocytic Vitamin B^{12} deficiency Thrombocytosis Low albumin Elevated serum antibody levels (adjunctive, prognostic)
Genetic testing	Nod2 Single Nucleotide Polymorphisms
Stool analysis	Gross blood in stool Fecal leukocytes Elevated calprotectin, lactoferrin Absence of enteric infection
Imaging	Wall thickening Mucosal enhancement Small bowel inflammatory changes Skip lesions Deep ulcers Inflammation not limited to mucosa Strictures Fistula or sinus tract(enterocutaneous, entero- enteral, enterovescicular) Perianal disease Abscess, fistula, anal canal ulcer Creeping fat Intra-abdominal or psoas abscess
Endoscopy	Skip lesions Perianal involvement Anal canal involvement Anusitis, anal ulcer, anal stenosis Rectal sparing Discrete ulcerations Aphthous, stellate, confluent, linear, 'rake' Cobblestoning of mucosa Pseudopolyps Stricture Fistula Ileocecal valve deformity Ileal or Ileocecal valve ulceration
Pathology	Chronic inflammation Crypt distortion, crypt drop-put, crypt destruction Basal lymphoplasmacytosis Non-caseating granulomas (not from crypt destruction) Intra-epithelial lymphocytes Pyloric metaplasia Transmural inflammation (gross)

Figure 2.4. Clinical and diagnostic features supporting a diagnosis of Crohn's disease.

In addition, as the disease can affect any part of the GI tract, the presetting location of active CD is variable. Nonetheless, the frequency of each anatomic location is well-characterized by several classic population-based studies (Figure 2.5). Classically, isolated small bowel involvement is seen in approximately 33% of patients, 20% have isolated large bowel involvement, and 45% have concomitant small and large bowel involvement. Of the approximately 80% of patients with some degree of small bowel involvement, about 1/3 have isolated involvement of the terminal ileum [6]. Between 30-50% of CD patients will have perianal involvement at some point in their disease course, a manifestation seen more commonly in patients with colorectal involvement [21, 22]. In one population-based study, the cumulative frequency of fistula occurrence was 12% at 1 year, 21% at 10 years and 26% at 20 years [21]. Interestingly, the perianal manifestations can predate the appearance and diagnosis of luminal CD, in some cases by years [21-23]. Further, in 2-5% of patients it is the only disease manifestation at presentation [24, 25].

Study	Population locale	Base population N	Disease Location			
			Colon only	Ileo-colonic	Ileal	Any ileal
Nyhlin 1986 [28, 29]	Northern Sweden	510,000	20	32	48	80
Munkholm 1992 [4]	Copenhagen	550,000	30	33	29	64
Gower-Rosseau 1994 [30]	Northern France	4,514,000	19	48	11	59
Moum 1996 [31]	Southeast Norway	966,000	44	29	27	56
Lapidus 1997 [29]	Stockholm County	1.6 million	32	41	27	68
Loftus 1998 [32]	Olmstead County, MN	106,000	32	45	22	67
Bjornsson 2000 [33]	Iceland	266,000	51	31	18	49
Witte 2000 [34]	20 European Centers	?	38	31	29	60

Figure 2.5. Population-based studies of Crohn's disease location at diagnosis.

Between 5 and 15% have oral involvement, while gastroduodenal involvement is seen in 1-4% and is almost universally seen with disease locations in the small or large bowel [10, 11]. Esophageal involvement is rarely seen (0.2% in one series), and almost never without concomitant small or large bowel involvement [12]. Only about 1% have isolated jejunal involvement, though proximal bowel involvement appears more common in pediatric patients [26]. In 1998, a consensus phenotypic classification schema for both CD and Ulcerative colitis was outlined by the International Working Party for the World Congress of Gastroenterology and presented at their meeting in Vienna, Austria (Figure 2-6) [27]. The proposed system, now called the Vienna Classification, was based on three main factors: age at diagnosis, location of disease, and behavior of disease. Patients could be given one of several sub-classifications within each of the three variable sets. In hopes of standardization of phenotyping, location strata were formally defined in the Vienna classification in 1998. Colonic disease location represented any disease limited to the region between the proximal ascending colon to the rectum. Ileocolonic location was formally defined as involvement of the terminal ileum and any colon between the ascending colon and rectum. Ileum involvement was defined as less than 1/3 of the distal ileum with or without spillover into the cecum, while upper gastrointestinal tract represented any disease location proximal to the distal 1/3 of ileum, regardless of additional involvement of the terminal ileum or colon.

In the behavior domain, inflammatory behavior was CD without any complication at any point. Structuring behavior represented any constant luminal narrowing by radiologic, endoscopic or surgical pathologic method. Either pre-stenotic dilation or signs/symptoms of obstruction must be present for this diagnosis. Penetrating disease was defined as any occurrence of internal or perianal fistula, inflammatory masses or abscess (excluding postoperative,) regardless of the presence of a stricture. A 'high water mark' approach was utilized when determining a patient's behavior; while a patient could progress from inflammatory to stenotic to penetrating or inflammatory to penetrating, their phenotype could not move from penetrating to inflammatory.

The criteria were refined at the 2005 meeting in Montreal, Quebec (Figure 2.6) [28]. In the original Vienna classification, the appearance of any upper tract involvement superseded any other concomitant location, making this categorization more difficult to interpret. The Montreal update addressed this with the use of upper tract involvement as either a lone phenotypic location category OR as a modifier of disease at one of the other location phenotypes. The Vienna classification did not allow the discrimination between perianal fistula and fistula at other locations. As these represent different clinical presentations, the Montreal update has allowed for perianal disease to be a phenotypic modifier, allowing for differentiation between fistula in the perineum and other locations. A more recent proposed pediatric modification of the Montreal Classification (termed the Paris Classification) has subsequently been proposed to more accurately reflect the nuances of pediatric CD, incorporating the presence of growth delay as well as more detail in the sub-classification strata [29].

	Vienna	Montreal
Age at diagnosis	A1: <40 years A2: ≥ 40 years	A1: <17 years A2: 17-40 years A3 : >40 years
Location of disease	L1: ileal L2: colonic L3 ileocolonic L4: upper gastrointestinal tract disease	L1: ileal L2: colonic L3 ileocolonic L4*: isolated upper gastrointestinal tract disease
Behavior of disease	B1: inflammatory B2: stricturing B3: penetrating	B1: non-stricturing, non-penetrating B2: stricturing B3: peforating p: perianal disease modifier**

*L4 can be the only location or can be added as a secondary location to L1-3, denoting concomitant involvement of the upper tract.

**p modifier added when perianal disease is present.

Figure 2.6. Vienna/Montreal phenotypic classification of Crohn's disease.

		N	Colon only	IC	Ileal only	Upper	B1	B2	B3
Thia 2010 [41]	Olmstead County	306	45	19	32	0.4%	81	2	14
Henrikson 2007 [39]	Southeast Norway	200	46	26	27	4	61	28	12
Wolters 2006 [42]	20 European Centers	358	42	37	15	6	74	16	10
Veerle 2013 [43]	Southwest Denmark	201	36	39	21	4	69	19	12
Jess 2007 [44]	Copenhagen	2216	30-43	24-33	9-31	8-19			
Charpentier 2014 [45]	Northern France	367	65	26	9	6	78	17	5
Cosnes* 2002 [38]	Paris, France	2002					83	4	13
Louis* 2001 [40]	Liege, Belgium	297					74	11	15

*referral-based cohort.

Figure 2.7. Population-based studies of location and behavior at diagnosis (after Vienna).

Population-based studies following the introduction of the Vienna and Montreal classification revealed consistent distributions of disease as noted in the pre-Vienna era, but also provided baseline frequencies of disease behavior (Figure 2.7). It was clear that the majority of patients (>75%) at diagnosis had not yet developed of stricturing or perforating complications. However, both population and referral-based analyses with extended follow-up periods revealed that phenotypes change significantly over time. Approximately two-thirds developing stricturing or penetrating complication in as few as 5 years [30-33]. One analysis reported that 26% of patients classified as B1 at presentation developed complications within 90 days of diagnosis.

Laboratory Evaluation

Traditional Laboratories

Initial evaluation of the patient with CD will often include standard laboratory testing with hematologic and serum chemistry evaluations. Thrombocytosis, anemia, and hypoalbuminemia are relatively common findings. These are most helpful at ruling out a functional cause of symptoms, such as irritable bowel syndrome, but these particular lab abnormalities are not features of this diagnosis.

Anemia, while not specific for CD even in the presence of GI symptoms, can be seen in Crohn's from multiple causes. Chronic overt or occult GI blood loss as well as impaired absorption of iron from the proximal small bowel can result in a microcytic, iron-deficiency anemia. Poor absorption of folate or vitamin B12 due to active proximal and terminal ileal disease, respectively, can result in macrocytic anemias. Further, dietary deficiencies (related to reduced oral intake due to symptoms or patient self-regulation of diet in attempts to avoid symptoms) in any of the above could result in nutritional contributions to anemia.

Thrombocytosis is a nonspecific inflammatory response, which is often seen in CD patients with disease activity and tends to mirror disease activity indices but can also been seen as part of the normal hematopoietic response to acute blood loss or severe iron deficiency anemia [34]. Hypoalbuminemia is reflective of overall nutritional state and can result from protein losing enteropathy as well as malnutrition. It is also a negative acute-phase reactant and can be seen to decrease during periods of prolonged inflammation.

The inflammatory marker and acute-phase reactant, C-reactive protein (CRP,) has been shown to correlate with clinical, endoscopic and histologic CD activity [35, 36]. It has a short half-life, is readily available, results easily reproducible and has been utilized as a noninvasive marker of response to therapy and reduced inflammatory activity in CD therapeutic clinical trials. However, it remains normal in up to 25% of CD patients despite documented active ulceration at endoscopy, limiting its sensitivity and negative predictive value. Erythrocyte sedimentation rate (ESR) is a nonspecific marker of inflammation which has a longer half-life than CRP and does not as closely correlate with CD activity.

Stool Analysis

Stool biomarkers are a useful tool for IBD providers as they are specific to inflammation in the GI tract. Fecal calprotectin is a calcium- and zinc-bound protein found in neutrophils and its presence in feces is a result of neutrophil migration to the GI tract due to an inflammatory process [37]. Multiple studies have demonstrated a correlation between fecal calprotectin and clinical disease activity scores as well as endoscopic activity [38-41]. Studies have also demonstrated stronger correlation of fecal calprotectin to endoscopic scores in CD than other serum biomarkers [42, 43]. This makes fecal calprotectin a valuable objective marker of GI inflammation for clinicians to help differentiate clinical symptoms related to CD activity versus symptoms due to other causes such as irritable bowel syndrome. Fecal lactoferrin is an alternative fecal biomarker and is an iron binding glycoprotein found in neutrophils [44]. Therefore, its presence in feces is also a sign of GI- specific inflammation.

Studies have also demonstrated correlation of elevated fecal lactoferrin levels and endoscopically active CD at rates that are comparable to fecal calprotectin [45]. However, correlation with clinical disease activity scores has not been clearly demonstrated. In clinical practice, fecal calprotectin is more commonly used likely owing to more robust data supporting its use and fecal lactoferrin has not demonstrated any specific advantages to fecal calprotectin in terms of performance or cost. Fecal biomarkers are a helpful tool in both diagnosis and longitudinal monitoring in CD. However, providers must recognize that these are non-specific markers of GI inflammation and other diagnoses such as infection, malignancy, and NSAID use can also elevate these markers.

Serologic Testing

Over the past few decades, several serum immune markers have been described. These have been documented to be elevated at different frequencies and to differing degrees in patients with CD, UC and even those without IBD. The appearance and combination of markers in a given patient were felt to represent that patient's immune phenotype, which is in part genetically determined. At the start of the 21st century, these markers hold promise for use in the diagnosis of IBD, as well as the differentiation between CD and UC.

Several iterations of diagnostic serologic marker panels are commercially available. The presence of Serum Antibodies directed against *Saccharomyces cerevisiae* (ASCA) has been shown to be present in 44% of patients with a diagnosis of CD, and its appearance has a reported specificity of 87% for the same when compared to non-IBD controls [46]. This led it to be initially termed "the Crohn's antibody."

The finding of a perinuclear pattern of anti-neutrophil cytoplasmic antibody staining pattern (pANCA) has a 60% sensitivity and 75% specificity for a diagnosis of UC, prompting it to be termed "the UC antibody" [46]. Subsequent reports of combining a patient's ASCA and pANCA results noted 56% sensitivity, 94% specificity and 91% positive-predictive value in differentiating CD from healthy controls and 44% sensitivity, 97% specificity and 78% positive-predictive value in differentiating UC from healthy controls [47].

Attempts to improve the sensitivity and specificity of the ASCA/pANCA combination included the discovery and inclusion of additional markers (antibodies directed against cell surface sugars/glycans, exocrine pancreas tissue, the flagellin CBIr1, *Pseudomonas flourescens*, the outer membrane porin of *E. coli*) in the diagnostic panels. However, due to sensitivity and specificity limitations of the individual markers, the combination of markers has not dramatically improved the diagnostic accuracy. Even in test populations with a high prevalence of known IBD, the combination remains too inaccurate for clinical discrimination of CD.

As the group with recognized with CD is very different from the population seen prior to their diagnosis, the test characteristics are unacceptable to be utilized for anything other than very limited adjunctive diagnostic purposes. Perhaps more commonly, these tests lead to unnecessary confusion, if the results do not support the providers' clinical impressions [48]. Likewise, using the diagnostic panels to differentiate between CD and UC in patients with indeterminate IBD colitis (a diagnosis given to 10% of patients with IBD colitis due to the lack of reliable discriminating features to differentiate as CD colitis or UC) was poorly discriminatory and has limited use in this regard clinically [48, 49].

Currently, serologic markers of CD have the most robust data and are utilized for prognostic purposes. Cross-sectional studies have consistently reported an association between both the numerical sum and titer of positive serum antibodies from various diagnostic panels and the CD complications of internal penetrating and/or stricturing disease as well as need for resection surgery [50, 51]. Further, a longitudinal analysis of 536 pediatric patients noted similar findings as well as a more rapid time to development of complications in patients with higher immune reactivity burden prior to development of complications [48, 51]. Finally, the presence of ASCA antibodies has been found to be an independent risk factor for the development of CD subsequent to colectomy and ileal pouch anal anastomosis formation done for a diagnosis of Inflammatory Bowel Disease-Unclassified (IBD-U) or UC [52].

Genetic Testing

To date, 140 genetic loci associated with CD susceptibility have been identified. The most widely studied being nucleotide-binding oligomerization domain 2/caspase recruitment domain-containing protein 15 gene (NOD2/CARD15) [53]. Several studies have demonstrated an increased risk of surgery and development of stricturing or fistulizing complications in patients with mutations in the NOD2/CARD15 gene, especially if multiple mutations are present [54]. Other genes have been identified in various points of the inflammatory process in IBD such as microbial sensing (CARD9 and RIPK2), intestinal barrier function (C1orf106 and HNF4A), innate and adaptive immune signaling (NLRP7, IL18RAP, CD28, IFNG, PTPN22, STAT4, IL6ST, IL23R, RORC, and IL17RA), and fibrosis (OSMR and SMAD3) [55]. However, few specific gene variants have been identified that reliably help with diagnosis or predict disease course. Furthermore, the cost associated with these types of genetic testing is cumbersome and thus not currently useful in clinical practice.

Endoscopic Evaluation

While endoscopic findings alone are not sufficient to make a diagnosis of CD, they certainly play a central role. *Endoscopy is the single most vital and indispensable diagnostic test in establishing a diagnosis of CD.* Endoscopy can assist in the determination of degree of inflammatory activity and to document the extent and distribution of disease. In landmark CD studies, endoscopy documented findings consistent with CD 87% of the time [56]. Endoscopy, when combined with other diagnostic studies, can differentiate CD from UC in more than 85% of patients, a number which rises over time [57, 58].

When CD is suspected clinically, a full colonoscopic examination with assessment of the terminal ileum should be attempted in all patients.

The only exception to this rule is those CD patients with severe-fulminant colitis or toxic megacolon [59]. However, routine EGD is not considered necessary as part of diagnostic evaluation in all patients as patients with upper-tract CD usually have disease in the ileum, colon or perineum [59]. However, EGD is helpful in ruling out other disorders (Celiac disease, eosinophilic gastroenteritis, etc.), or in patients with negative colonoscopy and ileoscopy.

In addition to the visual documentation of characterizing findings, endoscopy may provide tissue for histologic analysis. The histologic hallmark of CD has been the non-caseating granuloma and in the appropriate setting can be supportive of the diagnosis of CD. However, granulomas are only found in 15-36% of biopsy specimens in CD patients, though some literature suggests higher frequencies in the duodenum and a generally higher yield with biopsies taken on the edge of ulcers [11, 60].

Sodium phosphate preparations and pre-procedural NSAIDs should be avoided given risk that these therapies may mimic the endoscopic findings of IBD [59]. Enteroscopy is not routinely performed. If abnormalities outside the reach of the standard EGD scope are noted on other diagnostic tests (cross-sectional imaging or wireless capsule endoscopy); intraoperative enteroscopy is utilized only in select cases [59].

As there are no endoscopic features that are specific for CD, so the results are interpreted in the context of other clinic-historical and diagnostic findings (Figure 2.8). Biopsy specimens should be obtained from areas of both visually appearing normal and abnormal mucosa, and specimens from each segment should be labeled separately [59]. Findings such as mucosal edema and erythema are common in segments of mild disease but extremely nonspecific.

Factor	Descriptor	Crohn's Disease	Ulcerative Colitis
Disease location	Perineum (fistula, abscess, large skin tags)	Y	N
	Anal canal (ulcers, stenosis, atypical fissure)	Y	N
	Terminal ileum	Y	Very rare backwash
Disease Distribution	Continuous	Y (rare)	Y
	Patchy	Y	N
	Rectal sparing	Y	N
Endoscopic Description	Aphthous ulcerations	Y	N
	Linear, stellate, deep or serpiginous ulcerations	Y	N
	Cobblestoning		
	Punctate erosions	Y	N
	Pseudopolyps	N	Y
	Stricture/stenosis	Y	Y
		Y	N (except malignancy)

Figure 2.8. Endoscopic features in Crohn's disease and ulcerative colitis.

The archetypal lesion for CD is aphthous ulceration, and can be found anywhere between mouth and anus in CD patients. These are small (<5mm) shallow white/yellow ovoid breaks in the mucosal surface with a thin surrounding halo of erythema. Initially, these lesions are surrounded by normal mucosa, and can occur individually or as part of a group. Aphthous ulcerations can enlarge concentrically and coalesce with other ulcerations to form larger stellate, irregular, linear 'rake-like' or serpiginous ulcerations. These are often deeper but frequently surrounded by relatively benign intervening mucosa. Over time, the intervening mucosa can be very edematous and erythematous, giving the appearance of nodular or polyp-like prominences between ulcerated areas of colon. This has been described as *cobblestoning*, a hallmark mucosal description of severely active CD. The ulcerated areas represent the recessed lines of mortar while the edematous intervening mucosal protuberances represent the raised stones or bricks between mortar lines.

The appearance of patchiness or discontinuity of the inflammatory process (abnormal areas interspersed with normal intervening mucosal areas) is another characteristic feature in CD. This may provide some degree of endoscopic discrimination from UC. A subtype of patchy inflammation is the concept of rectal sparing (seen in approximately 50% of patients with CD colitis) where the rectum is specifically spared the inflammatory appearance of other colon tissue [6]. Interestingly it is not uncommon to have proctitis symptoms (urgency, tenesmus) in CD colitis patients without endoscopic evidence of proctitis [6].

It should be noted that in approximately 10% of patients with IBD involving the colon, it is not possible to ascertain definitively whether the patient has Ulcerative colitis or CD using clinical, laboratory, radiologic, endoscopic and pathologic features [61]. This phenomenon, previously referred to as indeterminate colitis, has been re-termed IBD-unclassified (IBD-U) [62].

A few caveats to skip lesions should be mentioned. The first is that, once medical therapy is initiated in a patient with UC, differential mucosal healing can occur in nearly half of patients, leading to discontinuous inflammation where continuous inflammation was once present, leading to the suggestion of CD [63]. This phenomenon has been well-described when rectally-administered topically-acting therapies have been employed in patients with proctitis [63].

The second is the phenomenon referred to as a *periappendiceal* or *cecal patch*. This is a well-characterized finding of discontinuous active colitis limited to cecum and always involving the appendiceal orifice in UC patients with an otherwise healthy right colon. It has been described in as many as 75% of patients with left-sided UC [64]. As such, its finding should not alter the diagnosis for UC if that diagnosis is otherwise favored based on all the gathered clinical and diagnostic information.

Large anal skin tags, atypical (non-midline) or deep fissures, or evidence of perianal fistula or abscess in conjunction with an inflammatory colitis can assist in differentiating CD from UC.

It should be noted that involvement of the ileum, while an important differentiating variable between CD and UC, can occur in about 10% of UC patients. However, the inflammatory changes should be mild/superficial, limited to the very end of the terminal ileum, are often associated with a patulous ileocecal valve. These are described as being associated with active pancolonic inflammation (termed *backwash ileitis*) [65]. Conversely, ileitis in CD appears more typically as aphthous ileitis, frank ulcerations or stenoses –all without the requirement of active pancolonic inflammation.

The finding of focal gastritis is nonspecific and seen in >40% of CD, 12% of UC, and nearly 20% of healthy patients undergoing upper endoscopy. This finding is insufficient to label a patient with gastric involvement with CD in the absence of other more typical endoscopic (frank ulcers, fistula, stricture, cobblestoning) or pathologic (non-caseating granulomas) findings [66].

Wireless capsule endoscopy (WCE) has been used since 2001 as a method to assist in the diagnosis of suspected small bowel CD. The outpatient procedure involves ingestion of a wireless pill-shaped illumination/video camera device which takes 2-6 pictures per second over an 8-12 hour battery life. The photos are transferred via a sensor array on the patient (usually in belt form), with image transfer to a belt-mounted battery-operated recorder. The images are collated into a video file, which is then reviewed by the endoscopist after the data is download. Images and findings are similar to those obtained with enteroscopy or ileoscopy [67].

Given the risks in CD patients of active inflammation and /or fibrosis resulting in luminal stenosis, the main risk of WCE in patients with CD is that of capsule retention with potential for subsequent bowel obstruction and perforation. As such, it has been suggested that a pre-procedure small bowel imaging study or a delayed-dissolution barium-containing Patency

Capsule be performed. Further, WCE is contraindicated in CD patients with symptoms of small bowel obstruction or objective evidence of stricturing small bowel lesions.

Interestingly, while known CD has been shown to be a risk factor for WCE retention and perforation, suspected CD has been associated with lower retention rates [67]. As with endoscopy in general, the WCE findings of CD are nonspecific.

More recently, the use of balloon-assisted enteroscopy has shown efficacy in obtaining retained WCE and avoiding surgery [68]. Enteroscopy can also allow tissue sampling to assist in the verification of the diagnosis of CD. Ominous alternative diagnoses (i.e., lymphoma) may improve with CD-therapies giving false security of CD as the diagnosis. NSAID use, which is often surreptitious, has been shown to cause asymptomatic visible mucosal erosions similar to those seen in CD in asymptomatic patients undergoing WCE [69]. As such, WCE should be performed after NSAID avoidance for 4-6 weeks and findings on WCE should be verified with some type of tissue sampling, even surgical resection, in order to verify a diagnosis.

The diagnostic yield in patients with CD has been variable. Its use has been suggested as an alternative to cross-sectional imaging with CT or MRI enterography or in cases where endoscopic and radiologic assessments are negative despite high index of suspicion for small bowel Crohn's [67, 70].

Radiographic Evaluation

Radiographic techniques have improved over time. They have increasingly been employed as tools to assist in diagnosis and disease assessment in CD. While imaging alone cannot make a definitive diagnosis, it may help support the diagnosis and lead providers towards further tests such as endoscopy to confirm their suspicion.

Computed Tomography (CT)

CT is often the initial imaging test of choice for patients who present in the acute setting with symptoms of abdominal pain, diarrhea, or weight loss. CT findings suggestive of CD include bowel wall thickening (particularly in the terminal ileum), mural hyperenhancement, perienteric fat stranding, enteric wall thickening separated by areas of focally increased fat (creeping fat), hypervascular appearance of mesentery (comb sign), strictures, fistulas, or intraabdominal abscesses [71-73]. While these findings may be suggestive of CD, they are not specific and can be seen with other causes of enteritis or colitis, particularly infections.

CT enterography is an alternative imaging technique and is superior to standard CT techniques at evaluating the small bowel [74-76]. For these studies, the patient ingests a low density oral contrast which helps to distend the bowel and also receives IV contrast. Features of small bowel CD seen on CT enterography include segmental mural hyperenhancement, wall thickening, intramural edema, strictures, ulcerations, engorged vasa recta, fibrofatty proliferation, fistula tracts, and abscesses [77]. CT enterography is equivalent in terms of sensitivity and specificity to MR enterography, which will be discussed below [78]. However, the downside to CT enterography is radiation, which can be substantial over the course of a lifetime.

Magnetic Resonance Imaging (MRI)

MR enterography (MRE) has increasingly been used to evaluate small bowel CD and as mentioned above has similar accuracy to CT enterography. The features seen on MRE that are suggestive of CD are very similar to those seen in CT enterography [77]. MRE has the advantage of no ionizing radiation. However, the downside is that MRE can often take longer that CT and may not be as widely available in certain medical settings.

Traditional MRI abdomen is less frequently used in CD. However, MRI pelvis is considered the best imaging modality to assess perianal involvement in CD. MRI pelvis in combination with the Van Assche index is a helpful scoring system used to assess severity and treatment response of perianal CD [79]. The scoring system was first created in 2003 and later modified in 2017 [80, 81]. The modified Van Assche index includes extension, hyperintensity on T2-weighted fat saturated images, rectal wall involvement, inflammatory mass, and dominant feature and gives a score from 0-19.5.

Ultrasound

Intestinal ultrasound (IUS) has recently emerged as a non-invasive, real time imaging tool that can be used in point of care settings to assess CD activity. Currently, IUS is performed during clinic visits and takes approximately 15 minutes to complete [82]. No bowel preparation or contrast is needed to perform IUS. The provider typically evaluates the distal sigmoid colon through the terminal ileum [83]. More proximal segments of small bowel and the rectum can also be scanned, though may be more challenging to visualize. The features of active CD that are assessed via IUS include bowel wall thickness (BWT), hyperemia, focal disruption of bowel wall layers, and hypoechoic or hyperechoic changes in the layers representing a loss of bowel wall stratification [84-86]. BWT is the most important feature evaluated and cutoff of > 3 mm in any segment has been showed to correlate with active endoscopic disease, with a sensitivity and specificity of 88% and 93% respectively [87, 88]. There are several IUS activity scores that have been developed that can be calculated at the point of care and provide crucial data to make real time clinical decisions. Two common scoring systems used in CD are the Simple Ultrasound Score for Crohn's Disease (SUS-CD) and the Simple Ultrasound Activity Score for CD, both of which correlate well with the commonly used Simple Endoscopic Score for Crohn's Disease (SES-CD) [86, 89].

When comparing to other cross sectional imaging modalities such as CT or MRE, IUS has comparable accuracy in diagnosing CD related complications. In a large prospective trial of 284 patients, 233 with small bowel CD, IUS and MRE had similar sensitivity and specificity for detecting disease in the terminal ileum (92% and 84% respectively for IUS vs 97% and 96% for MRE) [90]. However, MRE was superior to IUS for determining small bowel disease extent (sensitivity of 80% for MRE vs 70% for IUS). Another study of 234 patients with CD from Italy demonstrated similar findings of comparable sensitivity and specificity of IUS compared to MRE (96% and 97% for IUS and 96% and 94% for MR enterography) [91]. MRE did appear more accurate for detecting extent of small bowel disease ($r = 0.69$) and fistula detection ($r = 0.67$), but comparable to IUS in detection of strictures ($r = 0.82$), and abscesses ($r = 0.88$).

While it is unlikely that IUS will completely replace endoscopy or other imaging modalities, it certainly has many benefits in CD management. The most important function is that it empowers providers to make major treatment decision during routine clinic visits. Another important advantage to other diagnostic tools is the ability to directly involve the patient in the procedure itself. Currently, one of the main disadvantages is the limited number of certified IUS training centers in the United States. However, the number of training opportunities is expected to rapidly expand over the next decade and thus providers will have greater ability to develop these skills.

Conclusion

The diagnosis of CD is complex due to the wide variability in patient presentations. Clinical symptoms may provide clues to diagnosis and have been codified with the Vienna classification and the Montreal update. Endoscopy remains the single best test for evaluation and management decisions. New diagnostic tools such as intestinal ultrasound and magnetic resonance enterography, hold substantial promise for the future, but the diagnosis of CD remains as much an art as a science.

References

[1] Loftus, E. V., Jr., Clinical epidemiology of inflammatory bowel disease: Incidence, prevalence, and environmental influences. *Gastroenterology*, 2004. 126(6): p. 1504-17.

[2] Mekhjian, H. S., et al., Clinical features and natural history of Crohn's disease. *Gastroenterology,* 1979. 77(4 Pt 2): p. 898-906.

[3] Steinhardt, H.J., et al., European Cooperative Crohn's Disease Study (ECCDS): clinical features and natural history. *Digestion*, 1985. 31(2-3): p. 97-108.

[4] Munkholm, P., et al., Incidence and prevalence of Crohn's disease in the county of Copenhagen, 1962-87: a sixfold increase in incidence. *Scand J Gastroenterol*, 1992. 27(7): p. 609-14.

[5] Podolsky, D. K., Inflammatory bowel disease. *N Engl J Med,* 2002. 347(6): p. 417-29.

[6] Farmer, R. G., W. A. Hawk, and R. B. Turnbull, Jr., Clinical patterns in Crohn's disease: a statistical study of 615 cases. *Gastroenterology*, 1975. 68(4 Pt 1): p. 627-35.

[7] Abraham, B. P., S. Mehta, and H.B. El-Serag, Natural history of pediatric-onset inflammatory bowel disease: a systematic review. *J Clin Gastroenterol,* 2012. 46(7): p. 581-9.

[8] Pimentel, M., et al., Identification of a prodromal period in Crohn's disease but not ulcerative colitis. *Am J Gastroenterol,* 2000. 95(12): p. 3458-62.

[9] Burgmann, T., et al., The Manitoba Inflammatory Bowel Disease Cohort Study: prolonged symptoms before diagnosis--how much is irritable bowel syndrome? *Clin Gastroenterol Hepatol*, 2006. 4(5): p. 614-20.

[10] Yamamoto, T., R. N. Allan, and M. R. Keighley, An audit of gastroduodenal Crohn disease: clinicopathologic features and management. *Scand J Gastroenterol,* 1999. 34(10): p. 1019-24.

[11] Nugent, F. W. and M. A. Roy, Duodenal Crohn's disease: an analysis of 89 cases. *Am J Gastroenterol,* 1989. 84(3): p. 249-54.

[12] Decker, G. A., et al., Crohn's disease of the esophagus: clinical features and outcomes. *Inflamm Bowel Dis*, 2001. 7(2): p. 113-9.

[13] Han, H., et al., Appendiceal Crohn's disease clinically presenting as acute appendicitis. *World J Clin Cases*, 2014. 2(12): p. 888-92.

[14] Weston, L. A., et al., Ileocolic resection for acute presentation of Crohn's disease of the ileum. *Dis Colon Rectum*, 1996. 39(8): p. 841-6.

[15] Greenstein, A. J., et al., Free perforation in Crohn's disease: I. A survey of 99 cases. *Am J Gastroenterol,* 1985. 80(9): p. 682-9.

[16] Lennard-Jones, J. E., Classification of inflammatory bowel disease. *Scand J Gastroenterol Suppl*, 1989. 170: p. 2-6; discussion 16-9.

[17] Shivananda, S., et al., Incidence of inflammatory bowel disease across Europe: is there a difference between north and south? Results of the European Collaborative Study on Inflammatory Bowel Disease (EC-IBD). *Gut*, 1996. 39(5): p. 690-7.

[18] Binder, V., et al., Incidence and prevalence of ulcerative colitis and Crohn's disease in the County of Copenhagen, 1962 to 1978. *Gastroenterology*, 1982. 83(3): p. 563-8.

[19] Lichtenstein, G. R., et al., Management of Crohn's disease in adults. *Am J Gastroenterol*, 2009. 104(2): p. 465-83; quiz 464, 484.

[20] Van Assche, G., et al., The second European evidence-based Consensus on the diagnosis and management of Crohn's disease: Special situations. *J Crohns Colitis*, 2010. 4(1): p. 63-101.

[21] Schwartz, D. A., et al., The natural history of fistulizing Crohn's disease in Olmsted County, Minnesota. *Gastroenterology*, 2002. 122(4): p. 875-80.

[22] Lapidus, A., et al., Clinical course of colorectal Crohn's disease: a 35-year follow-up study of 507 patients. *Gastroenterology*, 1998. 114(6): p. 1151-60.

[23] Lapidus, A., Crohn's disease in Stockholm County during 1990-2001: an epidemiological update. *World J Gastroenterol*, 2006. 12(1): p. 75-81.

[24] Munkholm, P., Crohn's disease--occurrence, course and prognosis. An epidemiologic cohort-study. *Dan Med Bull*, 1997. 44(3): p. 287-302.

[25] Lockhart-Mummery, H. E., Symposium. Crohn's disease: anal lesions. *Dis Colon Rectum*, 1975. 18(3): p. 200-2.

[26] Ruuska, T., et al., Prospective evaluation of upper gastrointestinal mucosal lesions in children with ulcerative colitis and Crohn's disease. *J Pediatr Gastroenterol Nutr*, 1994. 19(2): p. 181-6.

[27] Gasche, C., et al., A simple classification of Crohn's disease: report of the Working Party for the World Congresses of Gastroenterology, Vienna 1998. *Inflamm Bowel Dis*, 2000. 6(1): p. 8-15.

[28] Silverberg, M.S., et al., Toward an integrated clinical, molecular and serological classification of inflammatory bowel disease: report of a Working Party of the 2005 Montreal World Congress of Gastroenterology. *Can J Gastroenterol*, 2005. 19 Suppl A: p. 5A-36A.

[29] Levine, A., et al., Pediatric modification of the Montreal classification for inflammatory bowel disease: the Paris classification. *Inflamm Bowel Dis*, 2011. 17(6): p. 1314-21.

[30] Cosnes, J., et al., Long-term evolution of disease behavior of Crohn's disease. *Inflamm Bowel Dis,* 2002. 8(4): p. 244-50.

[31] Henriksen, M., et al., Change of diagnosis during the first five years after onset of inflammatory bowel disease: results of a prospective follow-up study (the IBSEN Study). *Scand J Gastroenterol*, 2006. 41(9): p. 1037-43.

[32] Louis, E., et al., Behaviour of Crohn's disease according to the Vienna classification: changing pattern over the course of the disease. *Gut*, 2001. 49(6): p. 777-82.

[33] Thia, K. T., et al., Risk factors associated with progression to intestinal complications of Crohn's disease in a population-based cohort. *Gastroenterology*, 2010. 139(4): p. 1147-55.

[34] Phillips, M. S. D., M. W., Platelet count in patients with Crohn's disease. *Br Med J (Clin Res Ed)*, 1983. 286(6381): p. 1895-6.

[35] Solem, C. A., et al., Correlation of C-reactive protein with clinical, endoscopic, histologic, and radiographic activity in inflammatory bowel disease. *Inflamm Bowel Dis*, 2005. 11(8): p. 707-12.

[36] Fagan, E. A., et al., Serum levels of C-reactive protein in Crohn's disease and ulcerative colitis. *Eur J Clin Invest*, 1982. 12(4): p. 351-9.

[37] Pathirana, W. G. W., et al., Faecal Calprotectin. *Clin Biochem Rev*, 2018. 39(3): p. 77-90.

[38] Lee, Y. W., et al., The usefulness of fecal calprotectin in assessing inflammatory bowel disease activity. *Korean J Intern Med*, 2019. 34(1): p. 72-80.

[39] D'Haens, G., et al., Fecal calprotectin is a surrogate marker for endoscopic lesions in inflammatory bowel disease. *Inflamm Bowel Dis*, 2012. 18(12): p. 2218-24.

[40] Vieira, A., et al., Inflammatory bowel disease activity assessed by fecal calprotectin and lactoferrin: correlation with laboratory parameters, clinical, endoscopic and histological indexes. *BMC Res Notes,* 2009. 2: p. 221.

[41] Sipponen, T., et al., Correlation of faecal calprotectin and lactoferrin with an endoscopic score for Crohn's disease and histological findings. *Aliment Pharmacol Ther*, 2008. 28(10): p. 1221-9.
[42] Schoepfer, A. M., et al., Fecal calprotectin correlates more closely with the Simple Endoscopic Score for Crohn's disease (SES-CD) than CRP, blood leukocytes, and the CDAI. *Am J Gastroenterol*, 2010. 105(1): p. 162-9.
[43] Lobaton, T., et al., A new rapid test for fecal calprotectin predicts endoscopic remission and postoperative recurrence in Crohn's disease. *J Crohns Colitis,* 2013. 7(12): p. e641-51.
[44] Kane, S. V., et al., Fecal lactoferrin is a sensitive and specific marker in identifying intestinal inflammation. *Am J Gastroenterol*, 2003. 98(6): p. 1309-14.
[45] Bohra, A., et al., The Utility of Faecal Calprotectin, Lactoferrin and Other Faecal Biomarkers in Discriminating Endoscopic Activity in Crohn's Disease: A Systematic Review and Meta-Analysis. *Biomedicines*, 2023. 11(5).
[46] Sandborn, W. J., et al., Evaluation of serologic disease markers in a population-based cohort of patients with ulcerative colitis and Crohn's disease. *Inflamm Bowel Dis*, 2001. 7(3): p. 192-201.
[47] Peeters, M., et al., Diagnostic value of anti-Saccharomyces cerevisiae and antineutrophil cytoplasmic autoantibodies in inflammatory bowel disease. *Am J Gastroenterol,* 2001. 96(3): p. 730-4.
[48] Prideaux, L., et al., Serological antibodies in inflammatory bowel disease: a systematic review. *Inflamm Bowel Dis*, 2012. 18(7): p. 1340-55.
[49] Joossens, S., et al., The value of serologic markers in indeterminate colitis: a prospective follow-up study. *Gastroenterology*, 2002. 122(5): p. 1242-7.
[50] Ferrante, M., et al., New serological markers in inflammatory bowel disease are associated with complicated disease behaviour. *Gut*, 2007. 56(10): p. 1394-403.
[51] Dubinsky, M. C., et al., Increased immune reactivity predicts aggressive complicating Crohn's disease in children. *Clin Gastroenterol Hepatol*, 2008. 6(10): p. 1105-11.
[52] Coukos, J. A., et al., ASCA IgG and CBir antibodies are associated with the development of Crohn's disease and fistulae following ileal pouch-anal anastomosis. *Dig Dis Sci*, 2012. 57(6): p. 1544-53.
[53] Jostins, L., et al., Host-microbe interactions have shaped the genetic architecture of inflammatory bowel disease. *Nature*, 2012. 491(7422): p. 119-24.
[54] Adler, J., et al., The prognostic power of the NOD2 genotype for complicated Crohn's disease: a meta-analysis. *Am J Gastroenterol*, 2011. 106(4): p. 699-712.
[55] Graham, D. B. and R. J. Xavier, Pathway paradigms revealed from the genetics of inflammatory bowel disease. *Nature*, 2020. 578(7796): p. 527-539.
[56] Lorenz-Meyer, H., et al., European Cooperative Crohn's Disease Study (ECCDS): colonoscopy. *Digestion*, 1985. 31(2-3): p. 109-19.
[57] Chutkan, R. K., E. Scherl, and J.D. Waye, Colonoscopy in inflammatory bowel disease. Gastrointest *Endosc Clin N Am*, 2002. 12(3): p. 463-83, viii.
[58] Pera, A., et al., Colonoscopy in inflammatory bowel disease. Diagnostic accuracy and proposal of an endoscopic score. *Gastroenterology*, 1987. 92(1): p. 181-5.
[59] Leighton, J. A., et al., ASGE guideline: endoscopy in the diagnosis and treatment of inflammatory bowel disease. *Gastrointest Endosc*, 2006. 63(4): p. 558-65.
[60] Potzi, R., et al., Diagnostic significance of endoscopic biopsy in Crohn's disease. *Endoscopy*, 1989. 21(2): p. 60-2.
[61] Tremaine, W. J., Is indeterminate colitis determinable? *Curr Gastroenterol Rep*, 2012. 14(2): p. 162-5.
[62] Geboes, K., et al., Indeterminate colitis: a review of the concept--what's in a name? *Inflamm Bowel Dis*, 2008. 14(6): p. 850-7.
[63] Bernstein, C. N., et al., Patchiness of mucosal inflammation in treated ulcerative colitis: a prospective study. *Gastrointest Endosc*, 1995. 42(3): p. 232-7.
[64] D'Haens, G., et al., Patchy cecal inflammation associated with distal ulcerative colitis: a prospective endoscopic study. *Am J Gastroenterol*, 1997. 92(8): p. 1275-9.
[65] Yamamoto, T., et al., Mucosal inflammation in the terminal ileum of ulcerative colitis patients: endoscopic findings and cytokine profiles. *Dig Liver Dis*, 2008. 40(4): p. 253-9.
[66] Parente, F., et al., Focal gastric inflammatory infiltrates in inflammatory bowel diseases: prevalence, immunohistochemical characteristics, and diagnostic role. *Am J Gastroenterol*, 2000. 95(3): p. 705-11.

[67] Van de Bruaene, C., D. De Looze, and P. Hindryckx, Small bowel capsule endoscopy: Where are we after almost 15 years of use? *World J Gastrointest Endosc*, 2015. 7(1): p. 13-36.
[68] Van Weyenberg, S. J., et al., Double-balloon endoscopy as the primary method for small-bowel video capsule endoscope retrieval. *Gastrointest Endosc*, 2010. 71(3): p. 535-41.
[69] Goldstein, J. L., et al., Video capsule endoscopy to prospectively assess small bowel injury with celecoxib, naproxen plus omeprazole, and placebo. *Clin Gastroenterol Hepatol*, 2005. 3(2): p. 133-41.
[70] Kornbluth, A., et al., ICCE consensus for inflammatory bowel disease. *Endoscopy*, 2005. 37(10): p. 1051-4.
[71] Gore, R. M., et al., CT features of ulcerative colitis and Crohn's disease. *AJR Am J Roentgenol*, 1996. 167(1): p. 3-15.
[72] Cicero, G. and S. Mazziotti, Crohn's disease at radiological imaging: focus on techniques and intestinal tract. *Intest Res*, 2021. 19(4): p. 365-378.
[73] Dua, A., V. Sharma, and P. Gupta, Dual energy computed tomography in Crohn's disease: a targeted review. *Expert Rev Gastroenterol Hepatol*, 2022. 16(8): p. 699-705.
[74] Fletcher, J. G., et al., New concepts in intestinal imaging for inflammatory bowel diseases. *Gastroenterology*, 2011. 140(6): p. 1795-806.
[75] Maaser, C., et al., ECCO-ESGAR Guideline for Diagnostic Assessment in IBD Part 1: Initial diagnosis, monitoring of known IBD, detection of complications. *J Crohns Colitis*, 2019. 13(2): p. 144-164.
[76] Bruining, D. H., et al., Computed tomography enterography detects intestinal wall changes and effects of treatment in patients with Crohn's disease. *Clin Gastroenterol Hepatol*, 2011. 9(8): p. 679-683 e1.
[77] Guglielmo, F. F., et al., Small Bowel Crohn Disease at CT and MR Enterography: Imaging Atlas and Glossary of Terms. *Radiographics*, 2020. 40(2): p. 354-375.
[78] Loftus, E. V., Using CT and MR Enterography to Diagnose and Monitor IBD. *Gastroenterol Hepatol* (N Y), 2010. 6(12): p. 754-6.
[79] van Rijn, K. L., et al., Evaluation of the modified Van Assche index for assessing response to anti-TNF therapy with MRI in perianal fistulizing Crohn's disease. *Clin Imaging*, 2020. 59(2): p. 179-187.
[80] Van Assche, G., et al., Magnetic resonance imaging of the effects of infliximab on perianal fistulizing Crohn's disease. *Am J Gastroenterol*, 2003. 98(2): p. 332-9.
[81] Samaan, M. A., et al., The development of a magnetic resonance imaging index for fistulising Crohn's disease. *Aliment Pharmacol Ther*, 2017. 46(5): p. 516-528.
[82] Dolinger, M. T. and M. Kayal, Intestinal ultrasound as a non-invasive tool to monitor inflammatory bowel disease activity and guide clinical decision making. *World J Gastroenterol*, 2023. 29(15): p. 2272-2282.
[83] Parente, F., et al., Role of early ultrasound in detecting inflammatory intestinal disorders and identifying their anatomical location within the bowel. *Aliment Pharmacol Ther*, 2003. 18(10): p. 1009-16.
[84] Yekeler, E., et al., Crohn disease activity evaluated by Doppler ultrasonography of the superior mesenteric artery and the affected small-bowel segments. *J Ultrasound Med*, 2005. 24(1): p. 59-65.
[85] Karoui, S., et al., Assessment of activity of Crohn's disease by Doppler sonography of superior mesenteric artery flow. *J Crohns Colitis*, 2010. 4(3): p. 334-40.
[86] Saevik, F., et al., Development and Validation of a Simple Ultrasound Activity Score for Crohn's Disease. *J Crohns Colitis*, 2021. 15(1): p. 115-124.
[87] Fraquelli, M., et al., Role of US in detection of Crohn disease: meta-analysis. *Radiology*, 2005. 236(1): p. 95-101.
[88] Dong, J., et al., Ultrasound as a diagnostic tool in detecting active Crohn's disease: a meta-analysis of prospective studies. *Eur Radiol*, 2014. 24(1): p. 26-33.
[89] Ripolles, T., et al., Evaluation of Crohn's Disease Activity: Development of an Ultrasound Score in a Multicenter Study. *Inflamm Bowel Dis,* 2021. 27(1): p. 145-154.
[90] Taylor, S. A., et al., Diagnostic accuracy of magnetic resonance enterography and small bowel ultrasound for the extent and activity of newly diagnosed and relapsed Crohn's disease (METRIC): a multicentre trial. *Lancet Gastroenterol Hepatol*, 2018. 3(8): p. 548-558.
[91] Castiglione, F., et al., Noninvasive diagnosis of small bowel Crohn's disease: direct comparison of bowel sonography and magnetic resonance enterography. *Inflamm Bowel Dis*, 2013. 19(5): p. 991-8.

Chapter 3

Nutrition

Sandra Quezada[1,*], MD, MS, AGAF
Runa Watkins[2], MD
Erin Zisman[3], MD
and Katayoun Eslami[4], MD
[1]Division of Gastroenterology and Hepatology, University of Maryland School of Medicine, Baltimore, Maryland, USA
[2]University of Maryland School of Medicine, Baltimore, Maryland, USA
[3]Internal Medicine, University of Maryland Medical Center, Baltimore, Maryland, USA
[4]Pediatric Gastroenterology, University of Maryland Medical Center, Baltimore, Maryland, USA

Abstract

Patients with inflammatory bowel disease are at risk for nutritional deficiencies which can be due to disease activity or bowel resection. It is important to identify those patients most at risk (such as those with small bowel disease location or resection), and screen for treatable deficiencies to prevent complications. Dietary interventions have been studied for the treatment of inflammatory bowel disease (IBD), and while some have been associated with symptomatic improvement, thus far, none appear superior to medical therapy. In addition, extensive small bowel involvement or resection can result in short gut syndrome. With less than 200 cm of functioning small bowel, these patients are at risk for dehydration and nutritional deficiencies. While enteral nutrition is always preferred, in certain cases this may be contraindicated, and parenteral nutritional is needed. Total parenteral nutrition (TPN) may be required, but carries its own risks including bloodstream infections, deep vein thromboses, and hepatobiliary disorders. This chapter will review nutritional deficiencies, the existing literature addressing efficacy of dietary intervention to treat IBD, common food intolerances, nutritional markers, short gut syndrome, and TPN administration in IBD.

Introduction

Patients with Crohn's disease (CD) are motivated to discuss dietary strategies to treat their inflammatory bowel disease (IBD). In fact, many believe diet incited their disease, and that it can be fully treated with appropriate dietary intervention [1]. In addition to recognizing the risk

* Corresponding Author's Email: Squezada@som.umaryland.edu

In: Surgery for Crohn's Disease. Second Edition
Editors: Stephen M. Kavic, Rebecca Brown and Kerri Lopez
ISBN: 979-8-89530-676-5

for nutritional deficiencies, questions about the safety and tolerability of certain food items are often raised by patients.

Advanced therapy for IBD involves rare but concerning side effects such as infection and malignancy. Understandably, many patients hope medications can be minimized or avoided altogether by following a recommended dietary regimen. Nutrition-related issues have also been the focus of scientific investigation, as the disease pathophysiology and its treatment raise important nutritional considerations for patients with CD.

Role of Diet

Studies investigating the role of diet in the development, progression, and management of inflammatory bowel disease have found significant associations between certain diets and incidence, as well as symptom burden. Despite the abundance of research evaluating diet in patients with IBD, the impact of most dietary interventions remains uncertain.

Multiple studies have evaluated the effects of the low-fermentable oligosaccharides, disaccharides, monosaccharides, and polyols (FODMAP) diet in IBD. The low FODMAP diet is an elimination diet that excludes specified fruits and vegetables, dairy, legumes, breads, nuts/seeds, and foods with high levels of sugar or sweeteners. In a randomized trial, patients with IBD and coexisting Irritable Bowel Syndrome (IBS)-like symptoms randomized to the low-FODMAP diet had improved symptoms as measured by the IBS symptom severity system, and improved quality of life compared to those on a regular diet [2]. While this diet appears safe for IBD patients, it has not consistently improved symptoms or objective markers of inflammation [3, 4]. In addition, it is important to note that some study populations include participants with concomitant IBS, suggesting the symptom benefit of the low FODMAP diet is in largest part due to its modulation of IBS symptoms. While studies thus far have yet to demonstrate that the low FODMAP diet has any impact on IBD flares or progression as indicated by objective markers, clinical, endoscopic, and histologic disease, it can be stated that careful patient selection, focusing on IBD patients with concomitant IBS can provide improvement to those best positioned to gain symptom benefit from this dietary intervention.

In addition to the FODMAP diet, the potential impact of the CD exclusion diet and specific carbohydrate diet (SCD) in patients with IBD has been explored. In two small prospective cohort studies, patients with CD who followed an exclusion diet, characterized by reduced disaccharides, saturated fats, emulsifiers (e.g., lecithin, guar gum, carboxymethylcellulose), and red, ultra-processed meats trended towards having increased induction and maintenance of remission [5, 6]. However, a statistically significant association was not established. The Mediterranean diet (MD) and the specific carbohydrate diet (SCD), characterized by minimal consumption of sugars, grains, and lactose, have been associated with improved IBD symptoms and quality of life scores [7-9]. One randomized trial compared symptomatic remission in patients who adhered to a SCD versus the MD and demonstrated clinical remission was achieved at 46.5% and 43% respectively, which is on par with remission rates achieved in biologic clinical trials. Of note, those enrolled in the study had mild to moderate disease activity and were allowed to continue immunomodulator or biologic therapies throughout study participation [10]. The SCD was not superior to the MD, thus this latter diet may be preferred for its improved compliance in light of its increased flexibility and reduced rigidity.

Fiber, gluten, and artificial sweeteners are also being investigated for potential roles in the development and symptom burden in IBD. High dietary fiber intake has been associated with reduced CD incidence and progression, however its association with ulcerative colitis (UC) remains uncertain [11, 12]. Several reports suggest gluten free diet (GFD) may improve IBD symptoms, but to date, no studies have shown that eliminating gluten reduces inflammation in patients with IBD [13].

Western dietary patterns with high intake of meat, fats, refined sugars, and ultra-processed foods have generally been associated with increased incidence of IBD [14], whereas high intake of fruits and vegetables is strongly associated with a reduced incidence of disease [1, 11]. One meta-analysis of 9 different studies including 1,491 patients with IBD found that a Western dietary pattern was associated with an increased risk of developing IBD (relative risk (RR) 1.92), and with the development of both CD (RR 1.72) and ulcerative colitis (RR 2.15) individually [14]. Moreover, a separate meta-analysis pooling 4 studies found an inverse relationship between vegetable consumption and risk of IBD, including both CD and UC, as well as a protective association between dietary intake of fruit and both subtypes of IBD [11]. Thus, while additional research is required to further explore potential differences in the effects of specific diets on the incidence and progression of IBD, adhering to a diet abundant in fruits and vegetables, while restricting intake of foods typically deemed unhealthy in the general population, appears beneficial for patients with IBD.

Diet impacts the microbiome, which is also being studied in IBD. Decreased abundance of certain bacterial species and reduced general diversity overall are described in patients with IBD [15]. Interestingly, while the low FODMAP, gluten-free, and exclusion diets may reduce abdominal symptoms, these may also negatively affect the gut microbiota. Thus, the impact of diet interventions on the microbiome must be studied along with their impact on the disease course of IBD and should be considered when designing nutritional guidelines [15]. As the role of the microbiome in IBD activity is further elucidated, this may also enhance our understanding of the impact of diet and guide further directions for studying diet in IBD.

Elemental diets have demonstrated efficacy in inducing clinical, endoscopic, and histologic remission in patients with IBD. Elemental diets are liquid chemical nutrition consisting of amino acids, simple digestible carbohydrates, and triglycerides. Their palatability leaves much to be desired, leading to difficulty with adherence, and therefore are most often administered via a self-inserted nasogastric tube nightly. One prospective pilot study assessing the effect of an elemental diet in twenty-eight patients with CD demonstrated that 71% of patients achieved clinical remission with reduction in CDAI by 150 points after 4 weeks of therapy [16]. Some side effects included diarrhea and abdominal colic, especially during the initiation phase, for which reason it is recommended to increase the concentration rate slowly over a 7-day period. Notably, there were no instances in which the side effects required interruption of therapy, and these were adequately managed with temporary reduction in formula concentration and infusion rates. Importantly, endoscopic and histologic improvement was noted, and those with endoscopic healing also demonstrated reduction in previously elevated inflammatory cytokines to levels equivalent to healthy controls.

"Half-elemental" diets that allow participants to consume half of their calories with regular diet address the difficulty with adherence to these diets and improve compliance [17]. One study conducted in Japan randomized fifty-one CD patients to half-elemental or full regular diet after remission was induced by one of four methods: 1) total enteral nutrition, 2) total parenteral nutrition, 3) steroids, or 4) infliximab. After a 2-year follow-up period, relapse rates were significantly lower in the half-elemental group compared to the regular diet group, with similar adherence rates and no adverse events reported. It should be noted, all participants were also placed on concomitant 5-aminosalicylate treatment, and those who entered the study on low dose azathioprine (50 mg/ day) were allowed to continue this during the study, though no other therapies were allowed.

There is ongoing research evaluating exclusive enteral nutrition (EEN) combined with the CD exclusion diet to improve adherence and reduce exposure to dietary components that negatively impact the microbiome. Both diets independently induced remission, and the combination of the two induced sustained remission in a significantly higher proportion of pediatric patients than EEN alone [18]. These promising results warrant further investigation of combination diets in adult IBD patients.

These studies support use of elemental diets to treat CD, although their physiologic mechanism is yet to be fully understood. Additionally, these diets are not shown to be more beneficial than standard therapy for treating IBD. Thus, they can be considered as combination treatment along with advanced therapy for individuals with mild to moderate disease presentations. A meta-analysis reviewing eight trials that compared elemental diets to steroid therapy found that corticosteroids were more effective than elemental diet in achieving symptom remission [19]. The provider must consider the potential adverse effects of steroid therapy. Ultimately, if standard therapies are contraindicated or undesirable, and the patient is motivated, existing literature suggests elemental diets may present a reasonable option for induction or maintenance of IBD, though studies in larger populations are needed.

Nutritional Deficiencies

Most macro- and micro-nutrients are absorbed in the small bowel. In particular, digestive enzymes at the duodenal brush border make enterocytes the absorption location for most vitamins and minerals, as well as fats, proteins and carbohydrates. An exception to this is the complex process by which vitamin B12 is extracted from diet, ending in the terminal ileum. Patients with CD are at greater risk than those with UC to develop nutritional deficiencies.

Iron deficiency is the most common form of anemia seen in patients with IBD. Cytokines such as IL-6 have been identified as playing an important role in the inflammatory state that increase production of hepcidin, a negative regulator of intestinal iron absorption [20]. Given its frequency in the IBD population, patients who report active symptoms such as fatigue and decreased exercise tolerance should be screened for iron deficiency and provided supplementation as needed. It should be noted that oral iron therapy can often be difficult to tolerate and may also be less effective due to impaired intestinal absorption. Therefore, a low threshold to utilize intravenous iron supplementation is recommended.

Additional common vitamin and mineral deficiencies that occur in patients with IBD include deficiencies in vitamin B12, zinc, and vitamin D. Vitamin B12 deficiency results in a macrocytic, megaloblastic anemia which can cause neurologic symptoms such as impaired sensation and proprioception, as well as memory deficits. Patients found to have anemia with elevated mean corpuscular volume (MCV) should be screened for B12 deficiency. Because this condition often coexists with iron deficiency, even patients with normal MCV should be screened if the red cell distribution width (RDW) is high (>15). This suggests a broad range of red cell size that may include microcytosis from iron deficiency and macrocytosis from B12 deficiency. It should be noted that macrocytosis can also be an effect of azathioprine and 6-MP, commonly used medications in the treatment of IBD. In fact, this can be used as a simple marker for thiopurine medication adherence.

Zinc deficiency is also commonly seen in IBD patients. It may present with oral manifestations such as stomatitis and angular cheilitis, dermatologic conditions such as xerosis and alopecia, and can cause diarrhea. It should be considered in patients with small bowel involvement of IBD who demonstrate these signs and symptoms.

Vitamin D deficiency is common [21]. One research group found that repletion of vitamin D can result in improved quality of life in IBD patients [22], supporting the need for routine vitamin D repletion when indicated. There is also an increasing body of evidence suggesting that vitamin D itself plays a role in the pathogenesis of IBD, however the underlying mechanisms have yet to be fully elucidated [23].

Vitamin D deficiency is particularly relevant in the IBD population given the increased risk of osteoporosis [24]. Steroid exposure increases this risk, however retrospective clinical studies have demonstrated that IBD itself confers risk, independent of steroid use. Consequently, it is recommended that patients with IBD incorporate calcium and vitamin D supplementation into their nutritional regimen. The American Gastroenterological Association and American College of Gastroenterology recommend that screening for osteoporosis with DEXA scanning be performed in IBD patients including post-menopausal women over age 65, those who have been treated with prolonged courses of steroids (greater than 3 months or with repeated courses), those with history of low trauma fractures, and those with hypogonadism [25].

Deficiencies in the remaining fat-soluble vitamins A, E, and K, are less common, but are likely to be seen in patients with co-existing fat malabsorption. Control of small bowel inflammation with appropriate therapy should improve deficiencies. Providers should remain cognizant of the potential for these deficiencies in patients. Since deficiency in vitamin and minerals is often a result of the inflammatory process, reevaluation of the need for supplementation after the inflammatory process has been controlled and the symptoms have abated is reasonable.

Food Intolerance

While there is some data supporting the notion that inflammatory bowel disease can either be treated or exacerbated by diet [26], evidence remains conflicting. While food items should not impact inflammatory disease activity, patients perceive a clear effect on symptoms. This reality makes diet an important factor to consider for patients' overall well-being, and a frequent topic of concern among patients.

Identifying dietary triggers of gastrointestinal symptoms can be a powerful tool for patients. In a Crohn's and Colitis Foundation of America (CCFA) internet-based cohort study, dietary patterns of 6,768 patients with IBD were reviewed [27]. These patients were subdivided into groups by disease type (CD or UC), and presence of ostomy (O) or pouch (P). Interestingly, among all four categories, striking similarities emerged for food triggers.

Yogurt, rice and bananas were the three food items most commonly identified as having a positive effect on symptoms among IBD patients. Another interesting finding in this study was that among patients with CD, those with ostomy consumed a more liberal diet.

This study highlights trends that can be discussed with patients who have been unsuccessful in identifying food triggers. Understanding these patterns allows patients to adjust their diet to avoid negative triggers and minimize symptom exacerbation. Another study evaluated dietary intake and beliefs among 147 adults aged 18-35 years with IBD. They found that while patients with IBD struggle to meet guidelines for fiber intake, whole grains, fruits, and vegetables, a large majority of patients believe that modifying their diet could reduce IBD symptoms [1]. It should be emphasized that symptom response to diet ultimately is a very individual experience, and it may be advisable to maintain a food diary to help patients recognize patterns that may be unique to them.

While we generally consider food intolerance to be not readily generalized, an exception to this rule occurs in the case of intestinal stricture. If a patient with obstructing CD presents with stricture, they may report symptoms such as post-prandial abdominal pain, distention, nausea, or vomiting. For patients with a constricted lumen, a low fiber, low residual diet is needed to prevent an acute obstruction.

The term "low residual diet" does not always carry meaning for patients. It is often helpful to refer to this as a "melt-in-your-mouth" diet. Such a regimen allows passage of soft and liquid substances through a narrowing. This includes avoiding grains, seeds, nuts, raw fruits, and vegetables.

Also, adhering to a "low fiber" diet seems counterintuitive for many patients, who have consistently been educated on the health benefits of a high fiber diet. Providers must clarify that, in the setting of stricture, fiber can cause exacerbation of symptoms, or even lead to bowel obstruction. Once the underlying stricture and associated disease activity is treated, patients should be able to resume a healthy diet with fruits and vegetables. For those who feel strongly about maintaining some fruits and vegetables in their diet despite stricture, they should be advised to consume these food items cooked and not raw, and preferably without the peel.

Nutritional Markers in IBD

Patients with IBD are at risk for facing nutritional deficiencies for multiple reasons [28]. These include malabsorption due to active disease or surgical resection, decreased oral intake, and intestinal losses. Commonly albumin is considered important, with some studies finding significantly higher albumin levels in IBD patients in remission compared to patients with moderate to severe symptoms [29]. However, this can be misleading, as albumin levels are often decreased as a consequence of inflammation. With a half-life of 20 days, albumin levels are slow to correct despite appropriate supplementation.

As a nutritional marker, prealbumin is superior to albumin in that it is not affected by hydration and has a short half-life (36 hours). Prealbumin can also be followed once or twice weekly as an indicator of improved status. Like albumin, prealbumin is a negative acute phase reactant and can be decreased in patients with chronic disease. There is conflicting data on using pre-albumin as a marker of nutrition, as both critical and chronic illness characterized by inflammation can result in the reprioritization of hepatic protein synthesis, resulting in lower serum levels of albumin and prealbumin [30]. In addition, it can be falsely elevated after an alcohol binge due to its leakage from damaged hepatocytes, and it is decreased by zinc deficiency, though not affected by vitamin deficiency. Despite these limitations, there are studies that demonstrate a correlation between prealbumin levels and health outcomes in renal disease and in the critical care setting [31].

Unfortunately, there is no single serologic marker that determines the nutritional status of patients with IBD. Clinicians must use a holistic approach including consideration of factors such as the dietary history, physical exam, laboratory parameters, and clinical judgment. Use of standard nutritional screening tools, such as the Nutritional Risk Score, the Malnutrition Universal Screening Tool, and the Subjective Global Assessment, have been suggested for use in identifying patients with IBD who are malnourished [32]. IBD-specific screening tools, such as the Saskatchewan Inflammatory Bowel Disease-Nutrition Risk Tool (SaskIBD-NR Tool), have also been developed to identify patients at risk of malnutrition to allow for earlier intervention. The SaskIBD-NR Tool assesses gastrointestinal signs reflecting the activity of IBD, unintentional weight loss, anorexia, intake of nutrients, and food restriction [33]. By factoring in these variables, patients are then stratified as low, medium, or high risk for malnutrition.

Food Insecurity in IBD

There are many studies evaluating the impact of social determinants of health including food insecurity on clinical outcomes of patients with IBD. In the 2015 National Health Interview Survey, three million adults with IBD were identified in the US, of which over 40% reported at least one negative social determinant of health, with 12% (1 in 8 patients) reporting both food insecurity and lack of social support [34]. These patients were also more likely to experience financial hardship and cost-related medication non-adherence. Social barriers including financial strain and food insecurity have also been associated with greater disease activity in patients with IBD [35]. These findings support the need for routine assessment of social determinants of health, including food insecurity, in patients with IBD, given the already increased risk of malnutrition and vitamin deficiencies in this population. Future studies focusing on the implementation of interventions to reduce these barriers are also essential.

Conclusion

By using a comprehensive approach to assess a patient's nutritional status, including consideration of clinical factors and use of validated screening tools combined with objective markers including prealbumin and BMI, clinicians can identify which patients may benefit from additional nutritional supplementation. Given the important role of nutrition in wound healing, this may also help project surgical outcomes. Food intolerances are common, and identifying and avoiding these triggers can help reduce symptom exacerbation in IBD, but the impact of dietary interventions on the course of IBD remains unclear, thus standard medical therapy is required to treat this inflammatory process.

References

[1] Kamp KJ, Pennings B, Javelli D, Wyatt G, Given B. Dietary patterns, beliefs and behaviours among individuals with inflammatory bowel disease: a cross-sectional study. *J Hum Nutr Diet*. 2021 Apr;34(2):257-264. doi: 10.1111/jhn.12786. Epub 2020 Jun 14. PMID: 32536010; PMCID: PMC7736258.

[2] Pedersen N, Ankersen DV, Felding M, Wachmann H, Végh Z, Molzen L, Burisch J, Andersen JR, Munkholm P. Low-FODMAP diet reduces irritable bowel symptoms in patients with inflammatory bowel disease. *World J Gastroenterol*. 2017 May 14;23(18):3356-3366. doi: 10.3748/wjg.v23.i18.3356. PMID: 28566897; PMCID: PMC5434443.

[3] Bodini G., Zanella C., Crespi M., Pumo S. L., Demarzo M. G., Savarino E., Savarino V., Giannini E. G., A randomised, 6-wk trial of low FODMAP diet in patients with inflammatory bowel disease. *Nutrition.* 2019;67–68:110542. doi: 10.1016/j.nut.2019.06.023.

[4] Cox S., Prince A., Myers C., Irving P. M., Lindsay J. O., Lomer M. C., Whelan K. Fermentable carbohydrates [FODMAPs] exaccerbate functional gastrointestinal symptoms in patients with inflammatory bowel disease: A randomised, double-blind placebo-controlled, cross-over, re-challange trial. *J. Crohn's Colitis.* 2017;11:1420–1429. doi: 10.1093/ecco-jcc/jjx073.

[5] Szczubełek M, Pomorska K, Korólczyk-Kowalczyk M, Lewandowski K, Kaniewska M, Rydzewska G. Effectiveness of Crohn's Disease Exclusion Diet for Induction of Remission in Crohn's Disease Adult Patients. *Nutrients*. 2021 Nov 17;13(11):4112. doi: 10.3390/nu13114112. PMID: 34836367; PMCID: PMC8618677.

[6] Nitescu M, Istratescu D, Preda CM, Manuc TE, Louis E, Manuc M, Stroie T, Catrinoiu M, Tieranu CG, Badea LE, Tugui L, Andrei A, Diculescu MM. Role of an Exclusion Diet (Reduced Disaccharides, Saturated Fats, Emulsifiers, Red and Ultraprocessed Meats) in Maintaining the Remission of Chronic Inflammatory Bowel Diseases in Adults. *Medicina (Kaunas)*. 2023 Feb 9;59(2):329. doi: 10.3390/medicina59020329. PMID: 36837530; PMCID: PMC9959761.

[7] Jaber M, Altamimi M, Altamimi A, Cavaliere S, De Filippis F. Mediterranean diet diminishes the effects of Crohn's disease and improves its parameters: A systematic review. *Nutr Health*. 2022 May 25:2601060221102281. doi: 10.1177/02601060221102281. Epub ahead of print. PMID: 35611526.

[8] Comeche JM, Gutierrez-Hervás A, Tuells J, Altavilla C, Caballero P. Predefined Diets in Patients with Inflammatory Bowel Disease: Systematic Review and Meta-Analysis. *Nutrients*. 2020 Dec 26;13(1):52. doi: 10.3390/nu13010052. PMID: 33375314; PMCID: PMC7823473.

[9] Limketkai BN, Godoy-Brewer G, Parian AM, Noorian S, Krishna M, Shah ND, White J, Mullin GE. Dietary Interventions for the Treatment of Inflammatory Bowel Diseases: An Updated Systematic Review and Meta-analysis. *Clin Gastroenterol Hepatol*. 2023 Sep;21(10):2508-2525.e10. doi: 10.1016/j.cgh.2022.11.026. Epub 2022 Dec 5. PMID: 36470529.

[10] Lewis JD, Sandler RS, Brotherton C, Brensinger C, Li H, Kappelman MD, Daniel SG, Bittinger K, Albenberg L, Valentine JF, Hanson JS, Suskind DL, Meyer A, Compher CW, Bewtra M, Saxena A, Dobes A, Cohen BL, Flynn AD, Fischer M, Saha S, Swaminath A, Yacyshyn B, Scherl E, Horst S, Curtis JR, Braly K, Nessel L, McCauley M, McKeever L, Herfarth H; DINE-CD Study Group. A Randomized Trial Comparing the Specific Carbohydrate Diet to a Mediterranean Diet in Adults With Crohn's Disease. *Gastroenterology*. 2021 Sep;161(3):837-852.e9. doi: 10.1053/j.gastro.2021.05.047. Epub 2021 May 27. Erratum in: *Gastroenterology*. 2022 Nov;163(5):1473. PMID: 34052278; PMCID: PMC8396394.

[11] Milajerdi A, Ebrahimi-Daryani N, Dieleman LA, Larijani B, Esmaillzadeh A. Association of Dietary Fiber, Fruit, and Vegetable Consumption with Risk of Inflammatory Bowel Disease: A Systematic Review and Meta-Analysis. *Adv Nutr*. 2021 Jun 1;12(3):735-743. doi: 10.1093/advances/nmaa145. PMID: 33186988; PMCID: PMC8166559.

[12] Zhao M, Feng R, Ben-Horin S, Zhuang X, Tian Z, Li X, Ma R, Mao R, Qiu Y, Chen M. Systematic review with meta-analysis: environmental and dietary differences of inflammatory bowel disease in Eastern and Western populations. *Aliment Pharmacol Ther*. 2022 Feb;55(3):266-276. doi: 10.1111/apt.16703. Epub 2021 Nov 24. PMID: 34820868.

[13] Weaver KN, Herfarth H. Gluten-Free Diet in IBD: Time for a Recommendation? *Mol Nutr Food Res*. 2021 Mar;65(5):e1901274. doi: 10.1002/mnfr.201901274. Epub 2020 Jun 28. PMID: 32558265.

[14] Li T, Qiu Y, Yang HS, Li MY, Zhuang XJ, Zhang SH, Feng R, Chen BL, He Y, Zeng ZR, Chen MH. Systematic review and meta-analysis: Association of a pre-illness Western dietary pattern with the risk of developing inflammatory bowel disease. *J Dig Dis*. 2020 Jul;21(7):362-371. doi: 10.1111/1751-2980.12910. PMID: 32463159.

[15] Starz E, Wzorek K, Folwarski M, Kaźmierczak-Siedlecka K, Stachowska L, Przewłócka K, Stachowska E, Skonieczna-Żydecka K. The Modification of the Gut Microbiota via Selected Specific Diets in Patients with Crohn's Disease. *Nutrients*. 2021 Jun 22;13(7):2125. doi: 10.3390/nu13072125. PMID: 34206152; PMCID: PMC8308385.

[16] Yamamoto T, Nakahigashi M, Umegae S, Kitagawa T, Matsumoto K. Impact of elemental diet on mucosal inflammation in patients with active Crohn's disease: cytokine production and endoscopic and histological findings. *Inflamm Bowel Dis*. Jun 2005; 11(6):580-588.

[17] Takagi S, Utsunomiya K, Kuriyama S, et al. Effectiveness of an 'half elemental diet' as maintenance therapy for Crohn's disease: A randomized-controlled trial. *Aliment Pharmacol Ther*. Nov 1 2006; 24(9):1333-1340.

[18] Levine A., Wine E., Assa A., Sigall Boneh R., Shaoul R., Kori M., Cohen S., Peleg S., Shamaly H., On A. Crohn's Disease Exclusion Diet Plus Partial Enteral Nutrition Induces Sustained Remission in a Randomised Controlled Trial. *Gastroenterol*. 2019;157:440–450. doi: 10.1053/j.gastro.2019.04.021.

[19] Griffiths AM, Ohlsson A, Sherman PM, Sutherland LR. Meta-analysis of enteral nutrition as a primary treatment of active Crohn's disease. *Gastroenterol*. Apr 1995; 108(4):1056-1067.

[20] Langer AL, Ginzburg YZ. Role of hepcidin-ferroportin axis in the pathophysiology, diagnosis, and treatment of anemia of chronic inflammation. *Hemodial Int*. 2017 Jun;21 Suppl 1(Suppl 1):S37-S46. doi: 10.1111/hdi.12543. Epub 2017 Mar 22. PMID: 28328181; PMCID: PMC7732206.

[21] Fletcher J, Cooper SC, Ghosh S, Hewison M. The Role of Vitamin D in Inflammatory Bowel Disease: Mechanism to Management. *Nutrients*. 2019 May 7;11(5):1019. doi: 10.3390/nu11051019. PMID: 31067701; PMCID: PMC6566188.

[22] Zullow, Samantha; Rustgi, Ankur; Quezada, Sandra; et al. Risk Factors for Vitamin D Deficiency and Impact of Repletion in a Tertiary Care InflammatoryBowel Disease Population. Conference: Digestive Disease Week (DDW) Location: San Diego, CA Date: May 19-22, 2012 . *Gastroenterol*. Volume: 142 Issue: 5 Supplement: 1 Pages: S671-S671

[23] Vernia F, Valvano M, Longo S, Cesaro N, Viscido A, Latella G. Vitamin D in Inflammatory Bowel Diseases. Mechanisms of Action and Therapeutic Implications. *Nutrients*. 2022 Jan 9;14(2):269. doi: 10.3390/nu14020269. PMID: 35057450; PMCID: PMC8779654.

[24] Krela-Kaźmierczak I, Szymczak A, Łykowska-Szuber L, Eder P, Linke K. Osteoporosis in Gastrointestinal Diseases. *Adv Clin Exp Med*. 2016 Jan-Feb;25(1):185-90. doi: 10.17219/acem/33746. PMID: 26935513.

[25] Farraye F. A., Melmed G. Y., Lichtenstein G. R., Kane S. V. ACG clinical guideline: preventive care in inflammatory bowel disease. *Am J Gastroenterol*. 2017;112(2):241–258. doi: 10.1038/ajg.2016.537.

[26] Christensen C, Knudsen A, Arnesen EK, Hatlebakk JG, Sletten IS, Fadnes LT. Diet, Food, and Nutritional Exposures and Inflammatory Bowel Disease or Progression of Disease: an Umbrella Review. *Adv Nutr*. 2024 May;15(5):100219. doi: 10.1016/j.advnut.2024.100219. Epub 2024 Apr 8. PMID: 38599319; PMCID: PMC11063602.

[27] Cohen AB, Lee D, Long MD, Kappelman MD, Martin CF, Sandler RS, Lewis JD. Dietary patterns and self-reported associations of diet with symptoms of inflammatory bowel disease. *Dig Dis Sci*. 2013 May;58(5):1322-8. doi: 10.1007/s10620-012-2373-3. Epub 2012 Aug 26. PMID: 22923336; PMCID: PMC3552110.

[28] Pieczyńska J, Prescha A, Zabłocka-Słowińska K, Neubauer K, Smereka A, Grajeta H, Biernat J, Paradowski L. Occurrence of dietary risk factors in inflammatory bowel disease: Influence on the nutritional status of patients in clinical remission. *Adv Clin Exp Med*. 2019 May;28(5):587-592. doi: 10.17219/acem/78590. PMID: 30085433.

[29] Godala M, Gaszyńska E, Walczak K, Małecka-Wojciesko E. Evaluation of Albumin, Transferrin and Transthyretin in Inflammatory Bowel Disease Patients as Disease Activity and Nutritional Status

Biomarkers. *Nutrients*. 2023 Aug 7;15(15):3479. doi: 10.3390/nu15153479. PMID: 37571416; PMCID: PMC10421392.

[30] Evans DC, Corkins MR, Malone A, Miller S, Mogensen KM, Guenter P, Jensen GL; ASPEN Malnutrition Committee. The Use of Visceral Proteins as Nutrition Markers: An ASPEN Position Paper. *Nutr Clin Pract.* 2021 Feb;36(1):22-28. doi: 10.1002/ncp.10588. Epub 2020 Oct 30. Erratum in: *Nutr Clin Pract.* 2021 Aug;36(4):909. PMID: 33125793.

[31] Viganò C, Palermo A, Mulinacci G, Pirola L, Losco A, Meucci G, Saibeni S, Pastorelli L, Amato A, Gatti M, Cortelezzi C, Di Sabatino A, Morganti D, Boni F, Grasso G, Casella G, Casini V, Caprioli FA, Vecchi M, Bezzio C, Bergna I, Radaelli F, Mengoli C, Massironi S. Prevalence of Disease-Related Malnutrition and Micronutrients Deficit in Patients with Inflammatory Bowel Disease: A Multicentric Cross-Sectional Study by the GSMII (Inflammatory Bowel Disease Study Group). *Inflamm Bowel Dis.* 2023 Aug 3:izad146. doi: 10.1093/ibd/izad146. Epub ahead of print. PMID: 37536282.

[32] Jabłońska B, Mrowiec S. Nutritional Status and Its Detection in Patients with Inflammatory Bowel Diseases. *Nutrients*. 2023 Apr 20;15(8):1991. doi: 10.3390/nu15081991. PMID: 37111210; PMCID: PMC10143611.

[33] Haskey N, Peña-Sánchez JN, Jones JL, Fowler SA. Development of a screening tool to detect nutrition risk in patients with inflammatory bowel disease. *Asia Pac J Clin Nutr*. 2018;27(4):756-762. doi: 10.6133/apjcn.112017.01. PMID: 30045418.

[34] Nguyen NH, Khera R, Ohno-Machado L, Sandborn WJ, Singh S. Prevalence and Effects of Food Insecurity and Social Support on Financial Toxicity in and Healthcare Use by Patients With Inflammatory Bowel Diseases. *Clin Gastroenterol Hepatol*. 2021 Jul;19(7):1377-1386.e5. doi: 10.1016/j.cgh.2020.05.056. Epub 2020 Jun 9. PMID: 32526341; PMCID: PMC7987215.

[35] Damas OM, Kuftinec G, Khakoo NS, Morillo D, Quintero MA, Levitt J, Lopez J, Kerman DH, Abreu MT, Deshpande AR, Schwartz SJ, Palacio A. Social barriers influence inflammatory bowel disease (IBD) outcomes and disproportionally affect Hispanics and non-Hispanic Blacks with IBD. *Therap Adv Gastroenterol*. 2022 Mar 24;15:17562848221079162. doi: 10.1177/17562848221079162. Erratum in: *Therap Adv Gastroenterol*. 2022 Apr 22;15:17562848221097575. doi: 10.1177/17562848221097575. PMID: 35356362; PMCID: PMC8958706.

Chapter 4

Medical Management of Crohn's Disease

Joseph Clinton[1], MD
and Raymond K. Cross[2,*], MD, MS
[1]University of Maryland Medical Center, Baltimore, Maryland, USA
[2]University of Maryland School of Medicine, Baltimore, Maryland, USA

Abstract

The goal for medical management of Crohn's disease (CD) is ultimately to control symptoms and improve the patient's quality of life. A secondary goal is to minimize the effects of these therapies, including both short-term and long-term toxicity. Ideally, remission is evidenced by mucosal healing and reduction in biochemical markers of inflammation. Immunomodulators, including corticosteroids, are well-suited to manage acute inflammation. The latest agents, including the biologic class and small molecules, have shown efficacy in long term maintenance therapy in CD and are particularly suited for patients with moderate to severe disease. The decision about which therapy to choose must be made in an individualized manner for patients, factoring in clinical concerns such as disease severity and risk of disease progression as well as patient specific concerns such as safety data, costs, and patient preferences into the decision. Drug monitoring, disease monitoring, and endoscopic treatment are all necessary tools in the armamentarium of the gastroenterologist specializing in inflammatory bowel disease.

Introduction and Goals of Medical Therapy in Crohn's Disease

Inflammatory bowel disease (IBD), is comprised of Crohn's disease (CD) and ulcerative colitis (UC). It affects nearly three million people in the United States [1]. IBD is a chronic disease characterized by periodic exacerbations of disease ("flares") followed by symptom-free periods ("remission") [2, 3]. Symptoms include abdominal pain, diarrhea, bloody stools, fatigue, and extraintestinal manifestations of disease [4]. The symptoms have a significant negative impact on quality of life [5] and result in increased utilization of health care resources with significant direct and indirect health care costs [6, 7, 8].

The goal of treatment for patients with symptomatic CD is to induce remission as rapidly as possible, improve quality of life, avoid short- and long-term toxicity of medical therapy, achieve mucosal healing, prevent complications, and to decrease unnecessary utilization of

* Corresponding Author's Email: rcross@mdmercy.com

In: Surgery for Crohn's Disease. Second Edition
Editors: Stephen M. Kavic, Rebecca Brown and Kerri Lopez
ISBN: 979-8-89530-676-5

healthcare resources. As CD has a relapsing and remitting disease course, most patients will require long-term medical treatment to maintain remission. Despite advances in medical therapy, the disease course in CD varies considerably and thus there has been increased emphasis on a personalized approach to medical therapy. We will discuss the goals of medical therapy, agents used, treatment strategies, and controversies in medical management.

Endpoints of Medical Therapy

Traditionally, most studies of medications for CD define a clinical response and remission using patient-reported outcome measures that combine subjective and objective data. The gold standard to assess disease activity and response to treatment has been the CD activity index (CDAI) [9]. However, there is growing evidence that the treatment target of symptom control alone does not change the natural course of the disease. Underlying inflammation may persist despite absence of symptoms [10, 11]. Therefore, the current approach to CD treatment focuses on a "treat to target" strategy. This was first introduced in 2015 in the Selecting Therapeutic Targets in Inflammatory Bowel Disease (STRIDE) program, and later updated in 2021 in STRIDE-II, by the International Organization for the Study of Inflammatory Bowel Diseases (IOIBD) [12, 13]. This initiative established clear goals for achieving disease remission, including early symptomatic improvement, improvement in biochemical markers, and later mucosal healing.

Mucosal healing, or endoscopic remission, has been difficult to achieve with traditional therapies. For example, despite achieving clinical remission in 93% of patients with CD, only 30% achieved mucosal healing after high doses steroids [14]. However, with increased utilization of biologic and small molecule therapies, mucosal healing has become a realistic target.

Although there are no prospective studies demonstrating that treating patients to the target of mucosal healing is associated with improved outcomes compared to treating patients based on symptoms, there is evidence that mucosal healing is associated with better clinical outcomes. Allez evaluated colectomy rates over time in patients with and without severe ulcerations at the baseline endoscopic assessment [15]. They found that colectomy rates were higher at one year and eight years post baseline in patients with severe endoscopic lesions (31% vs. 6% at 1 year and 62% vs. 18% at 8 years, respectively) [15]. Limketkai found that those patients with CD who were proactively monitored with endoscopy for mucosal healing assessment within six months of biologic therapy initiation, had reduced CD-related complications over two years [16]. This effect was primarily related to reduced corticosteroid utilization.

A prospective cohort study from Norway demonstrated that achievement of mucosal healing was associated with decreased disease activity and requirement for steroids [17]. Similarly, mucosal healing was the only factor after early combined immunosuppressive therapy that predicted sustained remission off of steroids and biologics [18]. Mucosal healing is also associated with a reduced need for surgery. In one study of 183 patients with CD, only 14% of patients with mucosal healing required surgery compared to 38% of patients without mucosal healing [19].

Mucosal healing is clearly an excellent prognostic factor associated with improved disease control. Yet the question remains if using mucosal healing as a treatment endpoint will improve patient outcomes. Prospective studies are needed to determine the optimal endpoint of treatment and to evaluate whether treating to a "higher bar" (i.e., mucosal healing) improves clinical outcomes.

Furthermore, achieving complete or near complete mucosal healing may not be achievable for all patients, particularly those with a higher inflammatory burden. For example, in the SONIC trial which compared patients treated with the combination of infliximab plus azathioprine versus infliximab or azathioprine alone, only 44% of patients in the combination group achieved mucosal healing at six months [20]. Similarly, the CALM trial included patients who were bio-naïve and had a median disease duration of 1 year, suggesting they may be more likely to respond to therapy [21]. Even in the tight control group which escalated therapy based on clinical or biochemical criteria rather than symptoms alone, only 46% of patients achieved mucosal healing (CDEIS <4) at 48 weeks.

Personalized Approach for Selecting Medical Therapy in Crohn's Disease

Historically, a "step up" approach to medical management of CD has been used. Treatment regimens were typically determined based on severity of symptoms. However, more recently a "top down" approach and "treat to target" strategy has increasingly been encouraged as it may lead to improved disease outcomes. A top-down treatment approach was compared to conventional step-up therapy. At six months, 60% of patients in the top-down group were in remission off of steroids compared to 36% respectively for the step-up group. Although no statistical differences were seen in the primary end-point after one year, significantly more patients in the top-down group experience mucosal healing than the step-up group (73 vs. 40%) [22]. This finding is not trivial, as follow up studies have demonstrated that mucosal healing at year two predicts improved disease control over time [23].

Though symptoms vary at time of diagnosis, the unfortunate trend in CD is the progressive development of stricturing or penetrating complications over time [24]. In most of the pivotal trials mentioned above, patients with complicated CD were excluded. Not surprisingly, retrospective studies have shown that patients with complicated disease do not respond as well to medical therapy [25]. Therefore, it is imperative to identify patients at the earliest state of disease where medical therapy is likely to be most effective. Although it is tempting to be more aggressive in order to prevent complications of disease, this would likely result in overtreatment of a significant number of patients that will not develop complications.

The provider is left with the challenge of determining which patients are at highest risk for complications of disease. Numerous clinical factors have been identified to predict a complicated disease course in patients with CD (Figure 4.8). Risk factors include younger age at disease onset, perianal and/or rectal involvement, early exposure to steroids, smoking, and ileal disease location [26, 27, 28].

Allez demonstrated that more severe endoscopic inflammation predicted the need for colectomy [15]. Others have shown that serological responses to microbial antigens predicts complicated CD and the need for surgery; however, these labs are not routinely assessed in clinical practice [29, 30]. Others have suggested that more extensive involvement including upper GI tract and the presence of multiple extraintestinal manifestations predicts a more severe disease course [31, 32]. However, the findings have been inconsistent in the literature and the correlation of upper GI involvement with severe CD remains controversial [33, 34, 35].

Early and aggressive therapy be considered in all CD patients, however, the potential benefits must be weighed against the additional risks of more aggressive therapy (Figure 4.6). An early aggressive treatment approach is probably not appropriate for patients with mild disease. For patients with moderate to severe disease, a shared decision-making approach is used to select the ideal management plan for each patient. Providers must be flexible in their approach to treatment if the initial management is not effective, changing or adding therapy expeditiously to control CD symptoms.

Pharmacologic Agents Used for Crohn's Disease

Antibiotics

Mechanism of Action

IBD is thought to arise from a dysregulated immune response against intestinal microbial flora in a genetically susceptible host [36]. As a result, use of antibiotics to alter the flora and decrease the immune response has been explored as a treatment approach in CD. Three antibiotics have been most studied for the treatment of CD: ciprofloxacin, metronidazole, and rifaximin.

Efficacy

A randomized, controlled trial compared ciprofloxacin, mesalamine, and placebo in patients with active CD. Ciprofloxacin was found to have similar efficacy to mesalamine in inducing remission and resulted in a significant reduction in CDAI scores compared to placebo [37]. Metronidazole reduces c reactive protein and disease activity scores in patients with CD compared to placebo; however, the effect was limited to patients with colonic involvement [38]. Compared to sulfasalazine, metronidazole appears to have a similar effect at reduction in disease activity scores [39]. However, the use of 5-Amino salicylic acid (5-ASA) derivatives is controversial and recent guidelines suggest against their use in CD. This will be discussed further in the following section.

Of course, antibiotics are also used to treat septic complications of CD such as intra-abdominal and perianal abscess. Antibiotics have also been shown to be a useful adjunct to immune suppressants in the treatment of perianal fistulizing disease [40]. This will be discussed in greater detail in Chapter 11.

In summary, antibiotics have a role in management of infectious complications of CD as well as adjunctive therapy in perianal fistulizing disease. However, they are not recommended as treatment for induction or maintenance of CD due to lack of efficacy and availability of more effective treatments.

IVb. 5-Aminosalicylates (5-ASA)

Mechanism of Action

5-ASAs remain a commonly prescribed treatment for CD [41]. Their use in UC is well established as an effective treatment for induction and maintenance of remission [42, 43].

However, data supporting their use in CD is controversial. 5-ASAs are thought to exert a localized anti-inflammatory effect by inhibiting conversion of arachidonic acid into metabolites (prostaglandins, leukotriene B_4, and platelet activity factor) [44].

Efficacy

There is significant controversy over the role of 5-ASA for the treatment of CD. Numerous older clinical trials have shown variable rates of induction of remission with 5-ASAs, generally in the range of 30-50%. A recent meta-analysis of three placebo-controlled trials found a statistically significant but modest treatment effect with mesalamine. Compared to placebo, the net difference in CDAI scores was -18 points after use of mesalamine (P = 0.04) [45]. Another earlier meta-analysis suggested that sulfasalazine was more likely to induce remission compared to placebo, though the effect was only seen in patients with isolated colitis [46].

However, more recent data suggests no benefit of 5-ASA compared to placebo. A large meta-analysis from 2011 of twenty-two 5-ASA trials in the treatment of CD did not find a treatment benefit compared to placebo for induction of remission [47]. Further, a Cochrane review from 2016 found no evidence to suggest that oral 5-ASA preparations are superior to placebo for the maintenance of medically-induced remission [48]. The American College of Gastroenterology recommends against the use of 5-ASAs in their most recent guidelines, citing a lack of evidence supporting their efficacy [49].

Side Effects and Dosing

The 5-ASA medications have very low toxicity, which is the main reason that many providers prefer them as a first line treatment in mild CD despite their modest therapeutic effect. The most common reported side effects for this class of medication include watery diarrhea, headache, nausea, rash, and abdominal pain [50]. Rarely these medications can be associated with pancreatitis, nephrotoxicity, pneumonitis, or a paradoxical colitis exacerbation [50, 51].

There are multiple different 5-ASA formulations. These formulations differ in how and where 5-ASA is released in the intestine (Figure 4.2). Ethylcellulose-encapsulated formulations have a time-dependent release of 5-ASA throughout the small intestine, with 5-ASA typically released initially in the jejunum (i.e., Pentasa®). Acrylate-coated formulations are pH-dependent and release 5-ASA when they are exposed to the pH between 6-7 present in the distal small bowel (i.e., Delzicol®, Asacol HD®, and Apriso®). Some 5-ASA formulations utilize a pH-dependent release with a multi-matrix to not only delay release but to extend release throughout the colon (i.e., Lialda®). Another type of 5-ASA formulation links 5-ASA with an azo bond to either sulfapyridine, an inert carrier, or another 5-ASA. These formulations remain inactive until bacterial azoreductases in the colon cleave the azo-bonds releasing 5-ASA (i.e., Azulfidine®, Diazo®, and Dipentum®).

In summary, we suggest against the routine use of 5-ASA in the management of CD, given lack of efficacy. There are a few exceptions including sulfasalazine which may be considered in the treatment of mild colonic CD. In addition, there are probably sub-sets of patients that respond to 5-ASA. In particular, CD patients that have more of a "UC-like" presentation with bloody diarrhea may be more likely to benefit from 5-ASA. When given at equal doses of 5-ASA, the individual agents are similar in efficacy. Most clinicians start at a moderate dose of 5-ASA (2.4 g of 5-ASA per day) and increase the dose if needed to achieve a complete remission.

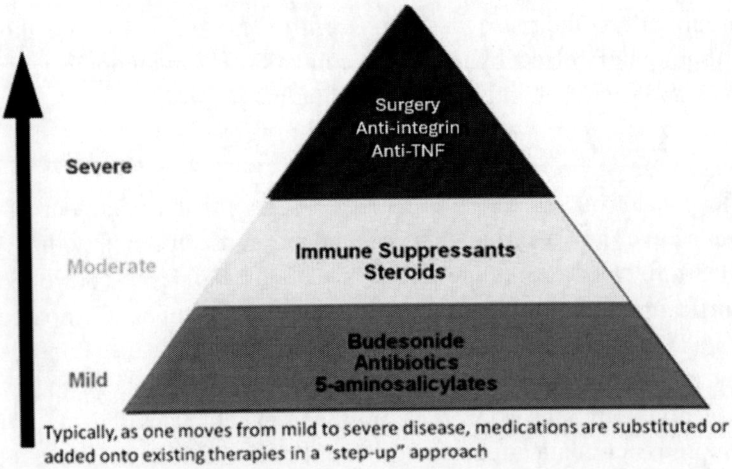

Figure 4.1. The "Step-Up" approach to medical treatment of Crohn's disease.

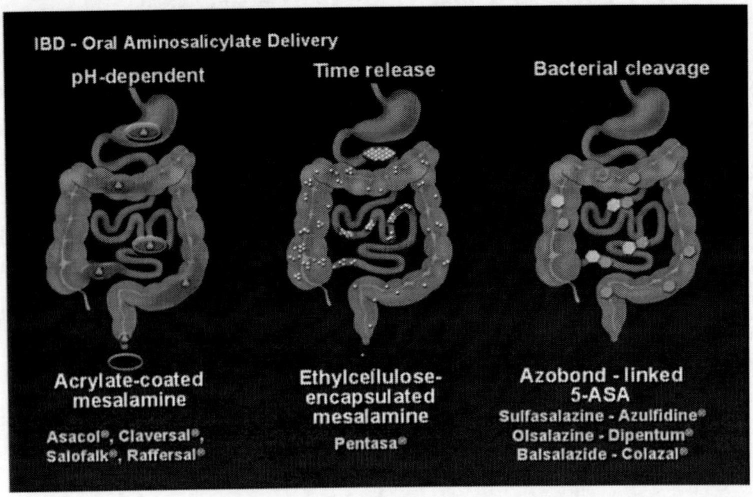

Figure 4.2. Principal locations of action for different formulations of 5-aminosalicylates.

Corticosteroids

Steroids have long been a mainstay of treatment in CD. In general, steroid treatment for CD is comprised of budesonide and systemic steroids. Budesonide is effective in inducing remission in CD and has fewer side effects than conventional steroids, though a meta-analysis of available studies showed it to be less efficacious than systemic steroids [52]. In the following section we will discuss the evidence behind the use of both types of therapy.

Budesonide

Mechanism of Action

Budesonide is a rapidly metabolized steroid that has low systemic effects due to first pass metabolism in the liver. It has a much lower rate of systemic side effects than conventional steroids, including minimal to no effect on bone mineral density [53, 54]. The common formulation facilities pH-dependent release in the terminal ileum with a topical effect in the terminal ileum and proximal colon [54]. A newer formulation approved for the treatment of UC adds multi-matrix technology to provide delayed and extended release throughout the colon [55].

Efficacy

Two randomized controlled trials demonstrated that budesonide was superior to placebo and mesalamine for induction of remission in mild to moderate ileocolonic CD. Rates of remission after use of budesonide in these studies ranged from 50-70% [56, 57]. When compared to systemic steroids, one controlled trial found budesonide to be nearly as effective in achieving remission [58]. However, a systematic review demonstrated that budesonide is less effective than systemic steroids. In addition, the meta-analysis confirmed that budesonide was superior to both placebo and mesalamine for induction of remission in CD [59].

Evidence for use of budesonide in maintenance of remission is limited. Low dose budesonide was not more effective than placebo at preventing relapses [60]. A planned meta-analysis of four trials confirmed that moderate dose budesonide prevents short-term relapse but provides no benefit after six months [61].

Systemic Steroids

Mechanism of Action

Corticosteroids are often first line therapy for induction of remission in patients with moderate to severe CD. They work via a systemic immunosuppressive and anti-inflammatory effect [54]. Although they may be necessary to induce a remission, long-term steroid treatment should be avoided because of the potential short and long-term adverse effects of these agents (Figure 4.3) [54].

Body system	Major side effects
Systemic	Cushingoid appearance (buffalo hump, moon facies, truncal obesity), weight gain
Skin	Bruising, skin thinning, striae
Eyes	Cataracts, glaucoma
Cardiovascular	Elevated blood pressure, increased risk of cardiovascular events
Musculoskeletal	Avascular necrosis, fractures, osteopenia/osteoporosis
Central Nervous System	Anxiety, confusion, delirium, depression, emotional lability, mania, psychosis
Endocrine	Exacerbation of diabetes hyperglycemia, hyperlipidemia
Infectious	Serious and opportunistic infections

Figure 4.3. Adverse effects of corticosteroids.

Efficacy

Oral steroids are extremely effective for treatment of moderate to severe CD with induction of remission rates between 50-60% and partial response to treatment in another 20-30% [62, 63]. However, the long-term outcomes after a course of prednisone are poor. A retrospective study reported on the results of CD patients treated with oral steroids. In the short-term, most patients responded to treatment. However, one year after receiving steroids, only one-third of patients were in clinical remission off of steroids, one third of patients were "steroid-dependent," and the other one third had undergone surgery [63]. Analyses of the available trials confirms that steroids are not effective in maintenance of remission compared to placebo over a two year time period [64]. Steroids have no role for maintenance of remission and steroid-dependence should not be confused as maintenance treatment.

Dosing and Side Effects
Systemic steroids are effective in inducing remission at a dose of 40 to 60 mg a day of prednisone or an IV corticosteroid equivalent in patients with severe flares [65]. Once remission is induced, steroids can then be tapered by 5mg a week until 10 mg of prednisone is reached, and then tapered by 5mg every other week.

There are numerous severe systemic side effects of steroids which have been listed by organ system in Figure 4.3. While long term side effects of corticosteroids are well documented, there is also increasing evidence that even short-term use can lead to significant adverse effects. Waljee and colleagues examined a retrospective cohort of patients treated with short term corticosteroids, defined as less than 30 days, for various conditions and found an increased risk of sepsis, venous thromboembolism, and fractures compared to non-steroid users [66].

In summary, budesonide may be used as a first-line treatment for patients with mild to moderate CD affecting the terminal ileum and right colon. Delayed and extended-release budesonide may be appropriate for patients with more extensive colonic involvement. Budesonide is effective as short-term maintenance therapy for CD as well. Systemic corticosteroids are reserved for patients with more severe disease or for those patients that do not respond to budesonide. It is recommended to transition patients to an immune suppressant or biologic after treatment with systemic steroids given the poor long-term efficacy and increased risk of adverse events associated with both short- and long-term use.

Immune Suppressants

Immune suppressants are the next category of medications in the typical "step up" approach to CD therapy and include azathioprine, 6-mercaptopurine, and methotrexate. Because the onset of action for these agents is slow, they are typically used to maintain remission after a course of corticosteroids or to facilitate steroid withdrawal in patients that are steroid-dependent.

Azathioprine and 6-Mercaptopurine

Mechanism of Action
Azathioprine (AZA) is a purine anti-metabolite that has anti-neoplastic and immune-modulating effects. It is a prodrug of 6-mercaptopurine (6-MP) which itself is broken down to an active metabolite 6-thioguanine nucleotides via a multistep enzymatic pathway that will be discussed in detail later in this chapter (Figure 4.4). These nucleotides then inhibit purine synthesis intracellularly, which likely inhibits DNA and RNA synthesis and T cell apoptosis [67].

Efficacy
AZA and 6-MP are not recommended as monotherapy for induction of remission in CD. Meta-analyses have demonstrated that AZA is not effective for induction of remission when used as monotherapy [68]. The reason for the lack of efficacy in induction of remission is the slow

onset of action. In one study, 72% of patients needed three months of treatment with 6-MP to demonstrate a clinical response [69].

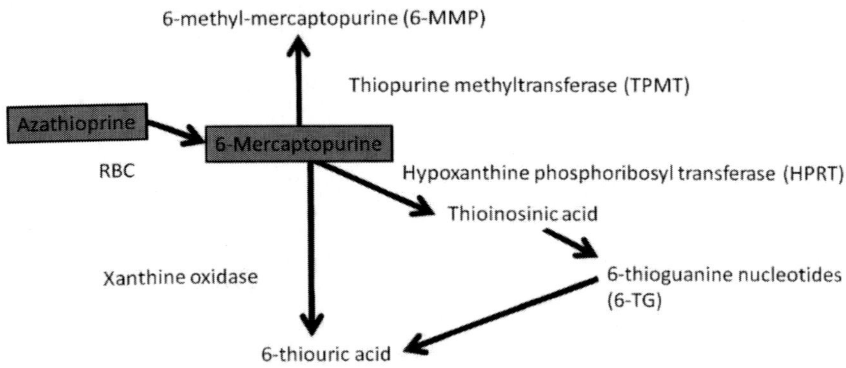

Figure 4.4. Metabolism of azathioprine and its relationship to 6-mercaptourine.

Conversely, AZA and 6-MP both have been shown to be effective in maintenance of remission, with the remission usually achieved with steroids or other rapid acting agents [70]. In one of the few trials directly comparing AZA to placebo for maintenance of remission, at fifteen months, 42% of AZA-treated patients had continued remission vs. 7% of patients who were transitioned to placebo [71]. A recent meta-analysis demonstrated an odds ratio for maintenance of remission of 2.3 and 3.3 for AZA and 6-MP respectively as well as an odds ratio for steroid sparing of 5.2 for AZA [70].

Side Effects and Dosing

Before starting AZA and 6-MP, the patient should be counseled extensively on the risks and benefits of treatment. Common reactions include myelosuppression, hepatotoxicity, nausea, vomiting, and fatigue. Less commonly, patients can develop a hypersensitivity reaction or pancreatitis. Many of the side effects occur within the first two months of starting therapy, although myelosuppression and hepatoxicity can occur at any time. Frequent monitoring is recommended initially, including complete blood counts and liver function tests. As an example, office visits with labs may be scheduled for weeks 2, 4 and 8 after starting treatment. Thereafter, monitoring frequency can be reduced [72].

6-MP and AZA are also associated with an increased risk of serious infection, opportunistic infection, non-melanoma skin cancer and hematologic malignancies [73, 74, 75]. Of special concern with use of 6-MP and AZA, especially in combination with anti-tumor necrosis factor (TNF) therapy is the development of hepatosplenic T-cell lymphoma. This is a rare and often fatal lymphoproliferative disorder. Of forty-one reported cases in the literature, twenty-three were on infliximab and thiopurine combination therapy, and seventeen were on thiopurine monotherapy [76]. Patients were predominately young men. The chance of developing this complication is very small and should not preclude use either as a primary or adjunctive therapy in patients with moderate to severe CD, but patients must be counseled regarding the risk prior to initiating therapy.

Methotrexate

Mechanism of Action

Methotrexate (MTX) is a competitive antagonist for folic acid. MTX blocks binding to dihydrofolate reductase, consequently inhibiting purine and pyrimidine synthesis [77]. Its exact mechanism of action in CD has not been clearly elucidated. It does not seem to produce a therapeutic effect due to folate antagonism as concurrent folate supplementation does not decrease effectiveness.

MTX was originally developed as a treatment for leukemia and subsequently used in rheumatoid arthritis and other autoimmune conditions. MTX has been used with increasing frequency for induction of remission, as a steroid-sparing agent in traditional step-up regimens, and in conjunction with an anti-TNF to decrease immunogenicity.

Efficacy

There is data supporting the use of MTX for induction of remission in CD. A landmark trial compared MTX to placebo in 141 patients with steroid-refractory CD. Twice the number of patients treated with MTX 25 mg intramuscularly weekly achieved remission compared to placebo (39% vs 19%) [78]. Orally dosed MTX has never been shown to have a statistically significant benefit when used as induction therapy in the available studies [79].

MTX has also been shown to be effective in the maintenance of remission when dosed via intramuscular (i.m.) injection at 15 mg weekly [80]. After successful induction therapy with MTX 25 mg i.m. weekly, MTX 15 mg i.m. weekly maintained remission in 65% of patients at 40 weeks as compared to 39% of placebo-treated patients [81]. It is not clear if these results would have been improved by continuing 25 mg i.m. weekly. As with other therapies for CD, retrospective studies have shown a gradual loss of response to MTX over time, with one review showing remission rates averaging only 43-63% by 36 months [82].

Side Effects and Dosing

MTX can be administered by the oral, subcutaneous, or intramuscular routes. Based on the lack of evidence of effect of oral MTX for induction of remission in CD, oral MTX is seldom used unless the MTX is being used solely to decrease immunogenicity. For induction and maintenance of remission either intramuscular or subcutaneous dosing can be employed. The optimal dose for maintenance is not certain.

MTX is metabolized by a first-pass effect through the liver and then eliminated by the kidneys. Adverse effects of MTX include nausea, vomiting, fatigue, headache, hair loss, hepatotoxicity, bone marrow suppression, acute lung injury, and pulmonary fibrosis (Table 3) [72]. Caution must be used in patients with chronic renal failure as elimination of MTX may be impaired with greater toxicity.

MTX was found to be associated with hepatotoxicity of nearly 25% when used in patients with rheumatologic disorders, particularly in psoriasis [83]. However, a prospective study in patients with IBD demonstrated little hepatotoxicity; nevertheless, periodic monitoring of liver enzymes is recommended [67, 84]. Besides regular assessment of transaminases (monthly for the first four months then every three months), patients should also undergo regular assessment of their complete blood count.

Supplemental folic acid, 1 mg po daily, should be prescribed to prevent or reduce side effects. Methotrexate is also associated with rare pulmonary complications, notably hypersensitivity pneumonitis. A baseline chest X-ray is recommended before initiating therapy. MTX is category X for pregnancy. Women are counseled to use two forms of birth control while taking MTX, and to avoid pregnancy for six months once MTX is discontinued [72].

Biologic Therapies

Biologic therapies are the next category of medications employed in the treatment of CD and most commonly prescribed for the induction and maintenance of moderate to severe disease. These agents are monoclonal antibodies that target various immune targets implicated in the pathogenesis of CD.

Anti-TNF Therapy

Anti-TNF agents are the mainstays of treatment of moderate to severe or treatment refractory CD. They remain one of the most frequently prescribed class of medications in CD due to abundance of clinical data collected over the past three decades supporting their efficacy. The first of these agents approved for use was infliximab (IFX), a chimeric monoclonal antibody to the TNFα receptor. The humanized antibodies adalimumab (ADA) and certolizumab pegol (CTZ) were subsequently approved for treatment of CD. Recently, CTZ has less commonly been prescribed compared to the other anti-TNF agents due to several studies suggesting relatively decreased efficacy. The following sections review the data behind usage of each of the three anti-TNF agents followed by a review of side effects and considerations of use of anti-TNF agents in general.

Infliximab

Efficacy

The first trial to evaluate the efficacy of IFX compared a single dose of IFX to placebo for induction of remission. Forty one percent of patients achieved clinical remission four weeks after IFX compared to 12% of placebo-treated patients [85]. A subsequent study compared IFX to placebo maintenance after three-dose induction with IFX at week 0, 2, and 6 in patients with moderate to severe luminal CD. Fifty eight percent of patients responded to open label IFX. IFX (at either 5 mg/kg or 10 mg/kg every 8 weeks) was superior to placebo for maintenance of remission [86].

IFX is also effective for treatment of fistulizing CD. Three dose induction therapy was more effective than placebo in reducing the number of fistula and achieving closure [87]. Similarly, maintenance IFX therapy every 8 weeks after three-dose induction therapy was more effective at maintaining fistula closure and response than placebo [88]. It is important to note that these trials were primarily comprised of patients with perianal fistula as opposed to enterocutaneous fistulas. It is likely that response rates to enterocutaneous fistulas are lower as these types of fistulas are often associated with an underlying intestinal stricture or severe transmural disease [25]. These studies will be discussed in greater detail in Chapter 11.

Adalimumab

Efficacy

ADA has been shown to be effective for induction of remission in IFX-naïve patients with a response and remission rates similar to IFX [89]. Similarly, ADA maintenance therapy (40 mg subcutaneously weekly or every other week) was more effective at maintaining remission after open-label induction therapy than placebo. Among open-label responders, about 40% of patients were in remission at one year compared to 12% of placebo treated patients [90].

Additionally, there is data to support use of ADA in patients with CD who lost response to or were intolerant of IFX. Twenty one percent of patients treated with ADA achieved remission after 4 weeks compared to only 7% of placebo-treated patients [91]. A subsequent open-label study demonstrated that 36% of IFX-exposed patients achieve remission at 6 months [92].

Certolizumab Pegol

Efficacy

CTZ has been shown to be superior to placebo for induction of a clinical response [93, 94]. However, when stratified by prior exposure to IFX, patients previously exposed to IFX did not have a statistically significant rate of clinical response or remission compared to placebo. Similarly to prior anti-TNF agents, CTZ maintenance therapy every four weeks was superior to placebo for maintenance of clinical response as well as clinical remission in patients that responded to open-label induction therapy [95].

There are currently no prospective trials comparing the efficacy of the three anti-TNF agents for induction or maintenance of remission. However, there are several meta-analyses that suggest no significant difference in the efficacy of IFX compared to ADA, but CTZ may be less likely to induce remission compared to the other two agents [96, 97, 98]. Therefore, CTZ is generally used as a second- or third-line agent in the class.

It is not recommended to electively switch between anti-TNF agents for non-medical reasons, as this may worsen outcomes. This was demonstrated in the SWITCH trial which included patients previously controlled on IFX and randomized them to continue IFX or switch to ADA [99]. The patients who switched to ADA were significantly more likely to develop loss of response compared to those that remained on IFX. However, switching to a second anti-TNF is possible in cases of failure or intolerance to a first anti-TNF. Determining which patients may benefit from a switch to an alternative anti-TNF is best made with knowledge of therapeutic drug levels: patients with loss of response and significant antidrug antibodies have a higher chance of responding to a switch within the anti-TNF class. In contrast, patients with therapeutic drug levels are best served by changing to a drug class with an alternative mechanism of action.

Side Effects and Dosing

IFX is dosed at 5 or 10 mg/kg intravenously at 0, 2, and 6 weeks for induction of remission. IFX maintenance dosing is 5 or 10 mg/kg infusions every 8 weeks. The dose can be increased, or the interval decreased if patients lose response to IFX. Loss of response to treatment is common, with nearly 40% of patients losing response to IFX over time, a phenomenon that is also seen with other anti-TNF agents [100, 101, 102].

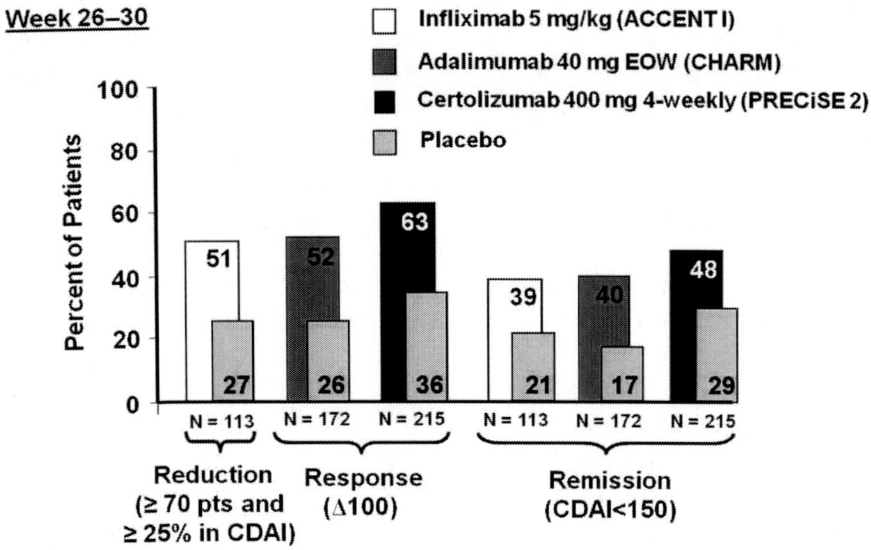

Figure 4.5. Comparative efficacies of the major anti-TNF agents, as illustrated by maintenance of remission.

System	Side Effect
Allergic/immunologic	Acute and delayed infusion reactions, injection site reactions
Skin	Eczema, psoriaform skin lesions, leukocytoclastic vasculitis, melanoma
Cardiac	Congestive heart failure
Infectious	Re-activation of latent infections (tuberculosis, hepatitis B, varicella), serious infections, opportunistic infections
Rheumatologic	Lupus-like reaction
Neurologic	Multiple sclerosis, peripheral neuropathy
Hematologic	Myelosuppression
Gastrointestinal	Drug-induced autoimmune hepatitis, hepatic failure

Figure 4.6. Side effects of anti-TNF therapy.

Recently, a subcutaneous formulation of IFX was evaluated compared to standard IV dosing for maintenance; the trial demonstrated non-inferiority of the subcutaneous and IV dosing [103]. The subcutaneous formulation is administered at a dose of 120 mg every two weeks starting at week 10 following induction. In observational studies, patients who switched from infusion to subcutaneous dosing had low rates of relapse and did not have increased risk of adverse events related to administration [104, 105].

ADA is dosed 160 mg subcutaneously at week 0, 80 mg at week 2, and 40 mg every 2 weeks for induction and 40 mg every 2 weeks for maintenance. As with IFX, if patients lose response to treatment, the interval of ADA dosing can be decreased or less commonly the dose of ADA is increased. CTZ is dosed 400 mg subcutaneously at weeks 0, 2, and 4 then every 4 weeks thereafter. Like IFX and ADA, the dose can be changed or increased in patients that lose response to treatment (200 or 400 mg subcutaneously every 2 weeks).

The side effects of anti-TNF agents include infusion or injection site reactions, serious systemic or opportunistic infections, paradoxical psoriasis, lupus and multiple sclerosis-like reactions, worsening heart failure, hepatotoxicity, lymphoma, and melanoma skin cancer (Figure 4.6) [72]. Infectious side effects of interest include reactivation of latent tuberculosis and hepatitis B, and invasive fungal infections. Therefore, it is recommended that before treatment is initiated, patients should have screening for hepatitis B and latent tuberculosis. Patients treated with anti-TNF should undergo monitoring by exam and laboratory analysis every 3-6 months to assess the ongoing efficacy and safety of treatment.

Anti-Integrin Agents

Anti-integrin agents, including vedolizumab (VDZ) and natalizumab (NTZ), are another class of biologic therapies which target leukocyte trafficking. The anti-integrin agents block the interaction between integrins on the surface of leukocytes and their ligands on the endothelium. This interaction prevents leukocytes from entering the mucosa and decreases the overall inflammatory response. NTZ blocks $\alpha 4\beta 1$ integrin in addition to $\alpha 4\beta 7$ whereas VDZ only blocks $\alpha 4\beta 7$, making the latter agent gut selective [106].

A randomized, controlled trial compared two doses of VDZ 300 mg at week 0 and 2 to placebo in patients with moderate to severe CD. After six weeks, remission and response rates were low in both groups although rates of clinical remission were higher in the VDZ group (15 vs. 7%, $p = 0.02$) [107]. A second induction study was conducted for anti-TNF exposed patients to determine if using an additional dose of VDZ at week six improved 10-week outcomes compared to placebo. This trial showed lower response and remission rates at week 6 as shown previously but demonstrated that remission rates increase to 27% at week 10 in the VDZ group (compared to 12% of placebo) [108]. In patients that responded to VDZ induction therapy, maintenance therapy with either VDZ 300 mg every 4 or 8 weeks maintained remission significantly better than placebo (36-39% compared to 22%) [107]. VDZ was approved by the FDA in May of 2014 for use in CD and UC.

A randomized, controlled trial demonstrated that 300 mg of NTZ at week 0, 4, and 8 induced a clinical response and remission in patients with moderate to severe CD compared to placebo (clinical response rate 48% vs. 32% for NTZ and placebo respectively, $p < 0.001$) [109]. A follow up study showed similar rates of response after infusions at week 0, 4, and 8 between NTZ and placebo-treated patients at 10 weeks (56 vs. 49% response rate for NTZ and placebo respectively, $p = 0.05$). However, sustained responses were higher over time in patients that continued NTZ every month compared to placebo (61 vs. 28%, $p < 0.001$) [110].

Side Effects and Dosing

VDZ is dosed at 300 mg intravenously at week 0, 2, and 6 then every 8 weeks thereafter. VDZ is now available as a subcutaneous injection for maintenance dosing following two phase 3 trials which demonstrated improved rates of clinical remission and clinical response compared to placebo in patients who responded to VDZ induction [111, 112]. Injection site reaction was the only new safety finding in patients treated with subcutaneous VDZ. NTZ is dosed at 300 mg intravenously every month.

In the initial studies, adverse events to NTZ [110] were similar to placebo. However, as use of NTZ increased for the treatment of multiple sclerosis and CD, several cases of progressive multifocal leukoencephalopathy (PML) were identified in patients undergoing treatment [113]. PML is a devastating demyelinating disorder that results from decreased central nervous system immune surveillance of the ubiquitous JC-polyoma-virus. It is thought that PML occurs in NTZ-treated patient because of inhibition of central nervous system leukocyte trafficking. It is estimated that the risk of PML is 1 per 1000 patients treated with

NTZ for a mean of 18 months [114]. Therefore, use of NTZ has been restricted to CD patients who have failed multiple other therapies.

The use of NTZ is now becoming increasingly limited to treatment of multiple sclerosis since the FDA approval of VDZ. Because VDZ is gut selective, it is thought that VDZ is not associated with PML. As such, routine assessment for JC polyoma virus before or after starting therapy is not recommended. Adverse effects of VDZ include headache, infusion reactions, hepatotoxicity, and nasopharyngitis [106]. There have been four cases of serious liver injury attributed to VDZ in long-term safety trials.

Anti-IL-12/23

The next class of biologic therapies includes Ustekinumab (UST) and Risankizumab (RIS), which target Interleukin-12 (IL-12) or combination IL-12 and Interleukin-23 (IL-23). UST was the first drug approved in this class and targets the p40 subunit on IL-12 and IL-23, which are pro-inflammatory cytokines on T cells, natural killer cells, and antigen-presenting cells [115]. In clinical trials, UST at a dose of 130 mg or 6 mg/kg had higher rates of clinical response at week 6 compared to patients treated with placebo (33-34% vs 22%, and 51-55% vs 29% respectively $p \leq 0.003$) [116]. For patients who responded to UST induction, those treated with either every 8- or 12-week maintenance UST dosing were significantly more likely to be in clinical remission at week 44 compared to placebo (53% and 49%, vs. 36% respectively, $p = 0.005$ and $p = 0.04$). Therefore, UST can be used either as first line therapy or as a second line agent in patients who previously failed other therapies, including anti-TNF.

RIS was more recently approved in 2022 for use in moderate to severe CD and targets the p19 subunit on IL-23, leading to decreased inflammation [117]. Two phase 3 clinical trials, RIS at doses of 600 mg or 1200 mg was significantly more likely to induce remission compared to placebo (45%, 42%, vs. 25% in the ADVANCE trial) and (42%, 40%, vs. 20% in the MOTIVATE trial) [118]. A subsequent maintenance trial including patients who responded to induction therapy found that patients treated with RIS maintenance therapy at 360 mg were more likely to be in clinical remission (52% vs 41%) and have endoscopic response (47% vs 22%) at one year compared to placebo [119].

In January 2024, The SEQUENCE trial was published which compared UST and RIS and is one of few available clinical trials that directly compared biologic therapies in a prospective study design [120]. The study included patients with moderate to severe CD who were previously treated with at least one anti-TNF and randomized them 1:1 to receive either RIS or UST induction therapy followed by maintenance therapy up to week 48. The authors found that patients treated with RIS were significantly more likely to achieve endoscopic remission (wk. 24: 29.4% vs 17.4%, $P = 0.001$; wk. 48: 31.8% vs 16.2%, $P < 0.0001$), mucosal healing (wk. 24: 25.1% vs 14.4%, $P < 0.01$; wk. 48: 30.2% vs 12.1%, $P < 0.0001$), and the composite endpoint of deep remission (wk. 24: 22.0% vs 10.2%, $P< 0.001$; wk. 48: 22.7% vs 10.9%, $P < 0.001$). There was no significant difference in terms of treatment related adverse events between the two drugs [120]. This study suggests that RIS should be positioned ahead of UST in patients with CD refractory to anti-TNF therapy.

Side Effects and Dosing

UST is dosed as a single IV induction dose of 260 mg, 390 mg, or 520 mg based on weight followed by 90 mg subcutaneous injection every eight weeks for maintenance dosing. RIS is dosed at 600 mg IV infusion at week 0, 4, and 8 for induction followed by a 180 mg or 360 mg subcutaneous injection every eight weeks thereafter for maintenance.

Both UST and RIS were well tolerated in clinical trials with low overall rates of adverse events. The main adverse events in clinical trials of UST were hypersensitivity reactions (<1%), nonmelanoma skin cancer (0.2%, similar to placebo), other malignancies (0.2%), and serious infections (2.3%, similar to placebo). A long-term safety study of patients with psoriasis treated with UST found low rates of malignancy (0.68/100 patient years (PY)), major cardiac events (0.33/100PY), serious infections (1.60/100PY), and overall mortality (0.46/100PY) [121].

The FORTIFY maintenance trial for RIS reported low rates of serious infections (3-4%), malignancy (1%), injection site reactions (5-6%), major cardiac events (1%), and hepatic events (3-4%) [119]. Similar to UST, long term safety data of patients with psoriasis treated with RIS showed low overall rates of serious infections (1.2 per 100 PY), nonmelanoma skin cancer (NMSC) (0.7 per 100 PY), malignant tumors excluding NMSC (0.5 per 100 PY), and major cardiac events (0.3 per 100 PY) [122].

Small Molecules

JAK Inhibitors

The next class of medications used in the treatment of CD is the JAK inhibitor class, which are oral small molecule medications. Currently, Upadacitinib (UPA) is the only JAK inhibitor approved for use in moderate to severe CD, which occurred in May 2023. UPA is a JAK-1 selective inhibitor that downregulates multiple pro-inflammatory cytokines including IL-2, IL-4, IL-6, IL-7, IL-9, IL-15, IL-21, and interferon gamma, which are involved in the pathogenesis of CD [123]. Both phase 3 induction trials, U-EXCEL and U-EXCEED, showed a statistically significant improvement in rates of clinical remission (49.5% vs. 29.1%, in U-EXCEL and 38.9% vs. 21.1%, in U-EXCEED, $p < 0.001$ for both comparisons) and endoscopic response (45.5% vs. 13.1% in U-EXCEL and 34.6% vs. 3.5% in U-EXCEED, $p < 0.001$ for both comparisons) for UPA compared to placebo [124]. Following this, the maintenance trial U-ENDURE included patients who had clinical response to UPA induction and randomized them to receive 15 mg UPA daily, 30 mg UPA daily, or placebo. Again, there was a statistically significant difference in rates of clinical remission (37% vs 48% vs 15.1%, $p < 0.001$ for both comparisons), and endoscopic response (28% vs 40% vs 7%, $p < 0.001$ for both comparisons) [124]. Notably, 45% of patients in U-EXCEL and 75% of patients in U-ENDURE had previous failure to biologic therapy. UPA has increasingly become popular as a second line agent in the treatment of CD, owing to its efficacy in trials as well as a more practical route of administration.

Side Effects and Dosing

UPA is dosed at 45 mg orally once daily for 12 weeks for induction followed by 15 mg or 30 mg orally once daily thereafter for maintenance.

The main adverse effects seen in long term safety studies of UPA in the treatment of rheumatoid arthritis, psoriatic arthritis, ankylosing spondylitis, and atopic dermatitis were increased risk of herpes zoster infections, serious infections, non-melanoma skin cancer, and elevations in creatine phosphokinase levels [125]. In phase 3 CD clinical trials, similar findings of increased risk of herpes zoster infection, serious infections, and elevated creatine kinase levels were seen [124]. In the same trials, there was a dose-dependent effect with UPA for increased risk of herpes zoster infections, elevated liver enzymes, and neutropenia. There were also four cases of GI perforation in the induction trials and one case of perforation in all three treatment groups in the maintenance trial, though it is unclear it this was related to treatment of inherent progression of CD. Lastly, a large post-marketing trial which compared patients treated with another JAK inhibitor, tofacitinib, versus patients treated with an anti-TNF for rheumatoid arthritis found increased rates of major adverse cardiovascular events, thrombosis, and malignancies [126]. Of note, patients included in this study were above the age of 50, had at least one cardiovascular risk factor, and were on concurrent methotrexate. Importantly, patients under the age of 65 without a history of smoking were not at increased risk for cardiovascular events or malignancy. Likewise, patients without a history of thromboembolic events were not at increased risk for subsequent events either. The risks associated with tofacitinib have not been seen in long-term safety studies of UC patients treated with tofacitinib. Therefore, extrapolating data from the study of rheumatoid arthritis to patients with IBD should be done cautiously given differences in disease pathogenesis and demographics of the patient population affected as patients with rheumatoid arthritis are often older and have a greater number of comorbid conditions. However, use of JAK inhibitors in CD should be done with caution in patients who are older and with significant cardiovascular risk factors [127].

Combination Therapy

Combination therapy with an immune suppressant and anti-TNF agent has been explored as a treatment option that may have improved benefit compared to either therapy alone. The SONIC trial compared AZA, IFX, and AZA plus IFX in 508 recently diagnosed, treatment-naïve patients [128]. After six months, the combination of AZA and IFX was superior to either agent alone in achieving steroid-free remission. In addition, rates of mucosal healing were higher in the AZA plus IFX group compared to either monotherapy group. Adverse events were not different between groups [128]. A third study compared the addition of MTX to IFX in patients with CD undergoing treatment with steroids [129]. No differences in treatment failure were seen between the groups at week 50; however, the rate of treatment failure was approximately 30% in both groups suggesting that co-induction with steroids and IFX is a highly effective strategy.

The advantage of combination therapy is likely related to the possible synergy between treatments and a decrease in immunogenicity associated with concurrent immune suppression use. It has been well described that concurrent treatment with immune suppressants decrease the development of antibodies to anti-TNF agents, especially when dosing of the anti-TNF is episodic [86]. Development of antibodies can be seen to all of three of the anti-TNF agents with associated infusion/injection site reactions and loss of response to therapy [130, 131]. Immunogenicity was a problem after approval of IFX because IFX was given episodically which promotes antibody development and adverse reactions; however, immunogenicity can still occur with maintenance therapy [86, 132].

Based on these data, it would seem that all CD patients should be considered for combination treatment. However, this is clearly not the case for several reasons. First, combination therapy will result in over treatment in roughly 15% of patients. Second, prospective studies have not been done to assess whether addition of an immune suppressant to an anti-TNF in patients with a partial response to treatment results in similar outcomes. Combination therapy is also more expensive than monotherapy.

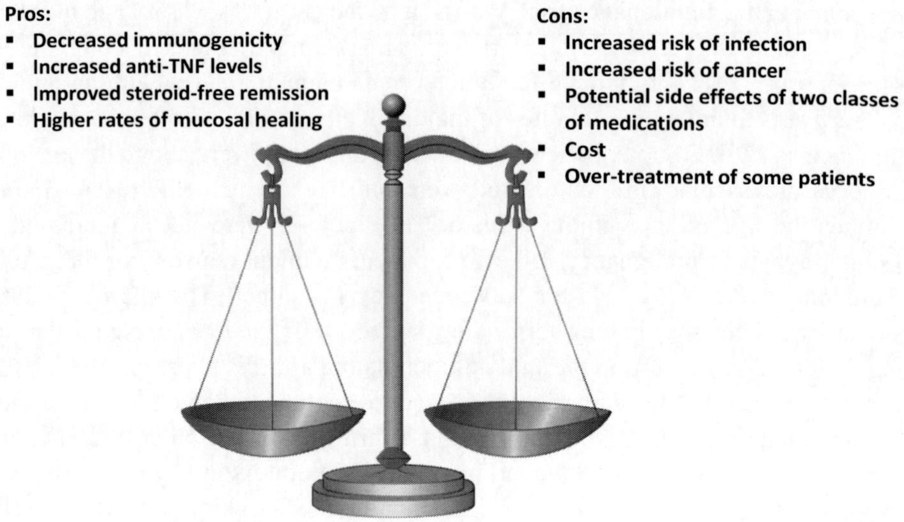

Figure 4.7. Advantages and disadvantages of combination therapy with immunosuppressants and anti-TNF therapy. A review of this material with the patient helps the clinician participate in shared decision-making.

Perhaps the most persuasive argument against combination therapy is the higher rate of adverse events associated with combination therapy. While there was not an increased rate of adverse events with use of combination therapy in the short-term trials, prospective and retrospective studies have demonstrated higher rates of opportunistic infections, nonmelanoma skin cancer, lymphoma and hepatosplenic T-cell lymphoma [73, 76, 133, 134]. Although the above studies have shown a higher relative risk of adverse effects of combination therapy, the absolute risks to patients are small. Therefore, the decision to use combination therapy should be a shared decision between the patient and provider (Figure 4.7).

Many providers try to avoid combination therapy (at least combination therapy with a thiopurine) in young men because of the increased risk of hepatosplenic T cell lymphoma. Many also try to avoid combination therapy in older patients where the risks of complication are higher [135]. Despite the risks of combination therapy, the American Gastroenterological Association recommends that anti-TNF drugs should be used in combination with thiopurines for treatment of CD (weak recommendation, moderate-quality evidence) [136].

De-Escalation of Therapy

Patients on combination therapy often achieve remission. Although this is the goal of therapy, and highly desirable, it raises the question of whether both agents are needed indefinitely for maintenance. After all, patients (and sometimes providers) are eager to minimize medications and to modify some of the risks of treatment including infection, opportunistic infection, and cancer.

Two studies have addressed the concept of treatment de-escalation. Patients with CD with controlled disease for ≥6 months were randomized to continue or the discontinue the immune suppressant with IFX [137]. The primary endpoint of the study was the proportions of patients that needed a change in IFX dose or interval or that stopped IFX during the two year follow up. There was no difference in loss of response to IFX over time between the groups. In addition, there was no difference in the rate of mucosal healing between groups. Patients that discontinued immune suppressant therapy had lower trough IFX levels compared to the combination therapy group (see therapeutic drug monitoring below) [137].

A subsequent study compared the rate of relapse after discontinuation of IFX in patients on concurrent immune suppressant therapy [138]. One hundred fifteen patients on concurrent therapy for one year and in steroid-free remission for 6 months underwent IFX withdrawal. After a median follow up of 28 months, 45% of patients relapsed. Predictors of relapse included male gender, no prior history of surgery, white blood cell count >6.0, hemoglobin ≤14.5 g/dL, c reactive protein ≥5.0 mg/L, and fecal calprotectin ≥300 mcg/g. Patients with no more than 2 of these factors had a 15% risk of relapse at one year. In relapsing patients, nearly 90% responded to reinfusion of IFX without adverse effects [138]. These results suggest that in patients with little evidence of active CD on IFX and immune suppressants, withdrawal of IFX can be considered.

In clinical practice, withdrawal of immune suppressant may be considered once patients have been in remission off steroids for one year. It is essential to share decision-making with patients, discussing the pros and cons of cessation of treatment. Most gastroenterologists pursue de-escalation of treatment in young men, older patients, and in those with possible adverse effects of therapy.

Therapeutic Drug Monitoring

One of the challenges faced in the medical management of CD is optimization of therapy when a patient has an inadequate response to, or loses response to, therapy. In the past, optimization of treatment was empiric. For example, if a patient lost response to IFX, the dose was increased from 5 mg/kg to 10 mg/kg or the interval was decreased (from 8 to 6 weeks). It is now possible to measure drug levels of thiopurines, IFX, ADA, CTZ, vedolizumab, and UST. In addition, measurement of anti-drug antibodies to biologics can be assessed. Here, we discuss measurement of drug levels and antibody levels of IFX and ADA as well as the evidence for using therapeutic drug levels in clinical practice as most of the evidence for therapeutic drug monitoring (TDM) comes from the anti-TNF class of biologics.

AZA is a pro-drug of 6-MP, to which it is non-enzymatically converted in red blood cells [139]. Three main enzymatic pathways are present to metabolize 6-MP. 6-MP is converted by thiopurine methyltransferase (TPMT) into the inactive 6-methyl mercaptopurine (6-MMP) and by xanthine oxidase into the inactive 6-thiouric acids. It is also converted by the enzyme hypoxanthine phosphoribosyl transferase (HPRT) into 6-thioguanine (6-TG), which acts as a purine antagonist to inhibit synthesis of protein, RNA and DNA (Figure 4.4).

There is important genetic variability in the enzyme expression of TPMT; it is absent in 0.3%, low in approximately 10%, and normal in about 90% [140]. In patients with absent and low TPMT activity, a much larger percentage of the drug is converted into active metabolites with a greatly increased risk of bone marrow suppression. Conversely, patients with high TPMT activity are more likely to produce higher levels of 6-MMP with increased risk for hepatotoxicity. It is thus recommended that TPMT enzyme activity is tested before initiating therapy with a thiopurine. Patients that have absent TPMT activity should not receive AZA or 6-MP. Those with low or intermediate activity should receive lower doses of 6-MP or AZA (0.5 mg/kg/day or 1.0 mg/kg/day respectively). Patients with normal to high activity should receive standard doses of 6-MP or AZA.

Once therapy has been initiated with a thiopurine, 6-TG and 6-MMP levels can be measured. While the levels correlate imperfectly to either clinical response or toxicity, they can be useful in a number of settings. Dubinsky found that a 6-TGN level of >235 pmol/8x10(8) erythrocytes was predictive of a clinical response in pediatric IBD patients whereas 6-MMP levels >5700 pmol/8x10(8) erythrocytes was predictive of hepatotoxicity [140]. Similarly, a study in adults demonstrated that a TPMT level <15.3 U/ml and a 6-TGN level of >292 pmol/8x10(8) erythrocytes correlated with a clinical response [141]. When these levels are drawn and are completely absent or low, it can be indicative of nonadherence with medication. Low 6-TGN levels in patients with inadequate clinical response can also be indicative of inadequate dose of the thiopurine. Increasing dosing based on 6-TGN levels can induce a response in patients who were previously not responding to therapy [142, 143]. It is prudent to select the dose of thiopurine based on TPMT enzyme activity testing. If patients do not respond to therapy after 8 weeks, 6-TGN and 6-MMP levels should be obtained. Others advocate for proactive measurement of levels after four weeks with adjustment to a therapeutic level if possible; this approach is also reasonable.

There are a number of commercially available assays to assess drug levels and anti-drug antibodies in patients on IFX and ADA. Prior retrospective studies have shown that anti-drug antibodies are associated with an increased rate of infusion reactions and loss of response [130]. Conversely, detectable trough levels of IFX and high trough levels of ADA have been shown to be associated with improved outcomes [144, 145].

A retrospective study from Mayo Clinic assessed the utility of IFX and antibody to IFX (ATI) in patients losing response to IFX [146]. They found that patients with undetectable IFX levels and no ATI had higher rates of response to dose escalation of IFX than patients with undetectable IFX levels and detectable ATI. Conversely, patients with detectable ATI and absent IFX were more likely to respond to a change in anti-TNF agents. Interestingly, patients with detectable IFX levels were often found to have no active inflammation to explain symptoms [146]. Similar findings were demonstrated with ADA [147].

Several studies have evaluated adjustment of IFX dosing based on proactive drug monitoring, before symptoms develop. One prospective randomized controlled trial evaluated patients with CD with stable responses to IFX maintenance therapy [148]. IFX doses were escalated or reduced based on a target trough concentration of 3-7 mcg/ml. The patients were then divided into two groups and had further dose adjustments based on continued target trough concentration monitoring versus clinical features. The study found that after initial dose escalation, there was a significant increase in clinical remission than before dose escalation (88% vs 65%; P = .020). In patients requiring dose reduction, there was a 28% reduction in drug cost from before dose reduction (P < .001). However, there was no significant difference in rates of clinical remission between the target trough concentration monitoring group versus clinical features group (69% vs 60%, p = .686). Another randomized controlled trial evaluated biologic naïve CD patients treated with combination IFX and an immunosuppressant and randomized them into groups in which IFX dosing was based on clinical symptoms, biomarkers, and serum IFX concentrations compared to clinical symptoms alone [149]. There was no significant difference between rates of corticosteroid free remission between the groups.

Younger age at disease onset
Perianal involvement
Early treatment with steroids
Cigarette smoking
Upper gastrointestinal tract, jejunal, and/or ileal disease location
Severe ulcerations on endoscopy
Serologic responses to microbial antigens
Multiple extraintestinal manifestations

Figure 4.8. Factors that predict a more complicated disease course in patients with Crohn's disease.

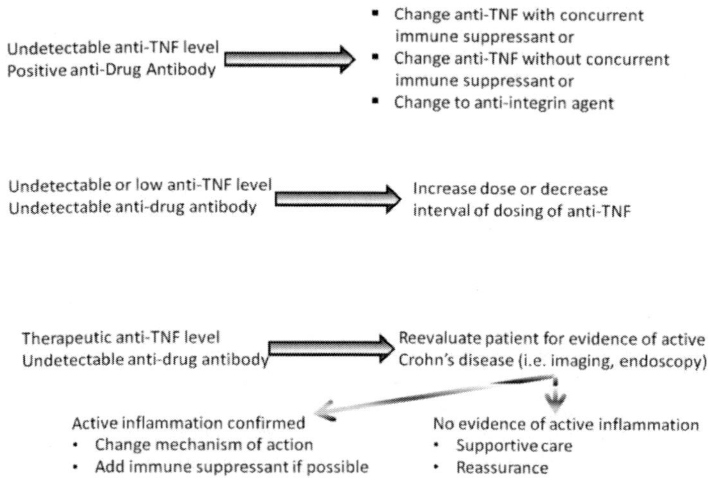

Figure 4.9. Algorithm for managing therapy based on anti-TNF and anti-drug antibody levels.

In regards to therapeutic drug monitoring with UST, one study found that a drug trough concentration of 2.3 mcg/mL at week 16 was associated with endoscopic response at 6 months [150]. Data from a real-world study from Dalal and colleagues evaluated CD patients undergoing dose escalation and found that 57.3% of patients at 12 months and 60.6% at 24 months achieved corticosteroid free clinical remission [151].

Given there is ongoing debate regarding the utility of proactive drug monitoring, Cheifetz published a comprehensive literature review and expert panel consensus statement in 2021 to help clarify and establish recommendations for therapeutic drug monitoring in CD [152]. The panel agreed that reactive drug monitoring should be used in all biologics for both primary nonresponse and secondary loss of response. They also recommended against discontinuing IFX or ADA until a target trough concentration of 10-15μg/ml is achieved. In regards to proactive drug monitoring, the panel recommended proactive TDM for anti-TNF post-induction and at least once in the maintenance phase of therapy. The panel felt that there was insufficient data to recommend the use of proactive drug monitoring in other biologics at this time. Last, they noted there was a need for more prospective and randomized controlled trials to determine which patients would benefit most from proactive drug monitoring, though there are promising areas of research including studies evaluating point of care assays and pharmacokinetic dashboards to personalize drug monitoring for individual patients and allow immediate changes in drug dosage.

In clinical practice, we agree with the expert panel's recommendation to use drug and anti-drug levels when patients either fail to respond to or lose response to IFX or ADA, a reactive drug monitoring approach. A useful algorithm is one proposed by Afif, and has been adapted by many practitioners (Figure 4.9) [146]. It is critical to reevaluate patients with therapeutic drug levels to confirm that active CD is present. In those patients, consider adding an immune suppressant in patients on anti-TNF monotherapy for synergy, or changing outside of the anti-TNF class. In addition, in patients that develop anti-drug antibodies, consider changing to another anti-TNF and also adding an immune suppressant to prevent future immunogenicity and loss of response to the second (or third) anti-TNF. We also agree with the panel recommendations for proactive drug monitoring post-induction and at least once during maintenance phase for anti-TNF therapy. Further studies are needed to determine if there is a role for proactive drug in other biologic therapies.

Comparing Advanced Therapies

With the multitude of advanced therapies available to treat CD, the provider is left with the difficult decision as to what therapy is "best" for a given patient. Despite the plethora of therapies available, primary nonresponse or loss of response remains common. Unfortunately, there are no diagnostic tests available to guide providers as to the ideal therapy and head-to-head prospective trials comparing advanced therapies are scarce. Therefore, much of our knowledge is from meta-analyses and expert opinion.

The SEAVUE trial is one of few head-to-head trials of biologic therapies in CD, which compared UST to ADA [153]. The trial included 386 patients who had failed conventional therapy but were biologic naïve. The patients were randomized to either UST or ADA induction therapy followed by maintenance therapy and the primary endpoint was clinical remission at one year. The study found no significant difference in rates of clinical remission at one year between UST and ADA (65% vs 61%, $p = 0.42$).

As mentioned previously, the recent SEQUENCE trial compared UST and RSK directly comparing patients treated with either UST or RIS induction followed by maintenance therapy up to 48 weeks [120]. The study found that patients treated with RIS were significantly more likely to achieve endoscopic remission, mucosal healing, and the composite endpoint of deep remission.

In 2021, Singh et al. published a systematic review and network meta-analysis of phase 2 and 3 randomized controlled trials of biologic therapies used in CD [154]. The group found that in biologic naïve patients, IFX monotherapy (odds ratio [OR] 4.53), combination IFX and azathioprine (OR 7.49), ADA (OR 3.01), and UST (OR 2.63) were significantly more likely to induce remission compared to CTZ. Combination therapy of IFX and azathioprine was significantly more likely to induce remission compared to VDZ (OR 3.76). The review also found that in biologic exposed patients, ADA after loss of response to IFX, and RIS, were significantly more likely to induce remission compared to VDZ (OR 2.82 and 2.10 respectively). The authors in this review concluded that IFX with azathioprine and ADA had the strongest evidence for first line therapy and ADA or RIS are preferred therapies in anti-TNF exposed patients [154].

Proposed Positioning of Advanced Therapies

Choosing the optimal therapy for every CD patient is challenging and it is unlikely that clinical trial data will provide guidance on every clinical scenario. However, providers should ideally tailor therapy towards the individual patient based on patient specific risk factors, costs, and patient preferences with the goal of clinical, biochemical, and endoscopic remission. In this section we propose a general treatment guideline for providers though noting that not every situation will be addressed and shared decision making should occur before making any treatment decision.

Biologic Naïve Patients

Anti-TNF therapy, primarily IFX and ADA, have the most clinical data supporting their efficacy in CD and therefore are appropriate for most patients with moderate to severe CD, provided the safety profile is acceptable to the patient. These medications, in particular IFX, should be considered as first line agents when treating patients with more severe disease features as well as specific phenotypes of CD including stricturing or penetrating complications, perianal disease, those with extraintestinal manifestations, and to prevent post-operative recurrence. Combination therapy with an immune suppressant should be considered in patients whom the safety profile is acceptable; an alternative would be to use monotherapy with proactive drug monitoring.

RIS, VDZ, and UST are reasonable first line therapies, particularly in patients with more moderate disease features. Although RIS appears to be superior to UST in terms of achieving endoscopic remission and mucosal healing in anti-TNF exposed patients, superiority in anti-TNF naïve patients has not been demonstrated. We recommend offering these biologic therapies as first line therapy in patients with more moderate disease features, while reserving anti-TNF therapy for patients with more severe disease features or specific phenotypes listed previously.

Data from clinical trials showed that UPA is effective in biologic naïve patients. However, it is only FDA approved for use in patients who have had inadequate response or intolerance to one or more anti-TNF medications and therefore not recommended as first line therapy.

Biologic Exposed Patients

Patients with primary nonresponse or loss of response to anti-TNF therapy are generally less likely to respond to other advanced therapies compared to patients who are biologic naïve. This is likely related to several factors including inherently more severe disease, underlying fibrosis leading to more complicated disease, and patient specific pharmacokinetics that may predispose to developing immunogenicity. One exception is RIS, which appears to be effective regardless of prior biologic exposure [154].

In patients who were treated with anti-TNF and subsequently lose response, switching to an alternative anti-TNF, RIS, or UPA has the most supporting evidence. In patients who lose response to initial anti-TNF due to immunogenicity, we recommend switching to an alternative anti-TNF along with an immune suppressant to prevent subsequent immunogenicity. Patients who lose response to anti-TNF therapy despite adequate drug levels should switch to a drug in a different class such as RIS or UPA. Both RIS and UPA were shown to be similarly effective in anti-TNF exposed patients in clinical trials. Despite sparse data directly comparing UPA to other biologic therapies, many experts suggest it should be positioned early in the treatment algorithm for patients with severe disease, particularly due to its rapid onset of action [155].

Endoscopic Therapy

As mentioned previously, development of complications such as stricture are common in patients with CD [24]. Strictures can be located anywhere within the gastrointestinal tract, but are most common at the terminal ileum or at sites of prior surgical resection [156, 157]. Symptoms can vary from acute, complete bowel obstruction requiring emergent surgery, to symptoms of intermittent obstruction such as postprandial abdominal pain, abdominal distention, borborygmi, nausea, vomiting, and weight loss.

In theory, strictures that are predominantly inflammatory may respond to medical therapy as described in the preceding sections. Fibrotic strictures, on the other hand, would be expected to require surgical intervention. However, a recent study demonstrated that most strictures have an inflammatory component as well as a fibro-stenotic component [158].

Endoscopic balloon dilation (EBD) is an alternative to surgery in patients with fibrostenotic strictures and an adjunct to medical therapy in patients with mixed strictures (See Chapter 5, Endoscopic Intervention). EBD may be especially useful in patients at risk for short gut syndrome with additional resections, in patients which surgery would be technically difficult, in patients at high-risk for complications from surgery, and in patients not yet mentally ready to accept surgery.

In a systematic review by Hassan, the technical success of EBD, typically defined as the ability of the colonoscopy to traverse the stricture after dilation, ranged between 70-100%, the clinical efficacy of EBD ranged from 40-100%, and the overall rate of major complications was 2% [159]. Variation in the reported data is likely due to variable techniques of dilation, selection of strictures that were dilated, and the skill level of the endoscopist [159]. Despite the high technical success rates of EBD, the need for repeat EBD ranges from 20 to 60% over time [160, 161, 162, 163]. Similarly, there is quite a bit of variation in the need for surgery during follow up after EBD from as low as 10% in a study by Scimeca and colleagues to 80% in a recent study [164, 165].

Patients with short strictures (<5 cm in length) may be offered EBD with or without changes in medical therapy given the excellent safety profile and short-term success. EBD is achieved by pneumatic balloon dilation through an endoscope with dilation of the stricture anywhere from 8 to 18 mm depending on the severity of the stricture. The inability to achieve a maximal balloon diameter of 18 mm predicts the need for repeat EBD over time [165]. Therefore, the endoscopist must plan serial dilations until achieving a luminal diameter of 18 mm if possible. If patients do not respond to serial EBD or if EBD is not technically successful, surgery is warranted. In addition, changes in medical therapy should be implemented if active inflammation is found in and around the stricture as recurrence of the stricture is likely without control of the inflammatory component.

Conclusion

CD is a complex disease whose natural history tends to progress to complications including stricturing and penetrating disease in most patients. As such, the majority of CD patients will eventually undergo surgery in their lifetime. The goals of medical therapy are to reduce symptoms, increase quality of life, reduce biochemical markers of inflammation, mucosal healing, and avoid short and long-term toxicity of therapy.

Before initiating medical therapy, the clinician must attempt to determine the cause of symptoms in patients with CD. It is important to understand that not all symptoms are from active CD inflammation. For example, diarrhea from loss of the ileocecal valve, small intestinal bacterial overgrowth, choleretic diarrhea, concurrent irritable bowel syndrome, *Clostridioides difficile* or other acute infections, and concurrent depression can all result in gastrointestinal symptoms. After appropriate diagnostics are completed and it is confirmed that the symptoms are from active inflammation, the first step is typically medical therapy although surgery for a short segment of ileal disease is reasonable. Recent data supports early aggressive medical therapy as there is increasing emphasis of clinical, biochemical, and endoscopic remission to prevent subsequent complications of the disease, rather than symptomatic improvement alone. However, therapy must be tailored to the individual patient and therefore aggressive therapy is likely not appropriate for all patients. When patients present with mild CD symptoms without clinical or serologic markers of a more severe disease course, it is reasonable to begin with less effective treatments such as a tapering course of budesonide, supportive care, or even a trial of dietary therapy. "Step up" therapy is then employed if patients fail to have clinical response or experience recurrent symptoms and/or inflammation despite use of these medications.

In patients with moderate to severe CD, early aggressive therapy with either biologic is appropriate, with consideration of combination therapy with an immune suppressant for patients with more severe disease presentations. Patients should be engaged in shared decision-making regarding the benefits and risks of the available advanced therapies to treat CD as well as the available comparative data supporting their individual efficacy and positioning with other therapies. Most patients with moderate to severe CD will need lifelong, maintenance therapy. However, providers can consider deescalating certain therapies with more significant adverse effects, particularly thiopurines. Anti-TNF remain the best studied and efficacious therapies available for CD, and are still recommended for use in patients with more severe disease presentations and phenotypes. Selecting therapy following anti-TNF must be done with a personalized approach as much as possible, accounting for efficacy, safety, costs, and patient preference. The use of therapeutic drug monitoring is encouraged at least in a "reactive" manner. However, proactive drug level monitoring is an alternative to combination therapy to prevent immunogenicity and to improve patient outcomes. Ideally, more head-to-head clinical trial data will become available that directly compares advanced therapies to help guide providers towards the "best" treatment for each patient. For now, providers must use available data and a shared decision-making approach with their patients to select the preferred therapy.

References

[1] Dahlhamer JM ZE, Ward BW, Wheaton AG, Croft JB. Prevalence of Inflammatory Bowel Disease Among Adults Aged ≥18 Years — United States, 2015. *MMWR Morb Mortal Wkly Rep.* 2016(65):1166–9.

[2] Loftus EV, Jr., Schoenfeld P, Sandborn WJ. The epidemiology and natural history of Crohn's disease in population-based patient cohorts from North America: a systematic review. *Aliment Pharmacol Ther*. 2002;16(1):51-60.

[3] Langholz E, Munkholm P, Davidsen M, Binder V. Course of ulcerative colitis: analysis of changes in disease activity over years. *Gastroenterology*. 1994;107(1):3-11.

[4] Sands BE. From symptom to diagnosis: clinical distinctions among various forms of intestinal inflammation. *Gastroenterology*. 2004;126(6):1518-32.

[5] Bernklev T, Jahnsen J, Lygren I, Henriksen M, Vatn M, Moum B. Health-related Quality of Life in Patients with Inflammatory Bowel Disease Measured with the Short Form-36: Psychometric Assessments and a Comparison with General Population Norms. *Inflamm Bowel Dis*. 2005;11(10):909-18.

[6] Gibson TB, Ng E, Ozminkowski RJ, Wang S, Burton WN, Goetzel RZ, et al. The direct and indirect cost burden of Crohn's disease and ulcerative colitis. *J Occup Environ Med*. 2008;50(11):1261-72.

[7] Longobardi T, Jacobs P, Bernstein CN. Work losses related to inflammatory bowel disease in the United States: results from the National Health Interview Survey. *Am J Gastroenterol*. 2003;98(5):1064-72.

[8] Kappelman MD, Rifas-Shiman SL, Porter C, Ollendorf DA, Sandler RS, Galanko JA, et al. Direct Health Care Costs of Crohn's Disease and Ulcerative Colitis in US Children and Adults. *Gastroenterology*. 2008.

[9] Best WR, Becktel JM, Singleton JW. Rederived values of the eight coefficients of the Crohn's Disease Activity Index (CDAI). *Gastroenterology*. 1979;77(4 Pt 2):843-6.

[10] Bouguen G, Levesque BG, Pola S, Evans E, Sandborn WJ. Endoscopic assessment and treating to target increase the likelihood of mucosal healing in patients with Crohn's disease. *Clin Gastroenterol Hepatol.* 2014;12(6):978-85.

[11] Colombel JF, Narula N, Peyrin-Biroulet L. Management Strategies to Improve Outcomes of Patients With Inflammatory Bowel Diseases. *Gastroenterology*. 2017;152(2):351-61 e5.

[12] Peyrin-Biroulet L, Sandborn W, Sands BE, Reinisch W, Bemelman W, Bryant RV, et al. Selecting Therapeutic Targets in Inflammatory Bowel Disease (STRIDE): Determining Therapeutic Goals for Treat-to-Target. *Am J Gastroenterol*. 2015;110(9):1324-38.

[13] Turner D, Ricciuto A, Lewis A, D'Amico F, Dhaliwal J, Griffiths AM, et al. STRIDE-II: An Update on the Selecting Therapeutic Targets in Inflammatory Bowel Disease (STRIDE) Initiative of the International Organization for the Study of IBD (IOIBD): Determining Therapeutic Goals for Treat-to-Target strategies in IBD. *Gastroenterology*. 2021;160(5):1570-83.

[14] Landi B, Anh TN, Cortot A, Soule JC, Rene E, Gendre JP, et al. Endoscopic monitoring of Crohn's disease treatment: a prospective, randomized clinical trial. The Groupe d'Etudes Therapeutiques des Affections Inflammatoires Digestives. *Gastroenterology*. 1992;102(5):1647-53.

[15] Allez M, Lemann M, Bonnet J, Cattan P, Jian R, Modigliani R. Long term outcome of patients with active Crohn's disease exhibiting extensive and deep ulcerations at colonoscopy. *Am J Gastroenterol.* 2002;97(4):947-53.

[16] Limketkai BN, Singh S, Jairath V, Sandborn WJ, Dulai PS. US Practice Patterns and Impact of Monitoring for Mucosal Inflammation After Biologic Initiation in Inflammatory Bowel Disease. *Inflamm Bowel Dis*. 2019;25(11):1828-37.

[17] Froslie KF, Jahnsen J, Moum BA, Vatn MH. Mucosal healing in inflammatory bowel disease: results from a Norwegian population-based cohort. *Gastroenterology*. 2007;133(2):412-22.

[18] Baert F, Moortgat L, Van Assche G, Caenepeel P, Vergauwe P, De Vos M, et al. Mucosal healing predicts sustained clinical remission in patients with early-stage Crohn's disease. *Gastroenterology*. 2010;138(2):463-8; quiz e10-1.

[19] Schnitzler F, Fidder H, Ferrante M, Noman M, Arijs I, Van Assche G, et al. Mucosal healing predicts long-term outcome of maintenance therapy with infliximab in Crohn's disease. *Inflamm Bowel Dis.* 2009;15(9):1295-301.

[20] Colombel JF, Sandborn WJ, Reinisch W, Mantzaris GJ, Kornbluth A, Rachmilewitz D, et al. Infliximab, azathioprine, or combination therapy for Crohn's disease. *N Engl J Med.* 2010;362(15): 1383-95.

[21] Colombel JF, Panaccione R, Bossuyt P, Lukas M, Baert F, Vanasek T, et al. Effect of tight control management on Crohn's disease (CALM): a multicentre, randomised, controlled phase 3 trial. Lancet. 2017;390(10114):2779-89.

[22] D'Haens G, Baert F, van Assche G, Caenepeel P, Vergauwe P, Tuynman H, et al. Early combined immunosuppression or conventional management in patients with newly diagnosed Crohn's disease: an open randomised trial. *Lancet.* 2008;371(9613):660-7.

[23] Baert F, Moortgat L, Van Assche G, Caenepeel P, Vergauwe P, De Vos M, et al. Mucosal healing predicts sustained clinical remission in patients with early-stage Crohn's disease. *Gastroenterology.* 2010;138(2):463-8; quiz e10-1.

[24] Cosnes J, Cattan S, Blain A, Beaugerie L, Carbonnel F, Parc R, et al. Long-term evolution of disease behavior of Crohn's disease. *Inflamm Bowel Dis.* 2002;8(4):244-50.

[25] Samimi R, Flasar MH, Kavic S, Tracy K, Cross RK. Outcome of medical treatment of stricturing and penetrating Crohn's disease: a retrospective study. *Inflamm Bowel Dis.* 2010;16(7):1187-94.

[26] Beaugerie L, Seksik P, Nion-Larmurier I, Gendre JP, Cosnes J. Predictors of Crohn's disease. *Gastroenterology.* 2006;130(3):650-6.

[27] Patil S, Rustgi A, Watson J, Betteridge J, Szeto W, Cheevers N, et al. Predictors of Disability in Patients with Crohn's Disease: 1612. *Official journal of the American College of Gastroenterology* | ACG. 2012;107:S651.

[28] Sands BE, Arsenault JE, Rosen MJ, Alsahli M, Bailen L, Banks P, et al. Risk of early surgery for Crohn's disease: implications for early treatment strategies. *Am J Gastroenterol.* 2003;98(12):2712-8.

[29] Mow WS, Vasiliauskas EA, Lin YC, Fleshner PR, Papadakis KA, Taylor KD, et al. Association of antibody responses to microbial antigens and complications of small bowel Crohn's disease. *Gastroenterology.* 2004;126(2):414-24.

[30] Dubinsky MC, Kugathasan S, Mei L, Picornell Y, Nebel J, Wrobel I, et al. Increased immune reactivity predicts aggressive complicating Crohn's disease in children. *Clin Gastroenterol Hepatol.* 2008;6(10):1105-11.

[31] Chow DK, Sung JJ, Wu JC, Tsoi KK, Leong RW, Chan FK. Upper gastrointestinal tract phenotype of Crohn's disease is associated with early surgery and further hospitalization. *Inflamm Bowel Dis.* 2009;15(4):551-7.

[32] Magro F, Rodrigues-Pinto E, Coelho R, Andrade P, Santos-Antunes J, Lopes S, et al. Is it possible to change phenotype progression in Crohn's disease in the era of immunomodulators? Predictive factors of phenotype progression. *Am J Gastroenterol.* 2014;109(7):1026-36.

[33] Crocco S, Martelossi S, Giurici N, Villanacci V, Ventura A. Upper gastrointestinal involvement in paediatric onset Crohn's disease: prevalence and clinical implications. *J Crohns Colitis.* 2012;6(1):51-5.

[34] Kim ES, Kwon Y, Choe YH, Kim MJ. Upper gastrointestinal tract involvement is more prevalent in Korean patients with pediatric Crohn's disease than in European patients. *Sci Rep.* 2020;10(1):19032.

[35] Greuter T, Piller A, Fournier N, Safroneeva E, Straumann A, Biedermann L, et al. Upper Gastrointestinal Tract Involvement in Crohn's Disease: Frequency, Risk Factors, and Disease Course. *J Crohns Colitis.* 2018;12(12):1399-409.

[36] Baumgart DC, Sandborn WJ. Crohn's disease. *Lancet.* 2012;380(9853):1590-605.

[37] Colombel JF, Lemann M, Cassagnou M, Bouhnik Y, Duclos B, Dupas JL, et al. A controlled trial comparing ciprofloxacin with mesalazine for the treatment of active Crohn's disease. Groupe d'Etudes Therapeutiques des Affections Inflammatoires Digestives (GETAID). *Am J Gastroenterol.* 1999;94(3):674-8.

[38] Sutherland L, Singleton J, Sessions J, Hanauer S, Krawitt E, Rankin G, et al. Double blind, placebo controlled trial of metronidazole in Crohn's disease. *Gut.* 1991;32(9):1071-5.

[39] Ursing B, Alm T, Barany F, Bergelin I, Ganrot-Norlin K, Hoevels J, et al. A comparative study of metronidazole and sulfasalazine for active Crohn's disease: the cooperative Crohn's disease study in Sweden. II. Result. *Gastroenterology*. 1982;83(3):550-62.

[40] Dejaco C, Harrer M, Waldhoer T, Miehsler W, Vogelsang H, Reinisch W. Antibiotics and azathioprine for the treatment of perianal fistulas in Crohn's disease. *Aliment Pharmacol Ther*. 2003;18(11-12):1113-20.

[41] Schoepfer AM, Bortolotti M, Pittet V, Mottet C, Gonvers JJ, Reich O, et al. The gap between scientific evidence and clinical practice: 5-aminosalicylates are frequently used for the treatment of Crohn's disease. *Aliment Pharmacol Ther*. 2014;40(8):930-7.

[42] Dignass A, Lindsay JO, Sturm A, Windsor A, Colombel JF, Allez M, et al. [Second European evidence-based consensus on the diagnosis and management of ulcerative colitis Part 2: Current management (Spanish version)]. *Rev Gastroenterol Mex*. 2015;80(1):32-73.

[43] Murray A, Nguyen TM, Parker CE, Feagan BG, MacDonald JK. Oral 5-aminosalicylic acid for induction of remission in ulcerative colitis. *Cochrane Database Syst Rev*. 2020;8(8):CD000543.

[44] Punchard NA, Greenfield SM, Thompson RP. Mechanism of action of 5-arninosalicylic acid. *Mediators Inflam*m. 1992;1(3):151-65.

[45] Hanauer SB SU. Oral Pentasa in the treatment of active Crohn's disease: A meta-analysis of double-blind, placebo-controlled trials. *Clinical Gastroenterology and Hepatology*. 2(5):379-88.

[46] Lim WC, Wang Y, MacDonald JK, Hanauer S. Aminosalicylates for induction of remission or response in Crohn's disease. *Cochrane Database Syst Rev*. 2016;7(7):CD008870.

[47] Ford AC KS, Khan KJ, Achkar JP, Talley NJ, Marshall JK, Moayyedi P. Efficacy of 5-aminosalicylates in Crohn's disease: systematic review and meta-analysis. *The American journal of gastroenterology*. 2011;106(4):617–29.

[48] Akobeng AK, Zhang D, Gordon M, MacDonald JK. Oral 5-aminosalicylic acid for maintenance of medically-induced remission in Crohn's disease. *Cochrane Database Syst Rev*. 2016;9(9):CD003715.

[49] Lichtenstein GR, Loftus EV, Isaacs KL, Regueiro MD, Gerson LB, Sands BE. ACG Clinical Guideline: Management of Crohn's Disease in Adults. *Am J Gastroenterol*. 2018;113(4):481-517.

[50] Ham M, Moss AC. Mesalamine in the treatment and maintenance of remission of ulcerative colitis. *Expert Rev Clin Pharmacol*. 2012;5(2):113-23.

[51] Sehgal P, Colombel JF, Aboubakr A, Narula N. Systematic review: safety of mesalazine in ulcerative colitis. *Aliment Pharmacol Ther*. 2018;47(12):1597-609.

[52] Seow CH BE, Griffiths AM, Otley AR, Steinhart AH. Budesonide for induction of remission in Crohn's disease. *Cochrane Database Syst Rev*. 2008;3:CD000296.

[53] Schoon EJ, Bollani S, Mills PR, Israeli E, Felsenberg D, Ljunghall S, et al. Bone mineral density in relation to efficacy and side effects of budesonide and prednisolone in Crohn's disease. *Clin Gastroenterol Hepatol*. 2005;3(2):113-21.

[54] Katz J. The Practical Use of Corticosteroids in the Treatment of Inflammatory Bowel Disease. Practical *Gastroenterology*. 2005;29(1):14-25.

[55] Sandborn WJ, Travis S, Moro L, Jones R, Gautille T, Bagin R, et al. Once-Daily Budesonide MMX(R) Extended-Release Tablets Induce Remission in Patients With Mild to Moderate Ulcerative Colitis: Results From the CORE I Study. *Gastroenterology*. 2012;143(5):1218-26 e2.

[56] Greenberg GR, Feagan BG, Martin F, Sutherland LR, Thomson AB, Williams CN, et al. Oral budesonide for active Crohn's disease. Canadian Inflammatory Bowel Disease Study Group. *N Engl J Med*. 1994;331(13):836-41.

[57] Thomsen OO, Cortot A, Jewell D, Wright JP, Winter T, Veloso FT, et al. Budesonide and mesalazine in active Crohn's disease: a comparison of the effects on quality of life. *Am J Gastroenterol*. 2002;97(3):649-53.

[58] Rutgeerts P, Lofberg R, Malchow H, Lamers C, Olaison G, Jewell D, et al. A comparison of budesonide with prednisolone for active Crohn's disease. *N Engl J Med*. 1994;331(13):842-5.

[59] Otley A, Steinhart AH. Budesonide for induction of remission in Crohn's disease. *Cochrane Database Syst Rev*. 2005(4):CD000296.

[60] Lofberg R, Rutgeerts P, Malchow H, Lamers C, Danielsson A, Olaison G, et al. Budesonide prolongs time to relapse in ileal and ileocaecal Crohn's disease. A placebo controlled one year study. *Gut.* 1996;39(1):82-6.

[61] Sandborn WJ, Lofberg R, Feagan BG, Hanauer SB, Campieri M, Greenberg GR. Budesonide for maintenance of remission in patients with Crohn's disease in medically induced remission: a predetermined pooled analysis of four randomized, double-blind, placebo-controlled trials. *Am J Gastroenterol*. 2005;100(8):1780-7.

[62] Munkholm P, Langholz E, Davidsen M, Binder V. Frequency of glucocorticoid resistance and dependency in Crohn's disease. *Gut*. 1994;35(3):360-2.

[63] Faubion WA, Jr., Loftus EV, Jr., Harmsen WS, Zinsmeister AR, Sandborn WJ. The natural history of corticosteroid therapy for inflammatory bowel disease: a population-based study. *Gastroenterology*. 2001;121(2):255-60.

[64] Steinhart AH EK, Griffiths AM, Modigliani R, Thomsen OO. Corticosteroids for maintenance of remission in Crohn's disease. *Cochrane Database Syst Rev*. 2003;4:CD000301.

[65] Benchimol EI, Seow CH, Steinhart AH, Griffiths AM. Traditional corticosteroids for induction of remission in Crohn's disease. *Cochrane Database Syst Rev*. 2008(2):CD006792.

[66] Waljee AK, Rogers MA, Lin P, Singal AG, Stein JD, Marks RM, et al. Short term use of oral corticosteroids and related harms among adults in the United States: population based cohort study. *BMJ*. 2017;357:j1415.

[67] Lichtenstein GR, Abreu MT, Cohen R, Tremaine W. American Gastroenterological Association Institute technical review on corticosteroids, immunomodulators, and infliximab in inflammatory bowel disease. *Gastroenterology*. 2006;130(3):940-87.

[68] Chande N, Tsoulis DJ, MacDonald JK. Azathioprine or 6-mercaptopurine for induction of remission in Crohn's disease. *Cochrane Database Syst Rev*. 2013;4:CD000545.

[69] Present DH, Korelitz BI, Wisch N, Glass JL, Sachar DB, Pasternack BS. Treatment of Crohn's disease with 6-mercaptopurine. A long-term, randomized, double-blind study. *N Engl J Med*. 1980;302(18): 981-7.

[70] Prefontaine E, Sutherland LR, Macdonald JK, Cepoiu M. Azathioprine or 6-mercaptopurine for maintenance of remission in Crohn's disease. *Cochrane Database Syst Rev*. 2009(1):CD000067.

[71] Candy S, Wright J, Gerber M, Adams G, Gerig M, Goodman R. A controlled double blind study of azathioprine in the management of Crohn's disease. *Gut*. 1995;37(5):674-8.

[72] McLean LP, Cross RK. Adverse events in IBD: to stop or continue immune suppressant and biologic treatment. *Expert Rev Gastroenterol Hepatol*. 2014;8(3):223-40.

[73] Siegel CA, Marden SM, Persing SM, Larson RJ, Sands BE. Risk of lymphoma associated with combination anti-tumor necrosis factor and immunomodulator therapy for the treatment of Crohn's disease: a meta-analysis. *Clin Gastroenterol Hepatol*. 2009;7(8):874-81.

[74] Beaugerie L, Brousse N, Bouvier AM, Colombel JF, Lemann M, Cosnes J, et al. Lymphoproliferative disorders in patients receiving thiopurines for inflammatory bowel disease: a prospective observational cohort study. *Lancet*. 2009;374(9701):1617-25.

[75] Peyrin-Biroulet L, Khosrotehrani K, Carrat F, Bouvier AM, Chevaux JB, Simon T, et al. Increased Risk For Non-Melanoma Skin Cancers In Patients Who Receive Thiopurines For Inflammatory Bowel Disease. *Gastroenterology*. 2011.

[76] Deepak P, Sifuentes H, Sherid M, Stobaugh D, Sadozai Y, Ehrenpreis ED. T-cell non-Hodgkin's lymphomas reported to the FDA AERS with tumor necrosis factor-alpha (TNF-alpha) inhibitors: results of the REFURBISH study. *Am J Gastroenterol*. 2013;108(1):99-105.

[77] Tian H, Cronstein BN. Understanding the mechanisms of action of methotrexate: implications for the treatment of rheumatoid arthritis. *Bulletin of the NYU hospital for joint diseases*. 2007;65(3):168-73.

[78] Feagan BG, Rochon J, Fedorak RN, Irvine EJ, Wild G, Sutherland L, et al. Methotrexate for the treatment of Crohn's disease. The North American Crohn's Study Group Investigators. *N Engl J Med*. 1995;332(5):292-7.

[79] McDonald JW, Wang Y, Tsoulis DJ, MacDonald JK, Feagan BG. Methotrexate for induction of remission in refractory Crohn's disease. *Cochrane Database Syst Rev*. 2014;8:CD003459.

[80] Patel V, Wang Y, MacDonald JK, McDonald JW, Chande N. Methotrexate for maintenance of remission in Crohn's disease. *Cochrane Database Syst Rev.* 2014;8:CD006884.

[81] Feagan BG, Fedorak RN, Irvine EJ, Wild G, Sutherland L, Steinhart AH, et al. A comparison of methotrexate with placebo for the maintenance of remission in Crohn's disease. North American Crohn's Study Group Investigators. *N Engl J Med.* 2000;342(22):1627-32.

[82] Hausmann J, Zabel K, Herrmann E, Schroder O. Methotrexate for maintenance of remission in chronic active Crohn's disease: long-term single-center experience and meta-analysis of observational studies. *Inflamm Bowel Dis.* 2010;16(7):1195-202.

[83] Zachariae H, Kragballe K, Sogaard H. Methotrexate induced liver cirrhosis. Studies including serial liver biopsies during continued treatment. *Br J Dermatol.* 1980;102(4):407-12.

[84] Te HS, Schiano TD, Kuan SF, Hanauer SB, Conjeevaram HS, Baker AL. Hepatic effects of long-term methotrexate use in the treatment of inflammatory bowel disease. *Am J Gastroenterol.* 2000;95(11):3150-6.

[85] Targan SR, Hanauer SB, van Deventer SJ, Mayer L, Present DH, Braakman T, et al. A short-term study of chimeric monoclonal antibody cA2 to tumor necrosis factor alpha for Crohn's disease. Crohn's Disease cA2 Study Group. *N Engl J Med.* 1997;337(15):1029-35.

[86] Hanauer SB, Feagan BG, Lichtenstein GR, Mayer LF, Schreiber S, Colombel JF, et al. Maintenance infliximab for Crohn's disease: the ACCENT I randomised trial. *Lancet.* 2002;359(9317):1541-9.

[87] Present DH, Rutgeerts P, Targan S, Hanauer SB, Mayer L, van Hogezand RA, et al. Infliximab for the treatment of fistulas in patients with Crohn's disease. *N Engl J Med.* 1999;340(18):1398-405.

[88] Sands BE, Anderson FH, Bernstein CN, Chey WY, Feagan BG, Fedorak RN, et al. Infliximab maintenance therapy for fistulizing Crohn's disease. *N Engl J Med.* 2004;350(9):876-85.

[89] Hanauer SB, Sandborn WJ, Rutgeerts P, Fedorak RN, Lukas M, MacIntosh D, et al. Human anti-tumor necrosis factor monoclonal antibody (adalimumab) in Crohn's disease: the CLASSIC-I trial. *Gastroenterology.* 2006;130(2):323-33; quiz 591.

[90] Colombel JF, Sandborn WJ, Rutgeerts P, Enns R, Hanauer SB, Panaccione R, et al. Adalimumab for maintenance of clinical response and remission in patients with Crohn's disease: The CHARM trial. *Gastroenterology.* 2007;132(1):52-65.

[91] Sandborn WJ, Rutgeerts P, Enns R, Hanauer SB, Colombel JF, Panaccione R, et al. Adalimumab induction therapy for Crohn disease previously treated with infliximab: a randomized trial. *Ann Intern Med.* 2007;146(12):829-38.

[92] Panaccione R, Loftus EV, Jr., Binion D, McHugh K, Alam S, Chen N, et al. Efficacy and safety of adalimumab in Canadian patients with moderate to severe Crohn's disease: results of the Adalimumab in Canadian SubjeCts with ModErate to Severe Crohn's DiseaSe (ACCESS) trial. *Can J Gastroenterol.* 2011;25(8):419-25.

[93] Sandborn WJ, Feagan BG, Stoinov S, Honiball PJ, Rutgeerts P, Mason D, et al. Certolizumab pegol for the treatment of Crohn's disease. *N Engl J Med.* 2007;357(3):228-38.

[94] Sandborn WJ, Schreiber S, Feagan BG, Rutgeerts P, Younes ZH, Bloomfield R, et al. Certolizumab pegol for active Crohn's disease: a placebo-controlled, randomized trial. *Clin Gastroenterol Hepatol.* 2011;9(8):670-8 e3.

[95] Schreiber S, Khaliq-Kareemi M, Lawrance IC, Thomsen OO, Hanauer SB, McColm J, et al. Maintenance therapy with certolizumab pegol for Crohn's disease. *N Engl J Med.* 2007;357(3):239-50.

[96] Kestens C, van Oijen MG, Mulder CL, van Bodegraven AA, Dijkstra G, de Jong D, et al. Adalimumab and infliximab are equally effective for Crohn's disease in patients not previously treated with anti-tumor necrosis factor-alpha agents. *Clin Gastroenterol Hepatol.* 2013;11(7):826-31.

[97] Osterman MT, Haynes K, Delzell E, Zhang J, Bewtra M, Brensinger C, et al. Comparative effectiveness of infliximab and adalimumab for Crohn's disease. *Clin Gastroenterol Hepatol.* 2014;12(5):811-7 e3.

[98] Stidham RW, Lee TC, Higgins PD, Deshpande AR, Sussman DA, Singal AG, et al. Systematic review with network meta-analysis: the efficacy of anti-TNF agents for the treatment of Crohn's disease. *Aliment Pharmacol Ther.* 2014;39(12):1349-62.

[99] Van Assche G, Vermeire S, Ballet V, Gabriels F, Noman M, D'Haens G, et al. Switch to adalimumab in patients with Crohn's disease controlled by maintenance infliximab: prospective randomised SWITCH trial. *Gut*. 2012;61(2):229-34.

[100] Gisbert JP, Panes J. Loss of response and requirement of infliximab dose intensification in Crohn's disease: a review. *Am J Gastroenterol*. 2009;104(3):760-7.

[101] Billioud V, Sandborn WJ, Peyrin-Biroulet L. Loss of response and need for adalimumab dose intensification in Crohn's disease: a systematic review. *Am J Gastroenterol*. 2011;106(4):674-84.

[102] Sandborn WJ, Lee SD, Randall C, Gutierrez A, Schwartz DA, Ambarkhane S, et al. Long-term safety and efficacy of certolizumab pegol in the treatment of Crohn's disease: 7-year results from the PRECiSE 3 study. *Aliment Pharmacol Ther*. 2014;40(8):903-16.

[103] Schreiber S, Ben-Horin S, Leszczyszyn J, Dudkowiak R, Lahat A, Gawdis-Wojnarska B, et al. Randomized Controlled Trial: Subcutaneous vs Intravenous Infliximab CT-P13 Maintenance in Inflammatory Bowel Disease. *Gastroenterology*. 2021;160(7):2340-53.

[104] Bae JH, Park JB, Baek JE, Hong SW, Park SH, Yang DH, et al. Effectiveness of Switching to Subcutaneous Infliximab in Ulcerative Colitis Patients Experiencing Intravenous Infliximab Failure. *Gut Liver*. 2024.

[105] Jeffrey AW, Abu-Rgeef R, Picardo S, Menon S, So K, Venugopal K. Safety and efficacy of transitioning inflammatory bowel disease patients from intravenous to subcutaneous infliximab: a single-center real-world experience. *Ann Gastroenterol*. 2023;36(5):549-54.

[106] McLean LP, Shea-Donohue T, Cross RK. Vedolizumab for the treatment of ulcerative colitis and Crohn's disease. *Immunotherapy*. 2012;4(9):883-98.

[107] Sandborn WJ, Feagan BG, Rutgeerts P, Hanauer S, Colombel JF, Sands BE, et al. Vedolizumab as induction and maintenance therapy for Crohn's disease. *N Engl J Med*. 2013;369(8):711-21.

[108] Sands BE, Feagan BG, Rutgeerts P, Colombel JF, Sandborn WJ, Sy R, et al. Effects of vedolizumab induction therapy for patients with Crohn's disease in whom tumor necrosis factor antagonist treatment failed. *Gastroenterology*. 2014;147(3):618-27 e3.

[109] Targan SR, Feagan BG, Fedorak RN, Lashner BA, Panaccione R, Present DH, et al. Natalizumab for the treatment of active Crohn's disease: results of the ENCORE Trial. *Gastroenterology*. 2007;132(5):1672-83.

[110] Sandborn WJ, Colombel JF, Enns R, Feagan BG, Hanauer SB, Lawrance IC, et al. Natalizumab induction and maintenance therapy for Crohn's disease. *N Engl J Med*. 2005;353(18):1912-25.

[111] Sandborn WJ, Baert F, Danese S, Krznaric Z, Kobayashi T, Yao X, et al. Efficacy and Safety of Vedolizumab Subcutaneous Formulation in a Randomized Trial of Patients With Ulcerative Colitis. *Gastroenterology*. 2020;158(3):562-72 e12.

[112] Vermeire S, D'Haens G, Baert F, Danese S, Kobayashi T, Loftus EV, et al. Efficacy and Safety of Subcutaneous Vedolizumab in Patients With Moderately to Severely Active Crohn's Disease: Results From the VISIBLE 2 Randomised Trial. *J Crohns Colitis*. 2022;16(1):27-38.

[113] Van Assche G, Van Ranst M, Sciot R, Dubois B, Vermeire S, Noman M, et al. Progressive multifocal leukoencephalopathy after natalizumab therapy for Crohn's disease. *N Engl J Med*. 2005;353(4):362-8.

[114] Yousry TA, Major EO, Ryschkewitsch C, Fahle G, Fischer S, Hou J, et al. Evaluation of patients treated with natalizumab for progressive multifocal leukoencephalopathy. *N Engl J Med*. 2006;354(9):924-33.

[115] Benson JM, Peritt D, Scallon BJ, Heavner GA, Shealy DJ, Giles-Komar JM, et al. Discovery and mechanism of ustekinumab: a human monoclonal antibody targeting interleukin-12 and interleukin-23 for treatment of immune-mediated disorders. *MAbs*. 2011;3(6):535-45.

[116] Feagan BG, Sandborn WJ, Gasink C, Jacobstein D, Lang Y, Friedman JR, et al. Ustekinumab as Induction and Maintenance Therapy for Crohn's Disease. *N Engl J Med*. 2016;375(20):1946-60.

[117] Khader SA, Thirunavukkarasu S. The Tale of IL-12 and IL-23: A Paradigm Shift. *J Immunol*. 2019;202(3):629-30.

[118] D'Haens G, Panaccione R, Baert F, Bossuyt P, Colombel JF, Danese S, et al. Risankizumab as induction therapy for Crohn's disease: results from the phase 3 ADVANCE and MOTIVATE induction trials. *Lancet*. 2022;399(10340):2015-30.

[119] Ferrante M, Panaccione R, Baert F, Bossuyt P, Colombel JF, Danese S, et al. Risankizumab as maintenance therapy for moderately to severely active Crohn's disease: results from the multicentre, randomised, double-blind, placebo-controlled, withdrawal phase 3 FORTIFY maintenance trial. *Lancet*. 2022;399(10340):2031-46.

[120] Peyrin-Biroulet L, Bossuyt P, Regueiro M, Schreiber S, Gecse K, Irving P, et al. DOP10 Risankizumab Versus Ustekinumab for the Achievement of Endoscopic Outcomes in Patients With Moderate-to-Severe Crohn's Disease: Results From the Phase 3b SEQUENCE Trial. *Journal of Crohn's and Colitis*. 2024;18(Supplement_1):i90-i1.

[121] Papp KA, Strober B, Augustin M, Calabro S, Londhe A, Chevrier M, et al. PSOLAR: design, utility, and preliminary results of a prospective, international, disease-based registry of patients with psoriasis who are receiving, or are candidates for, conventional systemic treatments or biologic agents. *J Drugs Dermatol*. 2012;11(10):1210-7.

[122] Gordon KB, Lebwohl M, Papp KA, Bachelez H, Wu JJ, Langley RG, et al. Long-term safety of risankizumab from 17 clinical trials in patients with moderate-to-severe plaque psoriasis. *Br J Dermatol*. 2022;186(3):466-75.

[123] Parmentier JM, Voss J, Graff C, Schwartz A, Argiriadi M, Friedman M, et al. In vitro and in vivo characterization of the JAK1 selectivity of upadacitinib (ABT-494). *BMC Rheumatol*. 2018;2:23.

[124] Loftus EV, Jr., Panes J, Lacerda AP, Peyrin-Biroulet L, D'Haens G, Panaccione R, et al. Upadacitinib Induction and Maintenance Therapy for Crohn's Disease. *N Engl J Med*. 2023;388(21):1966-80.

[125] Burmester GR, Cohen SB, Winthrop KL, Nash P, Irvine AD, Deodhar A, et al. Safety profile of upadacitinib over 15 000 patient-years across rheumatoid arthritis, psoriatic arthritis, ankylosing spondylitis and atopic dermatitis. *RMD Open*. 2023;9(1).

[126] Ytterberg SR, Bhatt DL, Connell CA. Cardiovascular and Cancer Risk with Tofacitinib in Rheumatoid Arthritis. Reply. *N Engl J Med*. 2022;386(18):1768.

[127] Olivera PA, Dignass A, Dubinsky MC, Peretto G, Kotze PG, Dotan I, et al. Preventing and managing cardiovascular events in patients with inflammatory bowel diseases treated with small-molecule drugs, an international Delphi consensus. *Dig Liver Dis*. 2024.

[128] Colombel JF, Sandborn WJ, Reinisch W, Mantzaris GJ, Kornbluth A, Rachmilewitz D, et al. Infliximab, azathioprine, or combination therapy for Crohn's disease. *N Engl J Med*. 2010;362(15):1383-95.

[129] Feagan BG, McDonald JW, Panaccione R, Enns RA, Bernstein CN, Ponich TP, et al. Methotrexate in combination with infliximab is no more effective than infliximab alone in patients with Crohn's disease. *Gastroenterology*. 2014;146(3):681-8 e1.

[130] Baert F, Noman M, Vermeire S, Van Assche G, G DH, Carbonez A, et al. Influence of immunogenicity on the long-term efficacy of infliximab in Crohn's disease. *N Engl J Med*. 2003;348(7):601-8.

[131] Ordas I, Mould DR, Feagan BG, Sandborn WJ. Anti-TNF monoclonal antibodies in inflammatory bowel disease: pharmacokinetics-based dosing paradigms. *Clin Pharmacol Ther*. 2012;91(4):635-46.

[132] Kugathasan S, Levy MB, Saeian K, Vasilopoulos S, Kim JP, Prajapati D, et al. Infliximab retreatment in adults and children with Crohn's disease: risk factors for the development of delayed severe systemic reaction. *Am J Gastroenterol*. 2002;97(6):1408-14.

[133] Toruner M, Loftus EV, Jr., Harmsen WS, Zinsmeister AR, Orenstein R, Sandborn WJ, et al. Risk factors for opportunistic infections in patients with inflammatory bowel disease. *Gastroenterology*. 2008;134(4):929-36.

[134] Long MD, Herfarth HH, Pipkin CA, Porter CQ, Sandler RS, Kappelman MD. Increased risk for non-melanoma skin cancer in patients with inflammatory bowel disease. *Clin Gastroenterol Hepatol*. 2010;8(3):268-74.

[135] Cottone M, Kohn A, Daperno M, Armuzzi A, Guidi L, D'Inca R, et al. Advanced Age Is an Independent Risk Factor for Severe Infections and Mortality in Patients Given Anti-Tumor Necrosis Factor Therapy for Inflammatory Bowel Disease. *Clin Gastroenterol H*. 2011;9(1):30-5.

[136] Dassopoulos T, Sultan S, Falck-Ytter YT, Inadomi JM, Hanauer SB. American Gastroenterological Association Institute technical review on the use of thiopurines, methotrexate, and anti-TNF-alpha biologic drugs for the induction and maintenance of remission in inflammatory Crohn's disease. *Gastroenterology*. 2013;145(6):1464-78 e1-5.

[137] Van Assche G, Magdelaine-Beuzelin C, D'Haens G, Baert F, Noman M, Vermeire S, et al. Withdrawal of immunosuppression in Crohn's disease treated with scheduled infliximab maintenance: a randomized trial. *Gastroenterology*. 2008;134(7):1861-8.

[138] Louis E, Mary JY, Vernier-Massouille G, Grimaud JC, Bouhnik Y, Laharie D, et al. Maintenance of remission among patients with Crohn's disease on antimetabolite therapy after infliximab therapy is stopped. *Gastroenterology*. 2012;142(1):63-70 e5; quiz e31.

[139] Elion GB. The purine path to chemotherapy. *Science*. 1989;244(4900):41-7.

[140] Dubinsky MC, Lamothe S, Yang HY, Targan SR, Sinnett D, Theoret Y, et al. Pharmacogenomics and metabolite measurement for 6-mercaptopurine therapy in inflammatory bowel disease. *Gastroenterology*. 2000;118(4):705-13.

[141] Cuffari C, Dassopoulos T, Turnbough L, Thompson RE, Bayless TM. Thiopurine methyltransferase activity influences clinical response to azathioprine in inflammatory bowel disease. *Clin Gastroenterol Hepatol*. 2004;2(5):410-7.

[142] Cuffari C, Hunt S, Bayless T. Utilisation of erythrocyte 6-thioguanine metabolite levels to optimise azathioprine therapy in patients with inflammatory bowel disease. *Gut*. 2001;48(5):642-6.

[143] Haines ML, Ajlouni Y, Irving PM, Sparrow MP, Rose R, Gearry RB, et al. Clinical usefulness of therapeutic drug monitoring of thiopurines in patients with inadequately controlled inflammatory bowel disease. *Inflamm Bowel Dis*. 2010.

[144] Maser EA, Villela R, Silverberg MS, Greenberg GR. Association of trough serum infliximab to clinical outcome after scheduled maintenance treatment for Crohn's disease. Clin Gastroenterol Hepatol. 2006;4(10):1248-54.

[145] Mazor Y, Almog R, Kopylov U, Ben Hur D, Blatt A, Dahan A, et al. Adalimumab drug and antibody levels as predictors of clinical and laboratory response in patients with Crohn's disease. *Aliment Pharmacol Ther*. 2014;40(6):620-8.

[146] Afif W, Loftus EV, Jr., Faubion WA, Kane SV, Bruining DH, Hanson KA, et al. Clinical utility of measuring infliximab and human anti-chimeric antibody concentrations in patients with inflammatory bowel disease. *Am J Gastroenterol*. 2010;105(5):1133-9.

[147] Roblin X, Rinaudo M, Del Tedesco E, Phelip JM, Genin C, Peyrin-Biroulet L, et al. Development of an algorithm incorporating pharmacokinetics of adalimumab in inflammatory bowel diseases. *Am J Gastroenterol*. 2014;109(8):1250-6.

[148] Vande Casteele N, Ferrante M, Van Assche G, Ballet V, Compernolle G, Van Steen K, et al. Trough concentrations of infliximab guide dosing for patients with inflammatory bowel disease. *Gastroenterology*. 2015;148(7):1320-9 e3.

[149] D'Haens G, Vermeire S, Lambrecht G, Baert F, Bossuyt P, Pariente B, et al. Increasing Infliximab Dose Based on Symptoms, Biomarkers, and Serum Drug Concentrations Does Not Increase Clinical, Endoscopic, and Corticosteroid-Free Remission in Patients With Active Luminal Crohn's Disease. *Gastroenterology*. 2018;154(5):1343-51 e1.

[150] Verstockt B, Dreesen E, Noman M, Outtier A, Van den Berghe N, Aerden I, et al. Ustekinumab Exposure-outcome Analysis in Crohn's Disease Only in Part Explains Limited Endoscopic Remission Rates. *J Crohns Colitis*. 2019;13(7):864-72.

[151] Dalal RS, Pruce JC, Allegretti JR. Long-Term Outcomes After Ustekinumab Dose Intensification for Inflammatory Bowel Diseases. *Inflamm Bowel Dis*. 2023;29(5):830-3.

[152] Cheifetz AS, Abreu MT, Afif W, Cross RK, Dubinsky MC, Loftus EV, Jr., et al. A Comprehensive Literature Review and Expert Consensus Statement on Therapeutic Drug Monitoring of Biologics in Inflammatory Bowel Disease. *Am J Gastroenterol*. 2021;116(10):2014-25.

[153] Sands BE, Irving PM, Hoops T, Izanec JL, Gao LL, Gasink C, et al. Ustekinumab versus adalimumab for induction and maintenance therapy in biologic-naive patients with moderately to severely active Crohn's disease: a multicentre, randomised, double-blind, parallel-group, phase 3b trial. *Lancet*. 2022;399(10342):2200-11.

[154] Singh S, Murad MH, Fumery M, Sedano R, Jairath V, Panaccione R, et al. Comparative efficacy and safety of biologic therapies for moderate-to-severe Crohn's disease: a systematic review and network meta-analysis. *Lancet Gastroenterol Hepatol*. 2021;6(12):1002-14.

[155] Dignass A, Esters P, Flauaus C. Upadacitinib in Crohn's disease. *Expert Opin Pharmacother.* 2024;25(4):359-70.

[156] Freeman HJ. Natural history and clinical behavior of Crohn's disease extending beyond two decades. *J Clin Gastroenterol.* 2003;37(3):216-9.

[157] Rutgeerts P, Geboes K, Vantrappen G, Beyls J, Kerremans R, Hiele M. Predictability of the postoperative course of Crohn's disease. *Gastroenterology.* 1990;99(4):956-63.

[158] Adler J, Punglia DR, Dillman JR, Polydorides AD, Dave M, Al-Hawary MM, et al. Computed tomography enterography findings correlate with tissue inflammation, not fibrosis in resected small bowel Crohn's disease. *Inflamm Bowel Dis.* 2012;18(5):849-56.

[159] Hassan C, Zullo A, De Francesco V, Ierardi E, Giustini M, Pitidis A, et al. Systematic review: Endoscopic dilatation in Crohn's disease. *Aliment Pharmacol Ther.* 2007;26(11-12):1457-64.

[160] Ajlouni Y, Iser JH, Gibson PR. Endoscopic balloon dilatation of intestinal strictures in Crohn's disease: safe alternative to surgery. *J Gastroenterol Hepatol.* 2007;22(4):486-90.

[161] Gustavsson A, Magnuson A, Blomberg B, Andersson M, Halfvarson J, Tysk C. Endoscopic dilation is an efficacious and safe treatment of intestinal strictures in Crohn's disease. *Aliment Pharmacol Ther.* 2012;36(2):151-8.

[162] Sabate JM, Villarejo J, Bouhnik Y, Allez M, Gornet JM, Vahedi K, et al. Hydrostatic balloon dilatation of Crohn's strictures. *Aliment Pharmacol Ther.* 2003;18(4):409-13.

[163] Ferlitsch A, Reinisch W, Puspok A, Dejaco C, Schillinger M, Schofl R, et al. Safety and efficacy of endoscopic balloon dilation for treatment of Crohn's disease strictures. *Endoscopy.* 2006;38(5):483-7.

[164] Scimeca D, Mocciaro F, Cottone M, Montalbano LM, D'Amico G, Olivo M, et al. Efficacy and safety of endoscopic balloon dilation of symptomatic intestinal Crohn's disease strictures. *Dig Liver Dis.* 2011;43(2):121-5.

[165] Armbruster S, Ally M, Deising A, Jambaulikar G, Cross R. The Efficacy and Safety of Endoscopic Balloon Dilation in the Treatment of Stricturing Crohn's Disease. *American Journal of Gastroenterology.* 2013;108:S547-S.

Chapter 5

Endoscopic Intervention

Mohammad Bourmaf[1], MD
Kelvin Liao[1], MD
and Eric Goldberg[2,*], MD
[1]Internal Medicine, University of Medicine Medical Center, Baltimore, Maryland, USA
[2]University of Maryland School of Medicine, Baltimore, Maryland, USA

Introduction

Therapeutic endoscopy has slowly but progressively been bridging the gap between medicine and surgery. It is used for a wide variety of indications, including the management of Crohn's disease. In recent decades, interventional endoscopy has transformed the management of fistulas and strictures, two commonly encountered complications of CD. These minimally invasive techniques offer significant benefits over traditional surgical approaches, including reduced recovery times and fewer complications. This chapter will explore the latest advancements and techniques in the endoscopic management of Crohn's strictures and fistulas, highlighting the evolving role of therapeutic endoscopy in improving patient outcomes.

Stricturing Disease Background

Strictures of the small and large bowel are common complications of CD (see Figure 5.1). It is estimated that up to 70% of CD patients develop ileocolonic strictures within 10 years of disease diagnosis [1]. Furthermore, Crohn's patients suffering from bowel strictures have been demonstrated to be associated with higher rates of hospitalization, steroid dependence, repeated endoscopy and surgery, and higher healthcare costs [2].

Classification of strictures based on bowel tissue layer involvement is important in guiding selection of the most appropriate therapy [1]. Intraluminal strictures are most commonly the result of inflammatory polyps and therefore more amenable to endoscopic management. Intramural strictures are typically attributed to either muscle hypertrophy and hyperplasia or fibroblast and macrophage activation leading to tissue fibrosis. These strictures are similarly amenable to endoscopic therapy. Extraluminal constriction is an important third category and involves compression of the luminal space from expansion of mesenteric fat and lymph nodes.

* Corresponding Author's Email: egoldberg@som.umaryland.edu

In: Surgery for Crohn's Disease. Second Edition
Editors: Stephen M. Kavic, Rebecca Brown and Kerri Lopez
ISBN: 979-8-89530-676-5

These subset of strictures often necessitate a surgical rather than endoscopic approach due to their extra-luminal nature. A final subtype of Crohn's related stricture is anastomotic stricture which arises following bowel resection. This is in contrast to the prior three described subtypes which represent primary strictures. The incidence of anastomic strictures is estimated to be between 3-30% at median of 5 to 12 months following bowel anastomosis [3].

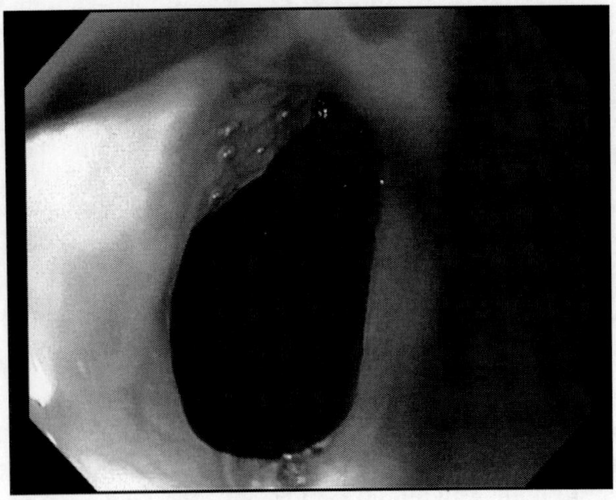

Figure 5.1. Endoscopic view of anastomotic stricture.

The main endoscopic approaches to management of Crohn's strictures are endoscopic balloon dilation, endoscopic stricturotomy and stricturoplasty, and endoscopic stenting. In general, most short strictures (less than 4-5cm) are amenable to endoscopic intervention. In most studies evaluating the efficacy of endoscopic intervention short-term efficacy is defined as the ability to traverse the stenotic area immediately after intervention. A large proportion of patients who receive endoscopic intervention will develop stricture recurrence. Therefore, long-term efficacy is commonly measured by time elapsed until repeat endoscopic or surgical intervention [4]. In the following sections we discuss for each of the endoscopic approaches their corresponding indications and contraindications, technical aspects, efficacy, and risks.

Endoscopic Balloon Dilation

The premise of endoscopic balloon dilation (EBD) in the management of stricturing CD involves generating intra-luminal pressure via water injection into either a through-the-scope (TTS) balloon or over-the-wire balloon. This serves to generate shear force which creates tears in mucosal and submucosal fibers in order to dilate strictures.

EBD is a viable, minimally invasive alternative to open or laparoscopic surgery in the treatment of Crohn's strictures. Indications for EBD include symptomatic Crohn's strictures less than 4 to 5cm. EBD is also favorable in strictures which cannot be traversed with a standard endoscope. Both primary and anastomotic strictures can be effectively treated with EBD. Similarly, both inflammatory and fibrotic strictures are amenable to treatment with EBD. Repeat EBD is indicated for re-stenosis of previously dilated strictures. However, in patients requiring more frequent intervention than every 3-12 months it may then be more appropriate to pursue more durable treatment with stricturotomy or stenting. Both these techniques will be discussed later in this chapter.

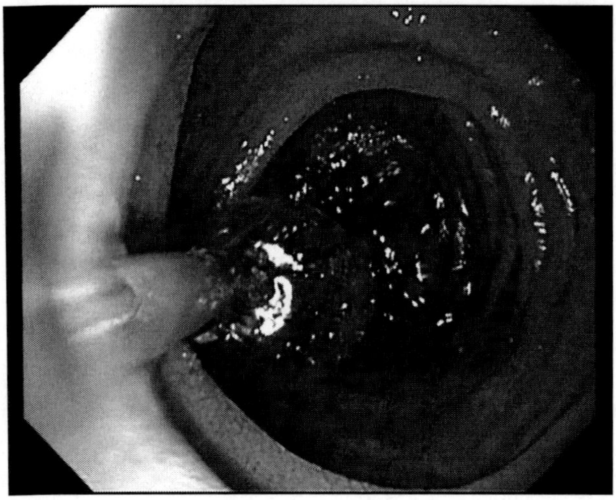

Figure 5.2. Balloon dilation of intestinal lumen.

Caution must be taken with EBD in the presence of deep ulcers, fistulous tracts, abscesses, or malignancy. In the setting of fistula and malignancy other treatments such as endoscopic stenting may be more appropriate. Finally, stenoses that involve severe curvature are unfavorable for EBD as it becomes increasingly difficult to uniformly dilate across any severe bends.

EBD can be performed anterograde or retrograde depending on stricture location within the GI tract. The aim is to traverse the stricture with a balloon catheter and then inflate to achieve stricture dilation. Through the scope (TTS) balloons are preferred as they allow direct visualization for the catheter passing through the stricture (See Figure 5.2). In cases where the stricture is too narrow to be endoscopically traversed, over-the-wire (OTW) balloon under fluoroscopic guidance can be considered. Once the stenosis is successfully traversed the balloon is insufflated and maintained in position to achieve adequate dilation to a pre-determined diameter. Graded dilation may be necessary in some cases of severe stricture. Choice of balloon diameter is left to the discretion of the endoscopist. Typically, we dilate to 3-5mm larger than the estimated luminal diameter of the stricture and then follow with serial dilations every few weeks with a goal of achieving a luminal diameter of 13-15mm.

To date there are no established standards for numerous key parameters regarding how EBD should be performed. Two of the most studied parameters include goal dilation diameter and steroid injection after dilation. A systematic review of 13 studies representing a total of 347 Crohn's patients undergoing TTS balloon stricture dilation found technical success ranging from 45% to 100% with no correlation to balloon size [5]. Dilation to 18mm, 20mm, and 25mm were present in the cases included in the systematic review. In two case series lower dilation pressure was felt to be a risk factor for need for earlier re-dilation [6, 7]. Conversely, at least one study has found that dilation to a larger diameter (25mm) is associated with increased rate of complications including perforation and hemorrhage [8]. Another key area of interest is the efficacy of steroid injection following dilation to reduce need for re-dilation. Evidence has been mixed with some studies demonstrating significantly longer time to re-dilation [9, 10] with steroid injection while another randomized controlled trial demonstrated significantly reduced time to re-dilation with steroid injection [11]. In light of this, current consensus guidelines from the Global Interventional Inflammatory Bowel Disease Group do not recommend the routine intralesional injection of steroids during EBD [12].

The efficacy of EBD in management of Crohn's stricture is conventionally measured in terms of both short-term technical success as well as need for re-intervention. A summary of 17 case series, each including 15 cases or more, demonstrated high rates of immediate technical success ranging from 79% to 100% [13]. Amongst these cases the rates of stenosis recurrence were also high and ranged from 24% to 76%. EBD has also been compared against surgical resection. Two retrospective studies found EBD to be associated with higher risk for further surgery and lower risk for adverse events when compared to surgical resection [14, 15]. While surgery may be the eventual endpoint in many patients with stricturing CD, EBD is an effective alternative which may delay time to surgery.

The major procedural risks associated with EBD include bowel perforation and bleeding. Most cases of perforation require surgical intervention. Across the 17-case series mentioned previously, rates of perforation were low ranging from 0% to 11% [13]. To minimize the risk of perforation we recommend a conservative dilation approach that is slow and steady rather than too aggressive. Bleeding is also a rare complication of EBD occurring in approximately 1% to 5% of cases [16].

Risk of clinical recurrence of stricture is also important to consider in EBD. Though results across studies vary, most reports have demonstrated a recurrence rate of approximately 30% - 60% at average follow-up of between 15 to 45 months [17].

Endoscopic Stricturotomy

The endoscopic needle-knife tool has long been used to perform incisions in the esophagus, pylorus, and duodenal papilla to dilate lumens and release strictures. The use of needle-knife and other cutting tools in the management of colonic strictures in CD is a relatively new development. However, the same principles apply as elsewhere in the gastrointestinal tract. Cuts are made through the scarred mucosal and submucosal fibers along the longitudinal intestinal axis resulting in dilation of the stricture and bowel lumen. The difference between stricturotomy and stricturoplasty is the use of clips to close the incised edges in stricturoplasty. However, from a practical standpoint these terms are used synonymously. For the purposes of this chapter, we will stick to using the term stricturotomy.

No guidelines have yet been established to dictate the indications or contraindications for endoscopic stricturotomy. Given stricturotomy is a more invasive procedure than balloon dilation and stenting it would be reasonable to view it as a second-line treatment for management of refractory or recurrent stricture after initial attempt with either balloon dilation or stenting. We prefer to utilize stricturotomy in areas of the GI tract with thicker walls, such as the rectum and anastomoses, to mitigate perforation risk.

As with other endoscopic modalities for the management of Crohn's related strictures pre-procedure planning is paramount and should involve cross sectional imaging to first determine the location and size of stricture. The endoscopic needle knife is then used to make precise cuts along the circumference of the stricture under direct visualization. Minimizing procedural bleeding by using endoscopic Doppler ultrasound to identify and avoid significant blood vessels within the stricture has also been described [17].

A recent case series by Lan et al. describes the short-term efficacy and safety of endoscopic stricturotomy used to treat 85 patients [18]. A total of 127 strictures were treated, 52 (41.6%) of which were endoscopically non-traversable prior to intervention. In all cases the scope was successfully passed through stricture immediately after stricturotomy. At median follow up at 0.9 years there were 13 (15.3%) patients who required stricture-related surgery. During this same follow up period there were 77 patients (60.6%) who required either additional stricturotomy, endoscopic balloon dilation, or both. Endoscopic stricturotomy may be an option for delaying need for surgery, however most patients require repeat intervention in order to achieve this.

Two additional retrospective studies by Lan et al. compare the efficacy of stricturotomy against endoscopic balloon dilation and surgical resection [19, 20]. The stricturotomy versus dilation study evaluated patients with ileocolonic anastomotic stricture. 21 patients were treated with stricturotomy and 164 treated with balloon dilation were included. Immediate technical success was achieved in 100% of patients treated with stricturotomy versus 89.5% of patients treated with dilation. 2 (9.5%) patients in the stricturotomy group required subsequent surgery versus 55 (33.5%) patients in the dilation group during median follow up at 0.8 years and 4.0 years, respectively. The authors concluded that stricturotomy appears more effective than balloon dilation in management of ileocolonic anastomotic Crohn's stricture.

The stricturotomy versus surgical resection study similarly evaluated patients with ileocolonic anastomotic strictures. They included 35 patients treated with stricturotomy and 147 treated with ileocolonic resection (ICR). No difference in surgery-free survival was found between the two groups based on Kaplan-Meier analysis ($p = 0.24$). They also report on several identified risk factors for decreased surgery free survival including preprocedural corticosteroids (Hazard Ratio (HR) 2.8, 95% Confidence Interval (CI): 1.0-8.1), multiple strictures (HR 4.9, 95% CI: 1.7-14.2), and increased disease-related hospitalizations (HR 4.0, 95% CI, 1.2-13.0) In this study stricturotomy demonstrated comparable surgery-free survival compared to ICR.

The major risks associated with endoscopic stricturotomy include bleeding and bowel perforation. Both events occur only rarely. In most cases bleeding has been observed within 4 days of procedure and at a rate of between 6.9% to 10.2% of procedures [18, 21]. Bowel perforation is an even rarer complication and has been reported at a rate of 1.1% (18). Compared to endoscopic balloon dilation, endoscopic stricturotomy carries a lower risk for perforation at the expense of a higher risk for bleeding [21].

Endoscopic Stenting

The evolution of various stent technologies in recent decades has expanded the role of endoscopic stenting in the management of Crohn's strictures. Fully covered self-expanding metal stents are now removable and have been FDA approved for a variety of benign indications. As with other techniques, the goal is to delay surgery and prioritize bowel preservation.

Typically stenting is preferred in cases in which balloon dilation is ineffective, such as in strictures longer than 4-5 cm or tortuous strictures which cannot be uniformly dilated [22].

One of the most important decisions to make in any endoscopic stenting procedure is the choice of stent. Stent material, diameter, and length all need to be considered prior to the procedure. There are three broad categories of endoscopic stents used in management of Crohn's strictures based on stent material: metal, plastic, and biodegradable. Regardless of material type, all stents are comprised of a fine tubular mesh that is packaged in a compressed form and contained within a device to facilitate delivery. Once deployed, the stents expand in a radial fashion and expand whatever lumen they are deployed within. The permanence of any stent is determined by the amount of plastic film overlying its mesh structure. Uncovered stents are intended to allow tissue ingrowth into the stent wall and are often used as palliative measures in malignant luminal obstruction with no intention for stent removal. In contrast, partially and fully covered stents are designed to be removed. Fully covered stents allow for greater ease of removal at the expense of greater likelihood for stent migration. Regarding stent diameter, the appropriate post-deployment diameter should be approximated from cross sectional imaging of the stricture obtained prior to procedure. The majority of bowel stents range from 10-20mm in diameter. Finally, the length of the stent should be 3-4cm longer than the length of stricture since expansion of the stent typically results in shortening ranging from 5% to 40% [22]. The ideal stent type and duration for management of Crohn's strictures is not known, however what is most commonly described in current literature is placement of either partially or totally covered self-expanding metal stents with retrieval times from one week to two months [23]. Stent retrieval is typically performed with either rat-toothed forceps or snares.

A recent meta-analysis by Giri et al. evaluated ten studies representing 170 patients with Crohn's related strictures who received endoscopic stents [24]. Technical success was defined as successful placement of the stent across the strictures as observed on fluoroscopy. Clinical success was defined as resolution of signs and symptoms amongst patients in whom technical success was achieved. The pooled technical success rate across all ten studies was found to be 98.2% (95% CI: 95.8-100, I^2 0.0%). Clinical success was only reported in nine of the ten studies and had a pooled rate of 71.3% (95% CI: 57.4-85.1, I^2 68.4%, p=0.001) with substantial heterogeneity among the studies. Rates of recurrence of signs and symptoms of stricture were also measured. Pooled recurrence rate was 40.1% (95% CI: 20.3-59.9, I^2 89.9%, p = 0.0001). Finally, need for surgical resection for indications other than immediate complication of stenting was measured across seven studies representing 66 patients. Pooled surgical resection rate was 8.6% (95% CI: 1.7-15.5, I^2 2.2%, p = 0.408). Overall, the authors conclude that there is good short-term benefit achieved with endoscopic stenting given high rates of technical and clinical success. The high rate of recurrence, though, suggests stenting is not yet a feasible long-term solution in a large portion of patients.

There are few comparative studies evaluating the safety and efficacy of endoscopic stenting versus other interventional modalities in the management of Crohn's related strictures. A recent randomized trial by Loras et al. compared endoscopic stenting to endoscopic balloon dilation in a cohort of 80 patients [25]. At 1 year, 51% of stent patients were free of further therapeutic intervention compared to 80% of balloon dilation patients (OR 3.9, 95% CI: 1.4-10.6), p = 0.006). There was one serious adverse event in each group and both events were bowel perforations. Another ongoing clinical trial currently enrolling patients aims to compare the safety and efficacy of endoscopic stenting versus surgical bowel resection [26]. Results from this trial and others will continue to help elucidate the most appropriate patients to select for endoscopic stenting in order to ensure the most favorable outcomes.

In a systematic review by Scotti et al. evaluating stent outcomes in eleven studies representing 173 patients the two most common complications were stent migration (29%) and post-procedure abdominal pain (15%) [27].

Stent migration may occur in either the proximal or distal direction relative to the stricture the stent has been placed in to. Fortunately, this is a rare complication with estimated occurrence of around 6% [28]. Stent retrieval in cases where the stricture must be traversed in order to reach the stent can be challenging. In some cases, surgical intervention may be needed to retrieve the stent. In some cases, distal stent migration may be considered an incident rather than complication since this event may indicate resolution of stenosis. Additionally distal migration of the stent aids in ease of eventual retrieval. However, distal migration is not always benign and may lead to impaction, perforation, and need for additional surgery.

Fistula Disease Background

Fistula disease is the most common presentation of penetrating CD [29]. The etiology of CD fistulas results from active disease or post-surgical complications such as anastomotic leaks.

There are a variety of fistulas characterized as internal and external, determined by the connection of bowel to another internal organ or the skin [30]. Internal fistulas include enteroenteric, enterocolonic, enterovesicular, and enterovaginal. External fistulas include enterocutaneous and perianal. A different subset of fistulas is those between a post-surgical pouch and intestine, bladder, and vagina [31]. There are also fistulas that develop in otherwise healthy appearing bowel and not likely to be caused by active CD [32].

It has been estimated that approximately 20-40% of patients with CD will develop fistula disease with one population-based study reporting 35% developing at least one fistula [33]. Perianal, enteroenteric, and rectovaginal fistulas are noted to be the most common locations of fistula disease in patients with CD [29].

The endoscopic modalities used to treat fistula disease in CD include endoscopic clipping, endoscopic suturing, endoscopic stenting, endoscopic fistulotomy, and endoscopic fistular injection [31]. The efficacy of these endoscopic therapies does not have the support of robust clinical trials and treatment choice is based on provider comfort and experience.

Endoscopic Clipping

Endoscopic clipping has various clinical uses in endoscopy, including bleeding control and perforations. There are two main modalities of endoscopic clipping, through-the-scope clips (TTSC) and over-the-scope clips (OTSC). The use of these clips in fistulizing CD is limited to a small case series of ten total patients with six having CD as the etiology. TTSCs are more frequently used in the control of gastrointestinal bleeding while OTSCs can cover a larger surface area and have more adherence power. Therefore, they are ideal for closing defects in the gastrointestinal tract, such as fistulas [29].

Fistula closure utilizing clips can be performed on any fistula reachable by a traditional endoscope (see Figure 5.3). The treatment of CD fistulas utilizing clips stems from experience closing post-gastrostomy gastrocutaneous fistulas. These types of fistulas require multi-modal therapy utilizing de-epithelization of the fistula tract followed by endoscopic clipping. The premise behind this method is that epithelized surfaces are smooth and do not stick well compared to de-epithelized surfaces. De-epithelization is typically performed with a rough cytology brush or thermal therapy with argon-plasma coagulation. For fistulas less than 5mm in diameter, TTSCs usually suffices. For fistulas larger than 5mm, OTSCs are preferred. These clips are often permanent and are not removed. Because of the large cap required to deploy an OTSC they typically cannot be deployed if there is co-existing stricturing disease.

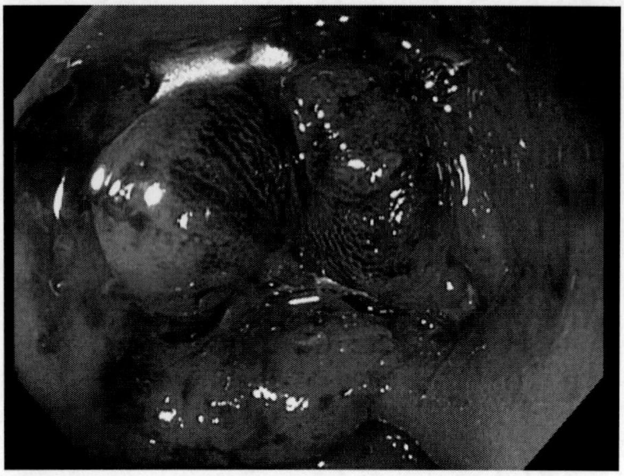

Figure 5.3. OVESCO clip of colonic stricture.

The efficacy of OTSC clipping for fistulizing CD is limited to one small case series. In this study, ten total patients were evaluated, six of those with CD. 70% of the patients were found to have permanent fistula closure with a median time from procedure of 72 days. One CD associated fistula in this study was found to have closure failure, with the OTSC spontaneously lost at day 40 [34]. The major adverse events associated with the use of OTSCs include perforation and bleeding. The use of APC during the de-epithelization process carries the risk of perforation, pneumoperitoneum, and subcutaneous gas bubbling [35].

Endoscopic Suturing

Endoscopic suturing is a technique that has emerged over the past decade. It has a wide variety of indications including closure of perforations, fixation of stents, endobariatric therapy, as well as gastrointestinal fistulas. Endoscopic suturing, while technically complicated, is becoming mainstream for interventional gastroenterology.

With respect to fistulas, the same premise for clipping applies. However, much larger fistulas can be treated with endoscopic suturing. Defects up to 3-4 cm can be closed with the endoscopic suturing device. Because of the large size of the device, it is only helpful for fistulas proximal in the upper gastrointestinal tract or distal in the colon. The most widely used endoscopic suturing device is the Overstitch by Apollo.

There are currently no studies evaluating the efficacy of suturing for fistulizing CD. There is minimal evidence that suturing is efficacious in non-IBD fistulas with one study demonstrating a clinical success rate of 55.6% with 24 total fistulas treated using endoscopic suturing [36]. The major adverse events associated with suturing include perforation and bleeding.

Endoscopic Stenting

Fully covered self-expandable metal stents (FCSEMS) have been successfully used for both benign and malignant indications. The advantage of the fully covered metal stent is that it allows for removal later since there is no tissue in-growth. Most benign indications are for gastrointestinal strictures; however, they are frequently used for fistulous disease especially in the esophagus, particularly for the management of tracheo-esophageal fistulas. Although there is limited data for CD fistulas, FCSEMS have been used for this indication [37].

The premise is that the stent occludes the fistula, limiting flow and allowing the tract to close. While there is anecdotal evidence of success there is also risk of stent-induced complications such as angulation related perforations and stent migration. We rarely use stents because of these complications but keep them in the treatment arsenal for select cases. In one case series of the use of FCSEMS in the management of CD fistulas, one patient was successfully managed via stenting while another needed to go on to surgery [37].

Endoscopic Fistulotomy

The premise of endoscopic fistulotomy is to open the fistula tract, clean debris/drain sources of potential infection, and close the fistula using endoscopic clips. This effectively helps prevent/treat infections associated with fistulas and subsequently closes tract to prevent future complications.

Endoscopic fistulotomy remains one of the best methods for treating simple fistulas associated with CD. Indications for fistulotomy include superficial, short, and fistulas associated with anastomotic leaks [29]. Though no absolute contraindication for endoscopic fistulotomy is present, only short and superficial fistulas are typically amenable to the endoscopic approach. These are predominately external fistulas, as noted above. Deeper and long fistulas are typically treated by surgical approaches or medical management.

An endoscope is passed to the area where the fistula resides (see Figure 5.4), after confirmation with imaging, typically fluoroscopy. A guidewire is used to traverse the fistula, followed by needle-knife fistulotomy. Any exposed debris or infection is cleaned and removed. After this is done, the fistula can be closed by different techniques including through-the-scope clips (TTSC), over-the-scope clips (OTSC), or endoscopic suturing.

There are some small studies demonstrating the efficacy of endoscopic fistulotomy. In one study, 89.6% of patients achieved complete resolution of the fistula, with 34.4% requiring only one session. Only three patients in the study required surgical intervention due to persistent fistula [38]. The major risks associated with endoscopic fistulotomy include bowel perforation by using the needle-knife to cut debris away from the fistula or during abscess drainage. Another major risk is bleeding, leading to hospitalization. In one small cohort study, only one patient in the 29 studied required transfusion due to bleeding post-fistulotomy. There were no perforations noted [38].

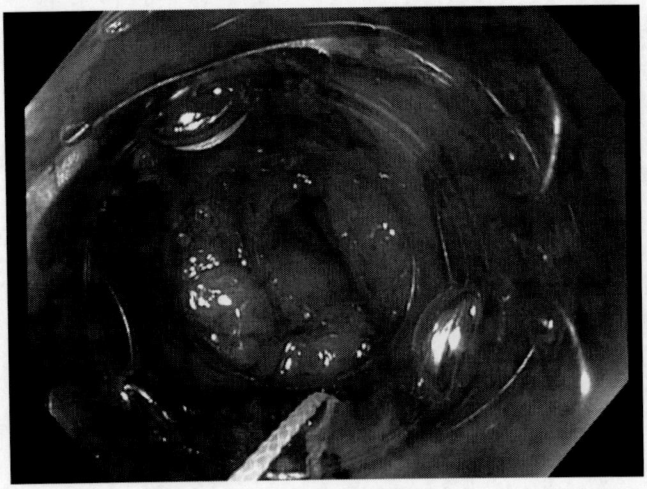

Figure 5.4. Colonic fistula seen from endoscopic viewpoint.

Endoscopic Fistular Injection

Endoscopic fistular injection uses different substances to treat IBD-related fistulas. These substances include fibrin glue, antibiotics such as doxycycline, 50% dextrose solutions, and even stem cells. The premise of this method is to induce local inflammation that results in fibrin discharge, and finally adhesion of the tissue surface that made the fistular tract [39].

Endoscopic injections to treat fistulas are typically limited to perianal disease. Fistulas in this area are subcategorized as simple or complex. Complex fistulas are "high" in terms of their anatomic location and associated with pain, perirectal abscesses, and multiple external openings [40]. The simple procedure of fistular injection is thought to be an effective method to treat complex fistulas as there is low morbidity associated with this procedure when comparing to other surgical methods.

There is no absolute contraindication to attempting endoscopic fistular injections to the author's knowledge. There are several studies that have evaluated the efficacy of injections for the treatment of fistulas in inflammatory bowel disease. One study demonstrated surgical treatments to have a higher healing rate when compared to the use of fibrin glue, though those results were not statistically significant. This study demonstrated a lower anal incontinence rate in patients who underwent fibrin injection compared to surgery, highlighting its lower morbidity [41]. A different study evaluated the use of stem cells in fistula treatment, showing 69.2% of patients had a reduction in the number of draining fistulas, with 56.3% of patients achieving complete closure [42]. Finally, a study comprised of 200 patients with perianal fistulas evaluated fibrin glue alone vs stem cells alone vs fibrin glue plus stem cells showed favorable healing rates for groups using stem cells at 24 - 26 weeks that improved at 1 year [43].

Endoscopic Management of Neoplasia in CD

Patients with CD are at an approximately 2 to 3-fold increased risk for colorectal cancer due to chronic inflammation which drives neoplastic progression [44]. This feared complication of inflammatory bowel disease is termed colitis-associated colorectal cancer (CAC). An entire textbook chapter can be devoted to the endoscopic management of CAC, which is beyond the scope of this chapter. However, a few paragraphs are warranted.

As with all colorectal cancers, primary prevention with screening and surveillance colonoscopy is a cornerstone in the overall clinical management of CAC. The majority of recent society guidelines recommend screening colonoscopy at 8-10 years after symptom onset followed by surveillance colonoscopy every 1-2 years depending on risk stratification.

Endoscopic intervention may be utilized to achieve removal of localized dysplasia. Visible, high-risk dysplastic lesions with distinct borders are removed with either endoscopic mucosal resection (EMR) or endoscopic submucosal dissection (ESD). EMR utilizes a blue dye lifting agent to delineate the boundaries of the lesion. Following this, an electrocautery snare is used to grasp and remove polyps limited to the mucosa and superficial submucosa. ESD is a more technically demanding procedure and uses a precise electrosurgical knife to perform dissection deeper into the submucosal layer of the bowel. ESD is often needed to remove large, flat lesions. Depth of invasion is also taken into consideration when choosing between EMR and ESD. Lesions which are suspected to invade below the superficial submucosa should be removed via ESD to facilitate full thickness submucosal resection.

Conclusion

The endoscopic management of Crohn's disease is currently being performed, with acceptable efficacy and safety profiles. However, it remains in the early stages of its application. Ongoing research and technological advancements are crucial to refining these techniques and expanding their utility. As improvements in endoscopic tools and methods continue, we anticipate significant progress in the development of even more effective and minimally invasive options. These advancements hold the potential to further reduce patient morbidity and improve quality of life. Continued collaboration between gastroenterologists, surgeons, and researchers will be essential to realize the full potential of therapeutic endoscopy in managing Crohn's disease.

References

[1] Lin, X., Wang, Y., Liu, Z., Lin, S., Tan, J., He, J., Hu, F., Wu, X., Ghosh, S., Chen, M., Liu, F., & Mao, R. (2022). Intestinal strictures in Crohn's disease: a 2021 update. *Ther Adv Gastroenterol*, 15, 17562848221104952. https://doi.org/10.1177/17562848221104951.

[2] Dehghan, M., Wong, G., Neuberger, E., Kin, C., Rieder, F., & Park, K. T. (2021). Worse outcomes and higher costs of care in fibrostenotic Crohn's disease: a real-world propensity-matched analysis in the USA. *BMJ Open Gastroenterol*, 8(1). https://doi.org/10.1136/bmjgast-2021-000781.

[3] Ismail, M. S., & Charabaty, A. (2022). Management of Crohn's stricture: medical, endoscopic and surgical therapies. *Frontline Gastroenterology*, 13(6), 524–530. https://doi.org/10.1136/flgastro-2021-101827.

[4] Sleiman, J., el Ouali, S., Qazi, T., Cohen, B., Steele, S. R., Baker, M. E., & Rieder, F. (2021). Prevention and Treatment of Stricturing Crohn's Disease - Perspectives and Challenges. *Exp Rev Gastroenterol Hepatol*, 15(4), 401–411. https://doi.org/10.1080/17474124.2021.1854732.

[5] Hassan, C., Zullo, A., de Francesco, V., Ierardi, E., Giustini, M., Pitidis, A., Taggi, F., Winn, S., & Morini, S. (2007). Systematic review: endoscopic dilatation in Crohn's disease. *Aliment Pharm Ther*, 26(11–12), 1457–1464. https://doi.org/10.1111/j.1365-2036.2007.03532.x.

[6] Sabaté, J. -M., Villarejo, J., Bouhnik, Y., Allez, M., Gornet, J. -M., Vahedi, K., Modigliani, R., & Lémann, M. (2003). Hydrostatic balloon dilatation of Crohn's strictures. *Aliment Pharm Ther*, 18(4), 409–413. https://doi.org/10.1046/j.1365-2036.2003.01715.x.

[7] Sabaté, J. -M., Villarejo, J., Bouhnik, Y., Allez, M., Gornet, J. -M., Vahedi, K., Modigliani, R., & Lémann, M. (2003). Hydrostatic balloon dilatation of Crohn's strictures. *Aliment Pharm Ther*, 18(4), 409–413. https://doi.org/10.1046/j.1365-2036.2003.01715.x.

[8] Gustavsson, A., Magnuson, A., Blomberg, B., Andersson, M., Halfvarson, J., & Tysk, C. (2012). Endoscopic dilation is an efficacious and safe treatment of intestinal strictures in <scp>C</scp> rohn's disease. *Aliment Pharm Ther*, 36(2), 151–158. https://doi.org/10.1111/j.1365-2036.2012.05146.x.

[9] Brooker, J. C., Beckett, C. G., Saunders, B. P., & Benson, M. J. (2003). Long-Acting Steroid Injection after Endoscopic Dilation of Anastomotic Crohn's Strictures May Improve the Outcome: A Retrospective Case Series. *Endoscopy*, 35(4), 333–337. https://doi.org/10.1055/s-2003-38145.

[10] di Nardo, G., Oliva, S., Passariello, M., Pallotta, N., Civitelli, F., Frediani, S., Gualdi, G., Gandullia, P., Mallardo, S., & Cucchiara, S. (2010). Intralesional steroid injection after endoscopic balloon dilation in pediatric Crohn's disease with stricture: a prospective, randomized, double-blind, controlled trial. *Gastrointest Endosc*, 72(6), 1201–1208. https://doi.org/10.1016/j.gie.2010.08.003.

[11] East, J. E., Brooker, J. C., Rutter, M. D., & Saunders, B. P. (2007). A Pilot Study of Intrastricture Steroid Versus Placebo Injection After Balloon Dilatation of Crohn's Strictures. *Clin Gastroenterol Hepatol*, 5(9), 1065–1069. https://doi.org/10.1016/j.cgh.2007.04.013.

[12] Shen, B., Kochhar, G., Navaneethan, U., Farraye, F. A., Schwartz, D. A., Iacucci, M., Bernstein, C. N., Dryden, G., Cross, R., Bruining, D. H., Kobayashi, T., Lukas, M., Shergill, A., Bortlik, M., Lan, N., Lukas, M., Tang, S.-J., Kotze, P. G., Kiran, R. P., … Sandborn, W. J. (2020). Practical guidelines on endoscopic treatment for Crohn's disease strictures: a consensus statement from the Global Interventional Inflammatory Bowel Disease Group. *Lancet Gastroenterol Hepatol*, 5(4), 393–405. https://doi.org/10.1016/S2468-1253(19)30366-8.

[13] Hirai, F. (2017). Current status of endoscopic balloon dilation for Crohn's disease. *Intest Res*, 15(2), 166–173. https://doi.org/10.5217/ir.2017.15.2.166.

[14] Lian, L., Stocchi, L., Remzi, F. H., & Shen, B. (2017). Comparison of Endoscopic Dilation vs Surgery for Anastomotic Stricture in Patients With Crohn's Disease Following Ileocolonic Resection. *Clin Gastroenterol Hepatol*, 15(8), 1226–1231. https://doi.org/10.1016/j.cgh.2016.10.030.

[15] Lan, N., Stocchi, L., Ashburn, J. H., Hull, T. L., Steele, S. R., Delaney, C. P., & Shen, B. (2018). Outcomes of Endoscopic Balloon Dilation vs Surgical Resection for Primary Ileocolic Strictures in Patients With Crohn's Disease. *Clin Gastroenterol Hepatol*, 16(8), 1260–1267. https://doi.org/10.1016/j.cgh.2018.02.035.

[16] Bharadwaj, S., Fleshner, P., & Shen, B. (2015). Therapeutic Armamentarium for Stricturing Crohn's Disease. *Inflam Bowel Dis*, 21(9), 2194–2213. https://doi.org/10.1097/MIB.0000000000000403.

[17] Attar, A. (2016). Stent for Crohn's disease strictures: Which one and when? Endoscopy International Open, 4(3), E309-10. https://doi.org/10.1055/s-0042-103417.

[18] Lan, N., & Shen, B. (2017). Endoscopic Stricturotomy with Needle Knife in the Treatment of Strictures from Inflammatory Bowel Disease. *Inflam Bowel Dis*, 23(4), 502–513. https://doi.org/10.1097/MIB.0000000000001044.

[19] Lan, N., & Shen, B. (2018). Endoscopic Stricturotomy Versus Balloon Dilation in the Treatment of Anastomotic Strictures in Crohn's Disease. *Inflam Bowel Dis*, 24(4), 897–907. https://doi.org/10.1093/ibd/izx085.

[20] Lan, N., Stocchi, L., Delaney, C. P., Hull, T. L., & Shen, B. (2019). Endoscopic stricturotomy versus ileocolonic resection in the treatment of ileocolonic anastomotic strictures in Crohn's disease. *Gastrointest Endosc*, 90(2), 259–268. https://doi.org/10.1016/j.gie.2019.01.021.

[21] Pokala, A., & Shen, B. (2020). Update of endoscopic management of Crohn's disease strictures. *Intest Res*, 18(1), 1–10. https://doi.org/10.5217/ir.2019.09158.
[22] Loras Alastruey, C., Andújar Murcia, X., & Esteve Comas, M. (2016). The role of stents in the treatment of Crohn's disease strictures. *Endosc Int Open*, 04(03), E301–E308. https://doi.org/10.1055/s-0042-101786..
[23] Navaneethan, U., Lourdusamy, V., Duvuru, S., Lourdusamy, D., Mehta, D., Raja, S., Murthy, S., & Sanaka, M. R. (2015). Timing of esophageal stent placement and outcomes in patients with esophageal perforation: a single-center experience. *Surg Endosc*, 29(3), 700–707. https://doi.org/10.1007/s00464-014-3724-2.
[24] Giri, S., Gopan, A., Sundaram, S., & Kale, A. (2022). Efficacy and Safety of Endoscopic Stenting for Crohn's Disease Related Strictures: A Systematic Review and Meta-analysis. *Korean J Gastroenterol*, 80(4), 177–185. https://doi.org/10.4166/kjg.2022.077.
[25] Loras, C., Andújar, X., Gornals, J. B., Sanchiz, V., Brullet, E., Sicilia, B., Martín-Arranz, M. D., Naranjo, A., Barrio, J., Dueñas, C., Foruny, J. R., Busquets, D., Monfort, D., Pineda, J. R., González-Huix, F., Pérez-Roldán, F., Pons, V., González, B., Reyes Moreno, J., … Esteve, M. (2022). Self-expandable metal stents versus endoscopic balloon dilation for the treatment of strictures in Crohn's disease (ProtDilat study): an open-label, multicentre, randomised trial. *Lancet Gastroenterol Hepatol*, 7(4), 332–341. https://doi.org/10.1016/S2468-1253(21)00386-1.
[26] Loras, C., Ruiz-Ramirez, P., Romero, J., Andújar, X., Bargallo, J., Bernardos, E., Boscá-Watts, M. M., Brugiotti, C., Brunet, E., Busquets, D., Cerrillo, E., Cortina, F. J., Díaz-Milanés, J. A., Dueñas, C., Farrés, R., Golda, T., González-Huix, F., Gornals, J. B., Guardiola, J., … Esteve, M. (2023). Endoscopic treatment (endoscopic balloon dilation/self-expandable metal stent) vs surgical resection for the treatment of de novo stenosis in Crohn's disease (ENDOCIR study): an open-label, multicentre, randomized trial. *Trials*, 24(1), 432. https://doi.org/10.1186/s13063-023-07447-1.
[27] Scotti, G. B., Lorenzetti, R., Aratari, A., Lamazza, A., Fiori, E., Papi, C., & Festa, S. (2023). Stricturing Crohn's disease: what is the role of endoscopic stenting? A systematic review. *Clin Endosc*, 56(6), 726–734. https://doi.org/10.5946/ce.2023.059.
[28] Chandan, S., Dhindsa, B. S., Khan, S. R., Deliwala, S., Kassab, L. L., Mohan, B. P., Chandan, O. C., Loras, C., Shen, B., & Kochhar, G. S. (2023). Endoscopic Stenting in Crohn's Disease-related Strictures: A Systematic Review and Meta-analysis of Outcomes. *Inflam Bowel Dis*, 29(7), 1145–1152. https://doi.org/10.1093/ibd/izac153.
[29] Lan N, Shen B. Endoscopic Therapy for Fistulas and Abscesses in Crohn's Disease. *Gastrointest Endosc Clin N Am.* 2022 Oct;32(4):733-746. doi: 10.1016/j.giec.2022.05.006. Epub 2022 Sep 7. PMID: 36202513.
[30] Wetwittayakhlang P, Al Khoury A, Hahn GD, Lakatos PL. The Optimal Management of Fistulizing Crohn's Disease: Evidence beyond Randomized Clinical Trials. *J Clin Med.* 2022 May 28;11(11):3045. doi: 10.3390/jcm11113045. PMID: 35683433.
[31] Shen B. Interventional inflammatory bowel disease: endoscopic therapy of complications of Crohn's disease. *Gastroenterol Rep (Oxf).* 2022 Sep 14;10:goac045. doi: 10.1093/gastro/goac045. PMID: 36120488.
[32] Poritz LS, Gagliano GA, McLeod RS, MacRae H, Cohen Z. Surgical management of entero and colocutaneous fistulae in Crohn's disease: 17 year's experience. *Int J Colorectal Dis.* 2004 Sep;19(5):481-5; discussion 486. doi: 10.1007/s00384-004-0580-x. Epub 2004 May 26. PMID: 15168043.
[33] Schwartz DA, Loftus EV Jr, Tremaine WJ, Panaccione R, Harmsen WS, Zinsmeister AR, Sandborn WJ. The natural history of fistulizing Crohn's disease in Olmsted County, Minnesota. *Gastroenterology.* 2002 Apr;122(4):875-80. doi: 10.1053/gast.2002.32362. PMID: 11910338.
[34] Mennigen R, Laukötter M, Senninger N, Rijcken E. The OTSC(®) proctology clip system for the closure of refractory anal fistulas. *Tech Coloproctol.* 2015 Apr;19(4):241-6. doi: 10.1007/s10151-015-1284-7. Epub 2015 Feb 26. PMID: 25715788.
[35] Sohail A, Khan A, Shah H, Rezko R. Use of Argon Plasma Coagulation and Endoscopic Hemoclips for Postsurgical Gastrointestinal Fistula. *Case Rep Gastrointest Med.* 2020 Nov 11;2020:8835437. doi: 10.1155/2020/8835437. PMID: 33224539.

[36] Callahan ZM, Su B, Kuchta K, Conaty E, Novak S, Linn J, Murad FM, Carbray J, Ujiki M. Endoscopic Suturing Results in High Technical and Clinical Success Rates for a Variety of Gastrointestinal Pathologies. *J Gastrointest Surg.* 2020 Feb;24(2):278-287. doi: 10.1007/s11605-019-04485-6. Epub 2019 Dec 10. PMID: 31823323.

[37] Cereatti F, Fiocca F, Dumont JL, Ceci V, Vergeau BM, Tuszynski T, Meduri B, Donatelli G. Fully covered self-expandable metal stent in the treatment of postsurgical colorectal diseases: outcome in 29 patients. *Therap Adv Gastroenterol.* 2016 Mar;9(2):180-8. doi: 10.1177/1756283X15610052. PMID: 26929780.

[38] Kochhar G, Shen B. Endoscopic fistulotomy in inflammatory bowel disease (with video). *Gastrointest Endosc*. 2018 Jul;88(1):87-94. doi: 10.1016/j.gie.2018.02.034. Epub 2018 Mar 6. PMID: 29501418.

[39] Neumann H, Neurath MF, Atreya R. Endoscopic Therapy in Inflammatory Bowel Diseases. *Viszeralmedizin*. 2015 Aug;31(4):280-6. doi: 10.1159/000435851. Epub 2015 Aug 4. PMID: 26557837.

[40] Sandborn WJ, Fazio VW, Feagan BG, Hanauer SB; American Gastroenterological Association Clinical Practice Committee. AGA technical review on perianal Crohn's disease. *Gastroenterology*. 2003 Nov;125(5):1508-30. doi: 10.1016/j.gastro.2003.08.025. PMID: 14598268.

[41] Cirocchi R, Farinella E, La Mura F, Cattorini L, Rossetti B, Milani D, Ricci P, Covarelli P, Coccetta M, Noya G, Sciannameo F. Fibrin glue in the treatment of anal fistula: a systematic review. *Ann Surg Innov Res*. 2009 Nov 14;3:12. doi: 10.1186/1750-1164-3-12. PMID: 19912660.

[42] de la Portilla F, Alba F, García-Olmo D, Herrerías JM, González FX, Galindo A. Expanded allogeneic adipose-derived stem cells (eASCs) for the treatment of complex perianal fistula in Crohn's disease: results from a multicenter phase I/IIa clinical trial. *Int J Colorectal Dis.* 2013 Mar;28(3):313-23. doi: 10.1007/s00384-012-1581-9. Epub 2012 Sep 29. PMID: 23053677.

[43] Herreros MD, Garcia-Arranz M, Guadalajara H, De-La-Quintana P, Garcia-Olmo D; FATT Collaborative Group. Autologous expanded adipose-derived stem cells for the treatment of complex cryptoglandular perianal fistulas: a phase III randomized clinical trial (FATT 1: fistula Advanced Therapy Trial 1) and long-term evaluation. *Dis Colon Rectum.* 2012 Jul;55(7):762-72. doi: 10.1097/DCR.0b013e318255364a. PMID: 22706128.

[44] Shah, S. C., & Itzkowitz, S. H. (2022). Colorectal Cancer in Inflammatory Bowel Disease: Mechanisms and Management. *Gastroenterology,* 162(3), 715-730.e3. https://doi.org/10.1053/j.gastro.2021.10.035.

Chapter 6

Extraintestinal Manifestations of Crohn's Disease

Rachael Belcher[1], MD
and Leon P. McLean[2,*], MD, PhD, MPH
[1]University of Maryland Medical Center, Baltimore, Maryland, USA
[2]Geisel School of Medicine at Dartmouth, Hanover, New Hampshire, USA

Abstract

In addition to luminal symptoms, patients with CD are at risk for developing a variety of symptoms unrelated to the gastrointestinal system. Extraintestinal manifestations may precede the diagnosis of IBD, creating diagnostic confusion. Patients should be queried about symptoms that could stem from more common EIMs such as arthralgias, aphthous ulceration, uveitis, pyoderma gangrenosum, and erythema nodosum. However, the clinician should remain mindful that EIMs can affect virtually any organ system and present with a variety of non-gastrointestinal symptoms. Treatment of IBD should improve certain EIMs such as aphthous stomatitis, EN, and Type I arthropathy. In cases where EIMs are suspected, expert consultation may be warranted.

Extraintestinal Manifestations

Extraintestinal manifestations (EIM) can be defined as "an inflammatory pathology in a patient with IBD that is located outside the gut and for which the pathogenesis is either dependent on extension/translocation of immune responses from the intestine, or is an independent inflammatory event perpetuated by IBD, or that shares a common environmental or genetic predisposition with IBD [1, 2]."

EIMs of Crohn's disease are common and can have a significant impact on patient quality of life. Symptoms stemming from EIMs can be more significant than symptoms from luminal disease and can develop prior to, concurrent with, or after the development of luminal symptoms. Although treatment of the underlying bowel disease can improve certain EIMs such as peripheral arthritis, oral ulcers, erythema nodosum, and episcleritis, other EIMs may require targeted therapy.

Up to 40% of IBD patients develop at least one EIM [3, 4]. Although virtually any organ system can be involved, musculoskeletal, dermatologic, and ocular EIMs are most common. In some patients, the presenting symptoms of IBD may be extraintestinal in nature, rather than

* Corresponding Author's Email: Leon.P.McLean@dartmouth.edu

In: Surgery for Crohn's Disease. Second Edition
Editors: Stephen M. Kavic, Rebecca Brown and Kerri Lopez
ISBN: 979-8-89530-676-5

relating to intestinal manifestations of CD [5]. Because diagnosing EIMs can be challenging, consultation with specialists may be warranted. In certain cases, treatment of the primary disease process (intestinal CD) may trigger or worsen EIMs. Clinicians should also consider whether the symptom of interest is a true EIM or, rather, an extraintestinal complication of the patient's bowel disease (e.g., enterocutaneous fistula).

Although EIMs associated with CD have been recognized for years, the factors that contribute to the development of these symptoms have not been determined for all conditions and may vary depending on the EIM in question [5]. Genetic factors likely play a role as concordance in the development of EIMs exists between both parent-child and sibling pairs [1]. Furthermore, certain IBD susceptibility loci such as NOD2/CARD15 may increase the risk of patients developing EIMs [1, 6]. The following section reviews clinical features and management options for EIMs associated with CD, and IBD more broadly.

Rheumatologic

Musculoskeletal symptoms are frequently encountered in patients with IBD, occurring in as many as 46% of patients, although the prevalence decreases with age [1, 5, 7-9]. Musculoskeletal EIMs are spondyloarthropathies and include IBD-related arthritis, psoriatic arthritis, ankylosing spondylitis (AS), enthesis-related arthritis, and reactive arthritis (Reiter's syndrome).

IBD arthropathies can be divided into peripheral or axial subtypes [10]. Peripheral arthropathies occur in 5 - 20% of IBD patients [1]. They are seronegative (rheumatoid factor negative), migrating, and transitory. Destruction of affected joints is uncommon; however, pain that can affect or limit activities of daily life is common. Symptoms may precede the diagnosis of IBD. Peripheral arthropathies can be subclassified into large joint pauci/oligo-articular (<5 joints) arthropathy (Type I) or small joint polyarticular (≥5 joints) arthropathy (Type II). Unlike peripheral arthropathies, axial arthropathies are associated with pain and stiffness in the lower back and/or sacroiliac joints [9, 10].

Peripheral Arthritis

Type I arthropathy affects five or fewer joints and is acute and self-limited, typically lasting less than 2 to 3 months [8, 10]. Large joints such as knees, ankles, hips, wrists, elbows, and shoulders are often affected. These symptoms may precede a diagnosis of IBD and often parallel IBD disease activity, particularly in patients with UC [8, 10]. Inflammation is present on synovial fluid analysis with cell count as high as 50,000 WBC/mm^3 [10]. HLA-B27 antigen is present in approximately one-quarter of patients [11]. Imaging is typically unremarkable with a diagnosis being made almost entirely on clinical grounds [11]. Treatment of Type I arthropathy is aimed at controlling IBD activity (i.e., treating underlying IBD) and may include colectomy in patients with UC or isolated colonic CD [8].

Type II arthropathy is chronic, lasting months to years, and affects five or more joints. The small joints of the upper extremities are often affected. Patients may develop pain, swelling, or effusions. Symptoms do not parallel IBD activity. Type II arthropathy may be slightly more common in CD than UC [10, 12, 13]. Imaging is also typically unremarkable. If erosive arthritis is detected consideration should be given to alternative diagnoses such as rheumatoid arthritis or psoriatic arthritis. As in Type I arthropathy, the diagnosis of Type II arthropathy is purely clinical. Treatment of Type II arthropathy may require agents directed against musculoskeletal symptoms. Options include COX-2 inhibitors (traditional NSAIDs may worsen IBD activity) [14], analgesics, physical therapy, and/or local steroid injection. Disease-modifying antirheumatic drugs (DMARDs) such as sulfasalazine and methotrexate (MTX) may also be employed in cases that do not respond to more conservative measures. Infliximab (IFX) may also be beneficial in refractory cases [8].

Type I and Type II arthropathies are now viewed as a spectrum of disease rather than distinct subtypes. Early in their disease course, patients may have fewer joints involved, with a greater proportion of joints affected over time.

Enthesitis and Dactylitis

Enthesitis (inflammation at tendon insertion site) and dactylitis (sausage like swelling of digit) may also occur in patients with IBD. Enthesitis, which is a peri-arthritis, occurs in 6 - 50% of IBD patients [15-17]. Enthesitis is associated with more substantial musculoskeletal pain. The diagnosis may not be apparent on clinical exam; however, early stages can be detected on ultrasound [1, 18, 19]. The Achilles tendon, plantar fascia, inferior patella, femoral greater trochanter, and the proximal humerus are commonly affected [20].

Dactylitis occurs in 2-4% of IBD patients [10]. The diagnosis of dactylitis is also clinical and is primarily based on physical exam. Clinical tools, such as the Leeds dactylitis instrument are used to measure disease severity and activity [10]. Immunomodulatory agents such as sulfasalazine or MTX may be required for treatment of enthesitis and dactylitis [8].

Axial Arthritis

Axial arthritis includes sacroilitis, inflammatory back pain (IBP), and AS, which overlap to some extent. Its prevalence ranges from 7 - 25% in patients with IBD. Sacroilitis may be asymptomatic or painful and is caused by inflammation of the sacroiliac joint. AS is diagnosed by radiographic evidence of sacroilitis with back pain or stiffness for greater than 3 months, which does not improve with rest, but does improve with exercise. Clinicians should be mindful that features of sacroiliitis can be observed on magnetic resonance enterography (MRE) [1]. Unlike AS, diagnosis of IBP does not require imaging [8]. Symptoms related to axial arthritis may precede symptoms stemming from IBD and are unrelated to underlying IBD activity [9].

Asymptomatic sacroilitis occurs in up to 50% of CD patients. Patients with symptomatic sacroilitis report pelvic pain at rest that improves with movement. Tenderness associated with pressure on the pelvic brim is suggestive of sacroilitis [5].

Inflammatory back pain is diagnosed clinically. The Calin criteria can be used to distinguish IBP from mechanical back pain and are fulfilled when 4 of the 5 following features are present: 1. Onset < 40 years of age, 2. Insidious onset, 3. Duration > 3 months, 4. Association with morning stiffness, 5. Improvement after exercise. The prevalence of IBP in IBD patients is approximately 20% [8, 10].

Ankylosing Spondylitis

The prevalence of AS in CD patients ranges from 1 - 10% and is unrelated to disease activity [8, 10]. AS associated with IBD has no gender predilection and a weaker association with HLA-B27 than sporadic AS [21]. Patients with AS report back pain as well as morning stiffness that improves with exercise. Imaging may demonstrate erosions, syndesmophytes, and bridging of the intervertebral discs giving the appearance of a "bamboo spine." AS is diagnosed using the modified New York criteria and requires the fulfillment of radiologic criteria in combination with clinical criteria (Figure 6.1). Treatment is similar to that for peripheral arthritis. Physical therapy may also be beneficial. The TNF-α antagonists IFX and adalimumab (ADA) are also effective for AS [22].

1.Low back pain > 3 months

Improved with exercise

Not relieved with rest

2.Limited lumbar motion

3.Reduced chest expansion

4.Bilateral grade > 2 sacroilitis on x-ray

5.Unilateral grade 3 or 4 sacroilitis on x-ray

AS: At least 1 from 1-3 as well as 4 or 5.

Figure 6.1. Modified New York criteria for ankylosing spondylitis.

Treatment of Musculoskeletal EIMs

The primary goal in treatment of patients with IBD is achieving clinical and endoscopic remission of the underlying bowel disease. Doing this can cause musculoskeletal symptoms to remit. However, musculoskeletal symptoms may remain even after endoscopic remission of a patient's luminal disease is achieved.

In cases where patients suffer from both luminal and musculoskeletal symptoms, therapies that target both conditions are most optimal. Agents that have the potential to treat both IBD and musculoskeletal disease include corticosteroids, sulfasalazine, methotrexate, TNF-α antagonists, ustekinumab (anti-IL-12/23), and the JAK inhibitors tofacitinib and upadacitinib. Although nonsteroidal anti-inflammatory drugs (NSAIDs) can be effective for the treatment of spondyloarthropathies, their use can increase diarrheal symptoms and promote the development of gastrointestinal erosions and ulcerations. Although risankizumab and guselkumab are both approved for the treatment of psoriatic arthritis, arthralgias have been observed in patients treated with anti-IL-23 agents [23-25].

Metabolic

Osteoporosis and Osteopenia

CD patients are at increased risk for developing osteopenia and osteoporosis although the reported prevalence varies in part due to factors such as age, disease duration, and study design [26, 27]. The prevalence of osteoporosis, defined as a T-score < -2.5, in CD patients is 17-41%. The prevalence of osteopenia, defined as a T-score between -1 and -2.5, is 22 - 67% [27, 28]. Factors that likely contribute to metabolic bone disease in CD patients include age, smoking, low body mass index, glucocorticoid use, vitamin deficiencies, calcium malabsorption, hypogonadism, and chronic inflammation [27]. CD patients have higher levels of proinflammatory cytokines, such as tumor necrosis factor-α, interleukin (IL)-1, IL-6, IL-7, and IL-17. These cytokines are thought to increase the ratio of receptor activator of nuclear factor-κB ligand (RANKL), an osteoclast activator, to osteoprotegerin (OPG), an osteoclast inhibitor, leading to increased bone resorption [29-31].

Patients with metabolic bone disease may be asymptomatic until a fracture occurs [13, 27]. A proportion of patients with fractures, particularly of the back, may be asymptomatic initially with the fracture detected only after pain develops. Fractures often occur after a fall and commonly affect the hip [13].

Assessment of CD patients for metabolic bone disease is recommended by professional societies [32, 33]. The American Gastroenterological Association (AGA) recommends dual X-ray absorptiometry (DEXA) scanning of patients with ≥ 1 risk factor for osteoporosis or fracture including history of prior fragility fracture, postmenopausal status, male >50 years, corticosteroid therapy > 3 months, or hypogonadism [32]. Bone mineral density (BMD) is expressed as a T-score or Z-score. The T-score is the number of standard deviations (SD) above or below the mean BMD for young adults whereas the Z-score is the number of SD above or below the mean BMD for age-matched controls. For peri-menopausal and post-menopausal women and men >50 years of age, osteoporosis is defined as a T-score of < -2.5 SD at the spine or hip with osteopenia defined as a T-score between -1 and -2.5 at these locations [34]. For pre-menopausal women and men <50, Z-scores are used with a value ≤ -2.0 indicating BMD is "below the expected range for age" [35]. If BMD is normal, DEXA may be repeated in 2-3 years, but this is reduced to one year in higher-risk patients. If BMD is abnormal, additional clinical and laboratory evaluation should be undertaken [27].

Treatment of metabolic bone disease focuses on fracture prevention. In general, patients should receive adequate calcium and vitamin D, avoid excess alcohol, stop smoking, and engage in weight-bearing exercise. Postmenopausal women and men >50 should receive 1200 - 1500 mg of calcium daily as well as 400 - 800 international units (IU) of vitamin D. Younger patients should receive at least 1000 mg of calcium daily. Patients who have undergone intestinal resection may require higher doses. Patients with hypogonadism should receive hormone replacement and men on long-term glucocorticoid therapy should have morning testosterone levels assessed with supplementation provided if hypogonadism is demonstrated. In addition, all patients receiving glucocorticoid therapy should receive calcium and vitamin D supplementation. Intestinal inflammation should be controlled by treating underlying IBD. Therapy with TNF-α antagonists have been shown to improve bone mineral density and alter serum markers of bone remodeling [36-38].

Recommendations for treatment of osteoporosis are extrapolated from studies in patients without CD. Antiosteoporotic therapy using bisphosphonates should be provided to patients with a fragility fracture, T-score of <-2.5, or a T-score of -2.5 to -1.0 on long-term glucocorticoid therapy with additional risk factors for fractures. Prophylaxis using bisphosphonates is appropriate in patients > 65 years of age at the initiation of glucocorticoid therapy or in patients < 65 years of age with a T-score < -1.5 who will receive glucocorticoid therapy for greater than 3 months [27, 32, 33].

Osteomalacia

Osteomalacia, which is defective mineralization of newly formed osteoid, is a distinct pathophysiologic process from osteoporosis, although both osteoporosis and osteomalacia result in low BMD [39]. In a study of 36 patients with CD who had undergone small bowel resection, 2 (6%) patients had findings suggestive of osteomalacia [40]. A separate study of 18 patients did not detect osteomalacia in IBD patients [41]. Osteomalacia is relatively common in patients with small intestinal resection, occurring in up to 40% of patients [13]. Overall, the frequency of osteomalacia co-existing with IBD is unclear but is likely small in those who have not undergone prior bowel resection.

Patients with osteomalacia are symptomatic and report generalized bone pain and muscle weakness. Hypocalcemia, hypophosphatemia, elevated parathyroid hormone concentrations, and elevated alkaline phosphatase, which can be used to distinguish osteomalacia from osteoporosis, exist. Vitamin D concentration is typically low. Pseudofractures, biconcave vertebrae, and a triradiate pelvis can be detected radiographically. Bone biopsy definitively establishes the diagnosis although this is infrequently performed [13, 39].

The mainstay of treatment is repletion of low vitamin D levels. Patients who have vitamin D deficiency should receive at least 1000 IU of vitamin D per day, although higher doses may be required if they suffer from co-existing malabsorptive processes. Vitamin D supplementation can be targeted to 25-hydroxy vitamin D level with a goal ≥ 25 ng/mL [13].

Growth Retardation in Children/Adolescents

Impairment of growth in pediatric IBD patients is recognized as one of the most serious complications of the disease and is reported in 15-40% of pediatric onset CD and 3-10% of pediatric onset UC [42-44]. Growth failure is characterized by delayed skeletal maturation as well as delayed onset of puberty. The Paris classification of impaired linear growth is defined by 1) height z-score at diagnosis or subsequently significantly less than expected height z-score (>2.0 using mid-parental height formula or >1.0 using pre-illness height z-score) or 2) reduction in height z-score since diagnosis ≥0.75 [45]. Growth failure is associated with malnutrition, which occurs secondary to decreased food intake and abdominal pain, malabsorption due to intestinal mucosal damage, corticosteroid administration, and growth hormone (GH) resistance due to inflammation [42]. Management of growth impairment is primarily directed at treatment of the underlying IBD. Strategies include immune suppressant therapy (AZA, 6MP, or MTX) alone or in combination with TNF-α antagonists, enteral nutrition in appropriately selected patients, and avoiding unnecessary corticosteroid use. For patients with advanced or refractory disease, surgical management should be considered [42].

Dermatologic

Cutaneous manifestations of IBD occur in approximately 6% of patients. Dermatologic EIMs include erythema nodosum (EN), pyoderma gangrenosum (PG), aphthous stomatitis, febrile neutrophilic dermatosis (Sweet's syndrome), and orofacial granulomatosis. Predictive factors involved in the development of cutaneous manifestations of IBD include female sex, CD, young age at diagnosis of IBD, presence of other EIMs, and distinctive genetic loci [46, 47]. The treatment of these conditions is generally empiric and includes topical therapy as well as use of immune suppressants and biologic agents. Achieving control of underlying IBD may cause symptoms associated with dermatologic EIMs to improve. Expert consultation with a dermatologist may be useful for the diagnosis and management of these conditions [9, 48].

Erythema Nodosum

EN is a form of panniculitis (inflammation of the subcutaneous fat tissue) that affects approximately 5% of patients with IBD. It is the most commonly observed cutaneous manifestation associated with IBD [13, 48-50]. In a study analyzing 2402 IBD patients, EN more commonly occurs in patients with CD than patients with UC (5.6% vs. 1.2%, $p < 0.0001$). In CD patients it is seen more often in those with isolated colonic involvement rather than ileal disease (OR = 4.7 [2.0-10.8]; $p = 0.0001$ [51]. Other conditions associated with EN include infections, sarcoidosis, rheumatologic disorders, drugs, autoimmune diseases, pregnancy, and malignancies. In greater than 50% of cases the cause is not identified. EN occurs in females more frequently than males.

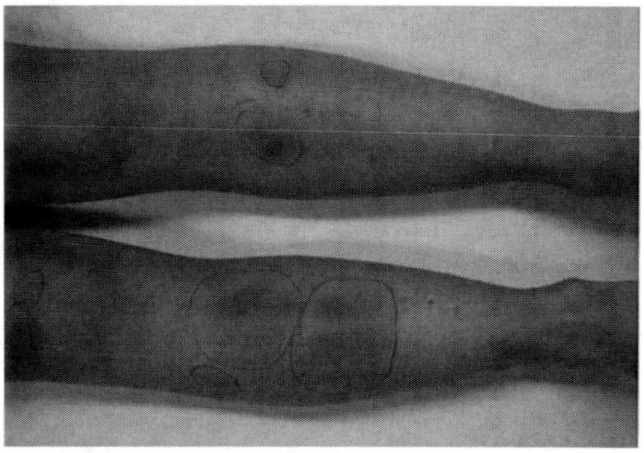

Figure 6.2. Erythema nodosum. Photograph by James Heilman, MD, distributed under a CC BY-SA 3.0 license.

EN nodules are multiple, painful, tender, deep red, warm, and usually occur symmetrically over the anterior legs and measure up to 5 cm in diameter (Figure 6.2). EN may also occur on the trunk, upper extremities, and face. They may transition to a yellow-tinged color similar to a bruise. EN does not scar or ulcerate. EN lesions may be accompanied by systemic symptoms, such as fever, malaise and arthralgia [52-55]. EN symptoms parallel disease activity, although it may precede the diagnosis of IBD by up to five years [52]. Diagnosis can be made based on their characteristic appearance. Biopsy is not required [13, 48].

Treatment for EN is supportive as lesions usually resolve spontaneously within 4 - 6 weeks. Patients with EN should be advised to elevate their legs and use compression stockings. EN usually improves as CD improves. Glucocorticoids, dapsone, and/or biologic therapy can be considered for patients with severe or refractory cases [13, 48, 56-58].

Pyoderma Gangrenosum

PG is a non-infectious, inflammatory, ulcerative skin disorder of unclear etiology. It is more severe than EN and is a type of neutrophilic dermatosis, which are conditions characterized by an influx of polymorphonuclear leukocytes that produce an inflammatory infiltrate. PG is associated with systemic illnesses in up to 50% of cases, such as CD, UC, arthritis, hematologic disorders, or malignancy. Several PG variants or subtypes exist including peristomal and drug-induced PG in addition to classic or ulcerative PG. PG affects up to 2% of patients with IBD [13, 48, 59]. PG in patients with IBD has been demonstrated to be associated with black African origin, familial history of UC, uninterrupted pancolitis as the initial location of IBD, and permanent stomas [51].

Classic PG presents with painful ulcerations usually located on the lower extremities, although lesions can also occur at any site. Classic PG is the most common subtype associated with IBD. It usually begins as a small papule or cluster of papules that devolve into a small ulcer. As the papules coalesce, necrosis occurs forming a larger deep ulcer with a violaceous border (Figure 6.3). The surrounding skin is typically erythematous and warm. Peristomal PG occurs around the stoma (Figure 6.4) after ileostomy or colostomy formation in IBD patients. This process is also observed in cancer patients. The appearance of peristomal PG is similar to that of classic PG. Drug-induced PG has been observed after gefitinib, pegfilgastrim, and propylthiouracil use. In addition to cutaneous features, patients may develop systemic symptoms and signs including fever, malaise, arthralgias, and myalgias [59].

Establishing a diagnosis of PG is based on both clinical and histologic features. Histologic findings are nonspecific and include epidermal necrosis, mixed inflammatory cell infiltrate, and lymphocytic vasculitis. Findings also vary depending on the age and location of the lesion. Biopsies permit infectious conditions to be ruled out as well as exclude other conditions that mimic PG [9, 13, 59].

No standardized treatment exists for PG. Local care should be provided including wet compresses, topical therapy including silver and antibacterial creams, and pain control. Topical medications used for PG include corticosteroids, cyclosporine, tacrolimus, and benzoyl peroxide. Local irradiation, electron beam therapy, and hyperbaric oxygen have also been utilized. Systemic therapy may be required in severe or refractory cases. Corticosteroids are considered first line treatment; however, TNF-α antagonist therapy, such as IFX, can be considered if rapid response to corticosteroids is not achieved [60]. Other treatments include antimicrobials such as dapsone or minocycline and immune suppressants such as cyclophosphamide, AZA, cyclosporine, mycophenolate mofetil, 6MP, MTX, and tacrolimus

[48]. In patients with peristomal PG, closure of the stoma can lead to resolution of the PG lesions [61].

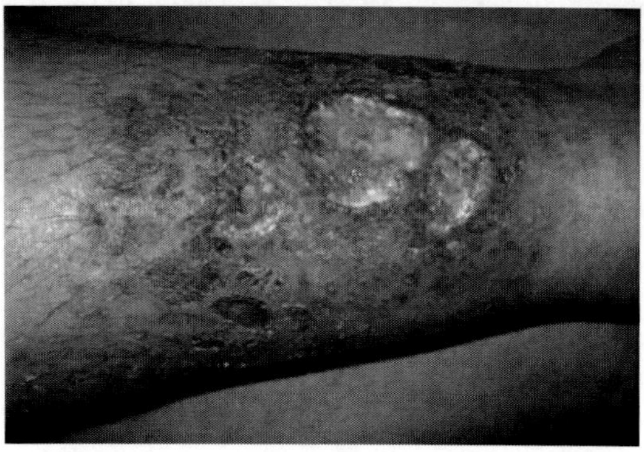

Figure 6.3. Pyoderma gangrenosum.

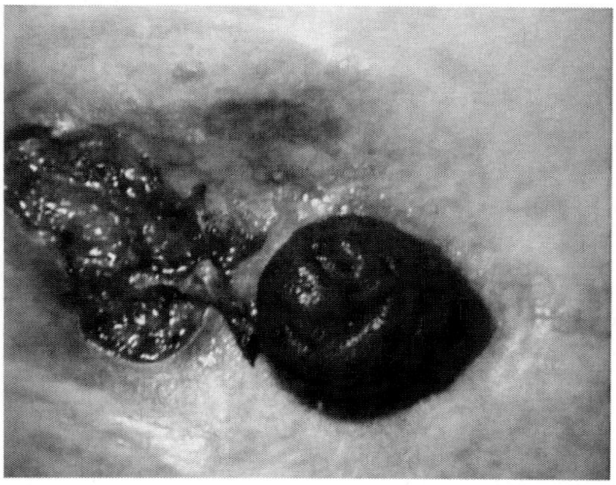

Figure 6.4. Peristomal pyoderma gangrenosum.

Metastatic Crohn's Disease

Metastatic CD is a cutaneous manifestation of CD in which erythematous, occasionally ulcerated, skin lesions occur. These lesions may occur anywhere, but are most commonly found on the extremities, flexures, and genitalia (Figure 6.5). The pathogenesis of metastatic CD is poorly understood. One theory is the unknown, possibly intestinal, antigens circulate to the dermis where they trigger a granulomatous response [62-64]. Another possible mechanism assumes type IV hypersensitivity reaction to an unknown antigen in the skin causes granuloma formation and vascular damage [63].

The prevalence of metastatic CD is unknown, although it is thought to occur rarely. Metastatic CD is infrequently seen in children and, when present, frequently occurs prior to the diagnosis of gastrointestinal CD [48]. Adults tend have a longer duration of metastatic CD lesions when compared to children [63, 65]. Metastatic CD is generally unrelated to severity of bowel disease, and surgical removal of bowel does not necessarily affect metastatic CD severity [63, 64, 66].

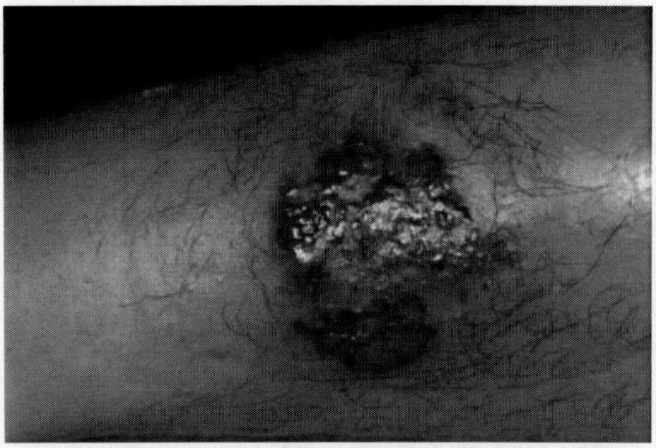

Figure 6.5. Metastatic Crohn's disease.

The diagnosis of metastatic CD requires the appropriate clinical context as well as histologic data (non-caseating granulomas) from a skin biopsy. The differential diagnosis includes PG, EN, Sweet's syndrome, fungal/mycobacterial infection, foreign body reaction, hidradenitis suppurativa, and sarcoidosis. Establishing the diagnosis can be challenging, particularly in patients who develop metastatic CD prior to intestinal CD [48].

Immune suppression in the mainstay of treatment. Oral and topical corticosteroids may be employed. Steroid-sparing agents such as AZA, cyclosporine, tacrolimus, or biologic agents may be required. Surgical therapy may be required in certain cases [13, 67].

Aphthous Stomatitis

Aphthous stomatitis is common in CD patients, affecting 4 - 20%. It also affects up to 15% of the non-IBD population. In patients with CD, stomatitis is often exacerbated during periods of symptomatic flares. Patients with aphthous stomatitis develop painful, shallow, round ulcers with an erythematous border located on the buccal mucosa, labial mucosa, floor of the mouth, or tongue. These lesions usually persist for two weeks or less and heal without scarring [9, 13, 68]. Aphthous stomatitis may become more severe in active disease; however, its presence does not correlate with disease activity [69].

Aphthous stomatitis is diagnosed based on history and clinical findings. Other disorders that have similar features include Behçet's disease, herpes, and coxsackievirus although patients with herpes or coxsackievirus initially develop vesicles, which do not occur in aphthous stomatitis [13].

Treatment is targeted at inducing remission of underlying IBD. Symptoms should be managed with topical analgesia using products such as viscous lidocaine. Topical steroids may promote healing. Amlexanox oral paste has been shown to accelerate healing [70]. Consideration can be given to systemic or intra-lesional glucocorticoids in particularly severe or refractory cases [13, 71].

Sweet's Syndrome

Sweet's syndrome was originally called an "acute febrile neutrophilic dermatosis" by Dr. Robert Sweet in 1964. At that time, he described a condition characterized by fever, elevated neutrophil count, and painful cutaneous lesions with a neutrophilic infiltrate in the upper dermis that responded rapidly to corticosteroid therapy. Tender, erythematous papules and nodules develop, often on the face, neck, and upper extremities (Figure 6.6). Lesions may occasionally exhibit central clearing. Pathergy, or long-lasting ulceration following minor trauma, may occur. Subcutaneous Sweet's syndrome is characterized by subcutaneous nodules, which may be seen on the lower extremities and can be mistaken for EN. Other symptoms include fever, arthralgias, malaise, headache, and myalgias. Sweet's syndrome occurs most often in women, those with colonic disease, and those with other extraintestinal features. In addition to IBD, Sweet's syndrome is also associated with pregnancy, cancer, and certain medications [5, 59, 60].

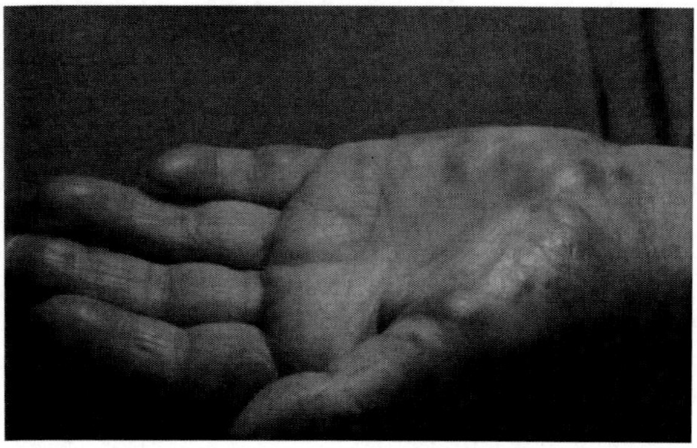

Figure 6.6. Sweet's syndrome, or acute febrile neutrophilic dermatosis.

The diagnosis of Sweet's syndrome is clinical. Diagnostic criteria have been proposed and include the presence of painful erythematous plaques or nodules, histopathologic evidence of a dense neutrophilic infiltrate without leukocytoclastic vasculitis, fever, and association with malignancy, inflammatory disease, or pregnancy among others [13, 72].

The treatment of choice for Sweet's syndrome is systemic corticosteroids. Other options include colchicine, potassium iodide, indomethacin, dapsone, cyclosporine, and TNF-α antagonists. Interleukin-1 antagonists have also been used, but further study is required before these agents can be recommended [13, 73].

Orofacial Granulomatosis

Orofacial granulomatosis (OFG) is a chronic inflammatory condition that is clinically characterized by recurrent, painless edema of the orofacial soft tissues. The most commonly affect area is the lips. Histological features include noncaseating giant cell granulomas and epithelioid histocytes [74-76]. Mellkersson-Rosenthal syndrome (MRS), which is a subtype of OFG, is characterized by a triad of symptoms, including recurrent facial palsy, orofacial edema, and fissured tongue (lingua plicata) [74, 77]. Between 8 and 46% of patients with OFG have

CD. The association is more common when OFG symptoms begin in childhood [75]. Treatment for OFG and MRS include oral steroids, intralesional steroid injections, and TNF-α antagonists [78]. Unfortunately, patients often continue to experience symptoms despite treatment [79]. Topical analgesic medications, beclomethasone mouthwash, and 5-ASA spray or ointment can be used for symptom relief [69]. Exclusion of cinnamon and benzoate from the diet improves symptoms in some patients [69].

Ophthalmologic

Ocular complications are associated with CD including uveitis, episcleritis, and iritis. Ocular EIMs occur in approximately 4-12% of IBD patients [80-82]. Even so, symptoms are often ignored or misunderstood by both patients and physicians. Many symptoms are nonspecific and include blurry vision, pain, photophobia, conjunctival or scleral injection, change in visual acuity, and teary or burning eyes. Because of this, ocular EIMs may be confused with other disorders. Ocular complications of CD can be serious and have the potential to cause blindness [83].

Uveitis

Uveitis is one of the most common ocular manifestations of IBD [80]. Uveitis is a condition in which the vascular coat of the eye is inflamed. Uveitis often occurs in the setting of arthralgias and/or cutaneous symptoms. In the anterior eye uveitis affects the iris and ciliary body, in the posterior eye the vitreous, choroid, or retina. Patients with anterior uveitis report a painful eye with blurring and photophobia. A ciliary flush, erythema most intense at the limbus with radiation outward, is characteristic of uveitis. Patients with posterior uveitis experience changes in visual acuity, floaters, scotomas, severe light sensitivity, ocular redness and even acute blindness [80]. Although posterior uveitis is less common, it is important to recognize symptoms because it can progress to permanent visual loss if left untreated [80, 84]. Uveitis occurs independent of gastrointestinal symptoms and may precede a diagnosis of IBD [83].

If uveitis is suspected prompt ophthalmologic evaluation should be obtained. Diagnosis is made by slit-lamp examination [83]. Anterior uveitis is treated with topical steroids and cycloplegic medications. Systemic steroids and/or immune suppressants may be required. TNF-α antagonists have also been used to treat uveitis. Posterior uveitis is treated with intraocular steroid injections followed by systemic immune suppression because steroid eye drops have poor penetration to posterior ocular structures [80]. Reports of improvement of uveitis in response to colectomy also exist [83].

Episcleritis

Episcleritis refers to inflammation of the episclera, the vascular plexus, and fibrous tissue layer found between the sclera (white of the eye) and the conjunctiva. Patients with episcleritis develop acute erythema of one or both eyes accompanied by irritation, pain, tenderness, or burning. Visual loss, photophobia, and loss of pupillary response to light do not occur. Conjunctivitis has a similar presentation, although the discomfort in episcleritis is more pronounced. On examination focal or diffuse areas of erythema can be seen within white areas of sclera [13, 83]. There is also injection that blanches with topical phenylephrine application [85].

Episcleritis parallels underlying CD activity. Treatment centers on inducing remission of underlying CD. In addition, cool compresses, topical lubricants and topical steroids may be used to provide symptomatic relief. NSAIDs may also offer relief but should be used with caution in patients with IBD [13, 83].

Scleritis

Scleritis is a rare EIM in patients with IBD. Unlike episcleritis, scleritis has the potential to impair vision. In patients with scleritis, the deep scleral vessels are injected in addition to the episcleral and conjunctival vessels. Patients most commonly report severe eye pain with associated tenderness.

Scleritis can be distinguished from episcleritis. In scleritis, the sclerae appear pink between the dilated surface vessels whereas in episcleritis the sclerae appear white. In addition, in episcleritis blood vessels blanch with topical application of phenylephrine due to their superficial location. This does not occur in scleritis. Additionally, patients with scleritis describe a deep boring pain of the eye upon wakening from sleep, which does not occur in episcleritis [83]. Scleritis can lead to retinal detachment, scleral perforation, and swelling of the optic nerve [86].

Aggressive treatment is required. Agents employed include systemic corticosteroids, NSAIDs, or immune suppressants. Although scleritis is not directly linked to IBD disease activity, the underlying IBD should also be treated. If scleritis is suspected immediate referral to an ophthalmologist is required [13, 83].

Hepatobiliary/Pancreatic

Primary Sclerosing Cholangitis

Primary sclerosing cholangitis (PSC) is an immune mediated disorder directed against the biliary tree. PSC is characterized by inflammation and fibrosis of the intrahepatic and/or extrahepatic ducts, leading to liver cirrhosis and end-stage liver disease [87]. PSC occurs in up to 5% of IBD patients and it is estimated that roughly 70% of patients with PSC have underlying IBD, most frequently UC [88-90]. PSC occurs more commonly in men than in women. Patients with PSC may develop jaundice, fatigue, weight loss, right upper quadrant pain, and/or pruritus. Even so, a large number of patients are asymptomatic and PSC is suspected based on elevated alkaline phosphatase on routine laboratory evaluation [13].

PSC may be diagnosed in the setting of an elevated alkaline phosphatase combined with cholangiographic abnormalities demonstrated on either MRCP or ERCP. If the diagnosis is unclear after cholangiography, liver biopsy can be pursued [5, 13, 91].

The only definitive therapy for PSC is orthotopic liver transplant. Survival is good, with a 5-year survival rate of 85 - 90%. Unfortunately, PSC recurs in the allograft in up to 20% of patients. Ursodeoxycholic acid does reduce colonic dysplasia and carcinoma [92], including both colorectal cancer and cholangiocarcinoma, but does not improve symptoms or mortality. If pruritus is present, cholestyramine can be administered [13, 92].

Liver function tests should be checked at least annually in all IBD patients, in part to screen for PSC [89]. Given the increased risk of cholangiocarcinoma (CCA), gallbladder carcinoma (GBC), and hepatocellular carcinoma (HCC) in IBD-PSC patients, most guidelines recommend screening IBD-PSC patients annually with CA 19-9 and biliary imaging [81, 89, 93-95].

Pancreatitis

Acute and chronic pancreatitis occur more frequently in CD patients than in the background population. IBD patients are at risk for "traditional" pancreatitis (i.e., gallstone or alcohol induced) as well as pancreatitis due to medication effect or autoimmune pancreatitis. Patients with IBD have a higher incidence of biliary lithiasis, particularly in cases with extensive ileal disease [96]. Drugs such as AZA and its active metabolite 6MP are well-known as causes of acute pancreatitis, with the effect occurring most commonly within the first few weeks of treatment [96].

Like other patients, CD patients with pancreatitis develop severe epigastric abdominal pain, often accompanied by nausea and vomiting. Patients should be queried regarding alcohol use, biliary tract disease, gallstones, family history of pancreatitis, medications, abdominal surgeries, abdominal trauma, and weight loss [13, 97-99].

Pancreatitis may be diagnosed in the presence of two of three characteristic features: abdominal pain characteristic of pancreatitis, amylase or lipase $\geq$3 times the upper limit of normal, or radiographic evidence of pancreatitis by CT scan. Potential culprit drugs (e.g., AZA, 6MP, 5-ASA) should be stopped. Biopsy is required to diagnose autoimmune pancreatitis [13].

Treatment is centered on aggressive rehydration and close monitoring. Culprit drugs, if present, should be stopped. Patients with end organ dysfunction should be managed in an intensive care unit. Enteral nutrition is favored over parenteral nutrition [13].

Hepatitis

Autoimmune hepatitis (AIH) is a rare, chronic, heterogenous liver disease characterized by abnormal liver tests, hypergammaglobulinemia, and autoantibodies, including antinuclear antibody (ANA), smooth muscle antibody, and anti-liver-kidney microsomal antibody [100, 101]. Clinical symptoms include fatigue, nausea, abdominal pain, jaundice, and acute hepatitis. Severe cases may progress to fulminant hepatic failure. Biopsy may be required to rule out additional or alternate causes of liver failure [102]. There is a known association between AIH and UC, with up to 16% of AIH patients having UC [100, 103]. AIH may also occur as a result of IBD therapies, particularly TNF-α antagonists [103]. Corticosteroids are used as the primary means to induce remission and may be continued at a lower dose as maintenance therapy [102]. Other agents such as AZA may be used along with prednisone to maintain remission. Patients with UC and concurrent AIH are more likely to fail AIH treatment and have persistent liver disease and liver lesions [103].

In addition to AIH, patients on immunosuppressive therapy for IBD are susceptible to reactivation of viral hepatitis. Reactivation of HBV can be seen with immune suppressants including corticosteroids, thiopurines, and advanced therapies [1, 100]. Therefore, patients with IBD should be screened for HBV with at least the following serologies: hepatitis B surface antigen (HBsAg), hepatitis B core antibody (HBcAb), hepatitis B surface antibody (HBsAb). Seronegative patients should undergo vaccination to achieve serological immune response [100]. Seropositive patients (HBsAg positive and/or HBcAb positive) should receive prophylactic treatment with nucleotide/nucleoside analogues prior to immunosuppressive treatment start and for at least 6 to 12 months after stopping immunosuppressants [104]. Cytomegalovirus and Epstein-Barr virus induced hepatitis in immunosuppressed IBD patients has also been described [1, 105].

Cardiovascular/Thromboembolic

Patients with IBD are at increased risk of developing cardiovascular disease (CVD) and venous thromboembolic events (VTEs), including deep vein thrombosis, pulmonary embolism and portal vein thrombosis [1, 106, 107]. Given the high morbidity and mortality associated with cardiovascular disease, it is important to understand the prevalence, risk factors, and treatment options for IBD-related CVD and VTE.

Cardiovascular Disease

Patients with IBD are at increased risk for atherosclerotic cardiovascular disease (ASCVD) such as myocardial infarction and stroke. This effect is most likely a consequence of chronic inflammation and disease activity. Possible mechanisms include endothelial dysfunction and platelet aggregation. Other factors which may contribute are lipid dysfunction, corticosteroid use, and gut microbiome abnormalities [1, 106, 108-110]. Elevated inflammatory markers, such as C-reactive protein, IL-6, and TNF-α, can lead to endothelial dysfunction and are frequently elevated in IBD patients [106].

Currently, there is limited evidence regarding optimal ASCVD prevention in patients with IBD [110]. Treatment should focus on risk reduction through screening for and treatment of CVD risk factors including obesity, diabetes, hypertension, dyslipidemia, and tobacco use. Further research is required to improve IBD-related CVD screening, preventative care, and treatment [110].

Deep Vein Thrombosis

Patients with CD are at increased risk of developing venous thromboembolism (VTE) [111, 112]. A meta-analysis evaluated 11 studies examining this topic and found that the relative risk (RR) for DVT and pulmonary embolism (PE) in IBD patients was 2.2 (95% CI 1.8

– 2.7) when compared to patients without IBD [112]. An earlier study examining ICD-9 codes of hospital discharges found that both UC (OR 1.9, 95% CI 1.7 – 2.0) and CD (OR 1.4, 95% CI 1.4 – 1.6) were associated with higher rates of VTE when compared to non-IBD patients. VTE in IBD patients was also associated with increased mortality (OR 1.5, 95% CI 1.8 – 3.4) and increased length of stay (11.7 vs. 6.1 days, $p < 0.00001$). Expenditures were also higher [13, 113].

Because of the increased risk of VTE and higher mortality associated with VTE in CD patients, all hospitalized IBD patients should receive unfractionated or low-molecular weight heparin for VTE prophylaxis unless clear contraindications, such as active GI bleeding, exist [13].

Portal Vein Thrombosis

The pro-inflammatory and hypercoagulable state associated with IBD is thought to increase the risk of portal vein thrombosis (PVT), mesenteric vein thrombosis and Budd-Chiari syndrome [100]. The estimated incidence of portal and mesenteric vein thrombosis in IBD patients is 0.17-2% [100, 114, 115]. Factors associated with increased thrombotic events include elevated platelet count, high fibrinogen, high factor V and factor VIII levels, greater extent of colonic disease, steroid use, and immobilization [100]. Patients with an active flare, post-surgical patients, particularly UC patients after proctocolectomy, and IBD patients with intra-abdominal infections are at highest risk for PVT [100, 116]. Prior history of VTE has been shown to be unrelated to the development of PVT in IBD patients [116].

PVT typically presents with non-specific abdominal pain. It is diagnosed with US, CT, or MRI [117]. Management of PVT is anti-coagulation (AC). A single center retrospective study examining the therapeutic efficacy of AC in IBD patients diagnosed with PVT demonstrated complete radiographic resolution of PVT in 71% of patients who started AC within 3 days of diagnosis. Of AC therapeutic options, patients receiving direct oral anti-coagulation (DOAC) therapy were significantly more likely to achieve complete radiographic resolution and require shortly treatment courses than patients taking warfarin [116]. Additionally, no patients receiving DOAC experienced major bleeding. Therefore, therapeutic anti-coagulation should be considered for all IBD patients with PVT, even in cases of prior gastrointestinal bleeding [100].

Perianal

Perianal Crohn's disease (PCD) is defined as inflammation at or close to the anus, including tags, fissures, fistulae, abscesses, or stenosis [118]. The reported incidence of PCD varies, from as low as 3.8% to as high as 61-80% [119]. PCD is not only common, but also can have a significant negative impact on quality of life, relationships, social life, and work life in CD patients [120].

Skin Tags

Anal skin tags are present in up to 37-70% of patients with CD and 25% of patients with UC [121, 122]. The are two main types of skin tags that occur in IBD patients. Type 1 skin tags are typically seen with CD and are large, edematous, hard, and cyanotic. Type 1 skin tags frequently occur during active disease and are thought to be due to lymphedema secondary to lymphatic obstruction. Type 2 skin tags are seen in CD and UC, and are flat, broad or narrow, soft, and painless [123]. Treatment should be directed at controlling intestinal inflammation [123]. Surgical resection is a therapeutic option for lesions that are particularly large or painful; however, should be avoided in patients with active proctitis as it increases the risk of nonhealing perianal wounds. Additionally, patients who undergo resection need detailed wound care and close follow up with their surgeon [121].

Anal Fissures

Anal fissures account for 21-35% of perianal lesions in CD. Fissures are primarily located posteriorly; however, multiple and/or lateral fissures can also occur [119]. Unlike patients without IBD, patients with IBD associated fissures are more likely to have normal resting anal sphincter pressure [119]. These lesions can heal spontaneously, but topical therapies include nitroglycerin, diltiazem, botulinum toxin, and local steroids. Surgical intervention via lateral internal sphincterotomy should be reserved for symptomatic and medically refractory patients without rectal disease and with internal sphincter muscle hypertonicity [121].

Abscesses and Fistulas (Perianal/Enterocutaneous)

Perianal fistulas and abscesses secondary to CD have an estimated incidence ranging between 4 and 80% [119, 121]. The wide range is likely due to variation in defining criteria. Patients with distal rectal disease have a 92% risk of developing perineal disease, compared to the 12% risk of patients with isolated ileal disease [124].

Perianal abscesses can lead to the development of perianal fistulas [119]. A fistula is defined as an abnormal communication between two epithelial surfaces. Perianal fistulas can be categorized as intersphincteric, transsphincteric, suprasphincteric, and extrasphincteric. Fistulas can also be classified as simple or complex [123]. A simple fistula is low (superficial intersphincteric or transsphincteric), confined to the anal canal, has a single external opening, and has no associated undrained perianal abscess. A complex fistula is high intersphincteric, transsphincteric, extrasphincteric or suprasphincteric, may have multiple external openings and may be associated with a perianal abscess. Additionally, complex fistulas may be associated with fistulas to adjacent organs, may be associated with the presence of an anorectal stricture, and may be associated with the presence of active rectal disease [123].

Symptoms of perianal abscesses and fistulas include persistent drainage, incontinence, pain, and decreased quality of life [124]. Diagnosis is achieved through a combination of exam under anesthesia, magnetic resonance imaging (MRI) of the pelvis with intravenous contrast, and/or endorectal ultrasound [121].

Treatment includes management of underlying IBD, particularly with immunosuppression and TNF-α antagonists [121, 123]. The presence of a perianal abscess requires incision and drainage, with or without placement of a drain for additional drainage over the next few days. Management of a perianal fistula depends on location, type of fistula and extent of disease. A simple perianal fistula without rectal disease activity can be managed with a fistulotomy [123]. Complex perianal fistulae may require prolonged drainage with a seton. In the absence of proctitis, endorectal advancement flaps have been used in the treatment of anal fistulae. In severe cases, fecal diversion with a loop ileostomy or colostomy may be required to allow the fistula to heal [123].

Genitourinary

Nephrolithiasis

CD patients are more likely to develop nephrolithiasis. The overall incidence of nephrolithiasis in IBD is approximately 10 - 20% versus 0.1% in the general population [125]. The risk is greatest in CD patients who have undergone bowel resection. Most kidney stones in IBD patients are comprised of calcium oxalate or uric acid. Normally, oxalate is bound to calcium and is poorly absorbed. In patients who have undergone ileal resection or who CD involving the ileum, bile salt absorption is impaired resulting in bile salt deficiency and fat malabsorption. Fat is then free to bind luminal calcium, decreasing the ability of calcium to bind oxalate. As a result, calcium absorption increases resulting in increased urinary oxalate excretion and oxalate stone formation. Urate stones develop because of increased intestinal fluid and bicarbonate loss. Concentrated, acidic urine is produced within which urate precipitates more readily, leading to the development of kidney stones [13, 126].

Patients with nephrolithiasis report intermittent colicky flank pain that may radiate to the lower abdomen or groin and is often associated with nausea or vomiting. Nephrolithiasis is likely when microscopic hematuria is detected in the setting of symptoms suggestive of renal colic. A CT scan without intravenous contrast may be obtained to demonstrate nephrolithiasis [13].

Treatment is similar to non-IBD patients and consists of hydration, pain control, and alkalization of urine. Potassium and magnesium supplementation may also reduce oxalate stone formation. Patients who do not respond to the above measures may require lithotripsy or percutaneous nephroureterolithotomy. Patients with oxalate stones should be counseled to follow a low oxalate diet [13, 127].

Glomerulonephritis

Glomerulonephritis encompasses a subset of renal diseases characterized by immune-mediated damage of the renal glomeruli [128]. IBD has been linked to various subtypes of glomerulonephritis, including immunoglobulin (Ig) A and IgM nephropathy, as well as membranous, mesangiocapillary, focal segmental and anti-glomerular basement membrane glomerulonephritis [129]. The prevalence of IgA nephropathy is higher in patients with IBD than those without and is a major cause of acute and chronic renal failure in IBD patients [130]. The correlation between IgA nephropathy and IBD is suspected to be genetic. Multiple loci involved in IgA nephropathy are associated with the development of IBD or maintenance of enteric mucosa [131]. Chronic immune stimulation and increased IgA production may also play a role [132].

IBD flares in patients with concurrent glomerulonephritis are associated with worse renal function [129, 130, 133]. Conversely, resolution of bowel inflammation is associated with improvement in renal function. Diagnosis of glomerulonephritis is made through analysis of laboratory data, primary creatinine, glomerular filtration rate, serum electrolytes, immunoglobins, autoantibodies, and urinalysis, as well as a renal biopsy [128]. Intermittent monitoring of patient's renal function with laboratory analysis is recommended in IBD patients [129].

Hydronephrosis

The incidence of hydronephrosis in patients with CD is approximately 6% [134]. CD patients with hydronephrosis can develop flank pain, hip pain, and/or urinary symptoms [135]. Hydronephrosis is diagnosed and graded by ultrasonography [134]. When evaluating hydronephrosis in CD patients, CT and/or intravenous pyelography can determine the level of obstruction and possible causes [135].

Development of hydronephrosis is thought to be secondary to intra-abdominal ureteral occlusion/stenosis from inflammation of the affected bowel into the retroperitoneum, fistulas, local abscesses and fibrosis [135, 136]. Obstruction most frequently occurs on the right-side at the level of the terminal ileum [135]. Left-sided hydronephrosis occurs with sigmoid colon or jejunal involvement and therefore the level of obstruction is more variable [135].

Management of hydronephrosis due to ureteric stenosis includes pulse-dose corticosteroids, percutaneous nephrostomy, and implantation of a ureteral catheter [134]. However, patients initially managed with stent placement may require intestinal resection with or without ureterolysis [136].

Fistulas (Colovesicular, Enterovesicular, Rectovaginal)

Similar to the increased incidence of enterocutaneous and perianal fistulas in IBD, patients are also susceptible to enterovesicular colovesicular, and rectovaginal fistulas [134, 137].

Enterovesical fistulas are the most common fistula affecting the urinary tract, likely due to the anatomical proximity of the ileum and bladder dome [138]. Common symptoms include pneumaturia, fecaluria, fever, urinary urgency, and abdominal pain [137]. The incidence of enterovesical fistula (EVF) in patients with CD is estimated at 2-8% [139, 140]. Fistulas arise from ulcerative disease that progresses to transmural fissures with subsequent penetration of the surrounding structures [140]. CD is recognized as the most common cause of enterovesicular fistulas and third most common cause of colovesicular fistulas [124, 137, 139, 141, 142].

Diagnosis of enterovesicular and colovesicular fistula is through cystoscopy, computed tomography, and MRI. Surgery is the mainstay of treatment and often involves resection of the involved bowel and bladder decompression with indwelling catheter to allow the bladder defect to heal primarily [140].

Anovaginal (AVF) and rectovaginal fistulas (RVF) account for 9% of fistulas in CD [124]. CD is the second most common cause of RVF after obstetrical trauma and is thought to be directly proportionate to the severity of colonic disease [143]. Symptoms include dyspareunia, perianal pain, vaginal irritation, and genitourinary infections [143, 144]. Diagnosis can be made through vaginal and/or rectal examination and contrast imaging studies. Medical treatment involves IBD-directed medications, such as corticosteroids, immunosuppressives, IFX, and antibiotics; however, medical therapies have high rates of recurrence [143]. Surgical intervention is often required and includes direct repair, fistulotomy, fibrin glue instillation, endorectal or vaginal advancement flap, abdominal procedures with colorectal or coloanal anastomosis, and epiplooplasty. The chosen surgical technique varies considerably based on the location of the fistula and extent of patient disease [140, 143, 145, 146].

Pulmonary

Pulmonary manifestations of IBD are rare but are becoming increasingly recognized by the medical community [1, 147]. Pulmonary manifestations may occur during active disease, independent of disease activity, and in post-colectomy patients [147-149].

Airway Disease

Studies have shown that patients with airway disease of the trachea and bronchioles are four times more likely to have IBD, with the relationship thought to be secondary to an inflammatory response [147, 150]. Symptoms include coughing, dyspnea, stridor and hoarseness. Computed tomography may demonstrate tracheal narrowing or circumferential tracheal wall thickening [149, 151].

Chronic bronchitis and bronchiectasis are strongly associated with UC and can frequently occur after colectomy [147, 151]. Patients report chronic productive cough and radiographical changes are visible on imaging studies [152].

Treatment for IBD-related airway disease includes inhaled and oral corticosteroids, with the former being more effective [147].

Lung Parenchymal Disease

Lung parenchymal disease associated with IBD is uncommon but tends to occur primarily in UC patients. Bronchiolitis Obliterans Organizing Pneumonia (BOOP) is the most common parenchymal manifestation of IBD. Treatment consists of systemic corticosteroids [147]. Eosinophilic pneumonia and nonspecific interstitial pneumonitis have also been reported to be associated with IBD [147].

Systemic

Systemic symptoms, particularly fatigue and pain, are frequently reported by IBD patients. These symptoms lead to profound decreases in health-related quality of life scales and can be very challenging to treat [1, 153].

Fatigue

Fatigue tends to be more common during active flares but can also occur during remission. Between 50 and 80% of IBD patients report fatigue [154, 155]. The relationship between fatigue and IBD is unclear; however, increased inflammatory markers, such as IL-6 levels, may play a role [156, 157]. Secondary factors such as malnutrition, anemia, sleep disturbance, and psychological comorbidities are other potential contributors to increased fatigue levels in IBD patients [158].

Currently there is no single effective treatment for IBD-related fatigue; however, psychosocial treatment and support has proven beneficial in some studies. One study found that cognitive behavioral therapy improved multiple somatic symptoms of depression, including fatigue, in adolescent patients with IBD [157]. Additionally, management of malnutrition with vitamin, particularly thiamine supplementation, and treatment of anemia has been demonstrated to decrease fatigue in IBD patients [157, 158].

Pain

Pain is common in UC and CD patients with up to 90% of patients reporting pain as a manifestation of their disease, without a significant difference between those with UC and those with CD [153, 159]. Of those with IBD-related pain, a majority report significantly lower health-related quality of life scores compared to those without pain [153]. Patients most commonly report abdominal pain (60%), followed by musculoskeletal pain of various locations. The presence of EIMs does not influence the occurrence rate of pain in IBD patients; however, this is an important factor in determining treatment [153, 159]. Management should be multidisciplinary and include treatment of the underlying disease along with physical therapy, pain medicine, psychiatry, and cognitive behavioral therapy [1].

Conclusion

EIMs are a group of diagnoses and pathologies that are due to either the direct effects of the inflammatory response of IBD, an independent inflammatory event instigated by IBD, or a common environmental or genetic predisposition linked to IBD. EIMs affect all organ systems leading to a wide array of potential symptoms and presentations in patients. While some EIMs tend to flare during disease activity, others are present during disease quiescence.

Various rheumatologic joint issues are common in IBD patients. Type I peripheral arthropathy affects less than 5 joints and usually presents in parallel to disease activity.

Conversely, type II peripheral arthropathy, axial arthritis, and ankylosing spondylitis are separate from disease activity. IBD-related arthritis is often successfully treated with medications that also treat IBD, such as TNF-α antagonists, ustekinumab, and other anti-inflammatory agents. The increased incidence of osteoporosis, osteopenia, osteomalacia, and growth retardation is thought to be secondary to the inflammatory activation seen in IBD disease activity leading to increased bone resorption and malnutrition.

Cutaneous and ocular EIMs that parallel disease activity includes erythema nodosum, aphthous stomatitis, Sweet's syndrome, orofacial granulomatosis, and episcleritis. Whereas metastatic CD, uveitis, and scleritis are not linked tot IBD activity. Cutaneous and ophthalmological EIMs can be treated with topical and systemic agents and can improve with remission of underlying IBD. However, the presence of visual changes in IBD patients should prompt immediate evaluation by an ophthalmologist.

Perianal manifestations are some of the most common EIMs in IBD patients. Anal skin tags and perianal abscesses and fistulas appear or worsen during periods of disease activity and are treated with controlling IBD targeted therapies, in conjunction with surgical management. On the other hand, perianal fissures will either resolve spontaneously or require intervention with local therapies, such as nitroglycerin or botulinum toxin injection.

Hepatobiliary, pancreatic, cardiovascular, genitourinary, and pulmonary EIMs occur less frequently than those listed above but should be considered when IBD patients present with elevated LFTs, VTEs, nephrolithiasis, or airway diseases.

Nonspecific symptoms such as fatigue and pain are some of the most commonly reported IBD EIMs and can significantly impact quality of life. However, research regarding causes and potential therapies for IBD-associated pain and fatigue is limited.

Approximately 40% of patients with IBD experience at least one EIM. Therefore, the ability to recognize and appropriately treat EIMs is critical for any clinician involved in the care of IBD patients. Health care providers should routinely query patients regarding symptoms associated with common EIMs, as many patients may not realize that their joint issues, skin changes, or other symptoms are secondary to their IBD. It is our practice to specifically question patients about joint, ocular, and dermatologic symptoms. Routine screening with laboratory analysis and imaging studies may also be necessary in some patients. Treatment of IBD disease activity may lead to regression of some EIMs; however, others require tailored treatment plans and consultation to other specialists.

References

[1] Rogler G, Singh A, Kavanaugh A, Rubin DT. Extraintestinal Manifestations of Inflammatory Bowel Disease: Current Concepts, Treatment, and Implications for Disease Management. *Gastroenterology*, 161(4), 1118-1132 (2021).

[2] Hedin CRH, Vavricka SR, Stagg AJ et al. The Pathogenesis of Extraintestinal Manifestations: Implications for IBD Research, Diagnosis, and Therapy. *Journal of Crohn's and Colitis*, 13(5), 541-554 (2018).

[3] Bernstein CN, Blanchard JF, Rawsthorne P, Yu N. The prevalence of extraintestinal diseases in inflammatory bowel disease: a population-based study. *The American journal of gastroenterology*, 96(4), 1116-1122 (2001).

[4] Su CG, Judge TA, Lichtenstein GR. Extraintestinal manifestations of inflammatory bowel disease. *Gastroenterology clinics of North America*, 31(1), 307-327 (2002).

[5] Ardizzone S, Puttini PS, Cassinotti A, Porro GB. Extraintestinal manifestations of inflammatory bowel disease. *Digestive and liver disease : official journal of the Italian Society of Gastroenterology and the Italian Association for the Study of the Liver*, 40 Suppl 2, S253-259 (2008).

[6] Orchard TR, Chua CN, Ahmad T, Cheng H, Welsh KI, Jewell DP. Uveitis and erythema nodosum in inflammatory bowel disease: clinical features and the role of HLA genes. *Gastroenterology*, 123(3), 714-718 (2002).

[7] Orchard TR, Wordsworth BP, Jewell DP. Peripheral arthropathies in inflammatory bowel disease: their articular distribution and natural history. *Gut*, 42(3), 387-391 (1998).

[8] Arvikar SL, Fisher MC. Inflammatory bowel disease associated arthropathy. *Current reviews in musculoskeletal medicine*, 4(3), 123-131 (2011).

[9] Patil SA, Cross RK. Update in the management of extraintestinal manifestations of inflammatory bowel disease. *Current gastroenterology reports*, 15(3), 314 (2013).

[10] Sheth T, Pitchumoni CS, Das KM. Musculoskeletal manifestations in inflammatory bowel disease: a revisit in search of immunopathophysiological mechanisms. *Journal of clinical gastroenterology*, 48(4), 308-317 (2014).

[11] Orchard TR, Thiyagaraja S, Welsh KI, Wordsworth BP, Hill Gaston JS, Jewell DP. Clinical phenotype is related to HLA genotype in the peripheral arthropathies of inflammatory bowel disease. *Gastroenterology*, 118(2), 274-278 (2000).

[12] Padovan M, Castellino G, Govoni M, Trotta F. The treatment of the rheumatological manifestations of the inflammatory bowel diseases. *Rheumatology international*, 26(11), 953-958 (2006).

[13] Larsen S, Bendtzen K, Nielsen OH. Extraintestinal manifestations of inflammatory bowel disease: epidemiology, diagnosis, and management. *Annals of medicine*, 42(2), 97-114 (2010).

[14] Ananthakrishnan AN, Higuchi LM, Huang ES et al. Aspirin, nonsteroidal anti-inflammatory drug use, and risk for Crohn disease and ulcerative colitis: a cohort study. *Annals of internal medicine*, 156(5), 350-359 (2012).

[15] de Vlam K, Mielants H, Cuvelier C, De Keyser F, Veys EM, De Vos M. Spondyloarthropathy is underestimated in inflammatory bowel disease: prevalence and HLA association. *The Journal of rheumatology*, 27(12), 2860-2865 (2000).

[16] Palm O, Moum B, Ongre A, Gran JT. Prevalence of ankylosing spondylitis and other spondyloarthropathies among patients with inflammatory bowel disease: a population study (the IBSEN study). *The Journal of rheumatology*, 29(3), 511-515 (2002).

[17] Turkcapar N, Toruner M, Soykan I et al. The prevalence of extraintestinal manifestations and HLA association in patients with inflammatory bowel disease. *Rheumatology international*, 26(7), 663-668 (2006).

[18] Horton DB, Sherry DD, Baldassano RN, Weiss PF. Enthesitis is an Extraintestinal Manifestation of Pediatric Inflammatory Bowel Disease. *Ann Paediatr Rheumatol*, 1(4) (2012).

[19] Sheth T, Pitchumoni CS, Das KM. Management of Musculoskeletal Manifestations in Inflammatory Bowel Disease. *Gastroenterol Res Pract*, 2015, 387891 (2015).

[20] Kataria RK, Brent LH. Spondyloarthropathies. *American family physician*, 69(12), 2853-2860 (2004).

[21] Jewell D. Do HLA antigens predict the occurrence of extraintestinal manifestations of IBD? *Inflammatory bowel diseases*, 14 Suppl 2, S28 (2008).

[22] van der Linden S, Valkenburg HA, Cats A. Evaluation of diagnostic criteria for ankylosing spondylitis. A proposal for modification of the New York criteria. *Arthritis and rheumatism*, 27(4), 361-368 (1984).

[23] Ferrante M, Panaccione R, Baert F et al. Risankizumab as maintenance therapy for moderately to severely active Crohn's disease: results from the multicentre, randomised, double-blind, placebo-controlled, withdrawal phase 3 FORTIFY maintenance trial. *Lancet*, 399(10340), 2031-2046 (2022).

[24] Sands BE, D'Haens G, Clemow DB et al. Two-Year Efficacy and Safety of Mirikizumab Following 104 Weeks of Continuous Treatment for Ulcerative Colitis: Results From the LUCENT-3 Open-Label Extension Study. *Inflamm Bowel Dis*, (2024).

[25] Sandborn WJ, D'Haens GR, Reinisch W et al. Guselkumab for the Treatment of Crohn's Disease: Induction Results From the Phase 2 GALAXI-1 Study. *Gastroenterology*, 162(6), 1650-1664 e1658 (2022).

[26] Rodriguez-Bores L, Barahona-Garrido J, Yamamoto-Furusho JK. Basic and clinical aspects of osteoporosis in inflammatory bowel disease. *World journal of gastroenterology : WJG*, 13(46), 6156-6165 (2007).

[27] Tigas S, Tsatsoulis A. Endocrine and metabolic manifestations in inflammatory bowel disease. *Annals of gastroenterology : quarterly publication of the Hellenic Society of Gastroenterology*, 25(1), 37-44 (2012).

[28] Lichtenstein GR, Sands BE, Pazianas M. Prevention and treatment of osteoporosis in inflammatory bowel disease. *Inflammatory bowel diseases*, 12(8), 797-813 (2006).

[29] Tilg H, Moschen AR, Kaser A, Pines A, Dotan I. Gut, inflammation and osteoporosis: basic and clinical concepts. *Gut*, 57(5), 684-694 (2008).

[30] Oh HJ, Ryu KH, Park BJ, Yoon BH. Osteoporosis and Osteoporotic Fractures in Gastrointestinal Disease. *J Bone Metab*, 25(4), 213-217 (2018).

[31] Boyce BF, Xing L. The RANKL/RANK/OPG pathway. *Curr Osteoporos Rep*, 5(3), 98-104 (2007).

[32] Bernstein CN, Leslie WD, Leboff MS. AGA technical review on osteoporosis in gastrointestinal diseases. *Gastroenterology*, 124(3), 795-841 (2003).

[33] Lewis N, Scott B. Guidelines for Osteoporosis in Inflammatory Bowel Disease and Coeliac Disease. (Ed.^(Eds) (British Society of Gastroenterology, London, 2007)

[34] Kanis JA, Melton LJ, 3rd, Christiansen C, Johnston CC, Khaltaev N. The diagnosis of osteoporosis. *Journal of bone and mineral research : the official journal of the American Society for Bone and Mineral Research*, 9(8), 1137-1141 (1994).

[35] Lewiecki EM. Premenopausal bone health assessment. *Current rheumatology reports*, 7(1), 46-52 (2005).

[36] Miheller P, Muzes G, Racz K et al. Changes of OPG and RANKL concentrations in Crohn's disease after infliximab therapy. *Inflamm Bowel Dis*, 13(11), 1379-1384 (2007).

[37] Franchimont N, Putzeys V, Collette J et al. Rapid improvement of bone metabolism after infliximab treatment in Crohn's disease. *Aliment Pharmacol Ther*, 20(6), 607-614 (2004).

[38] Abreu MT, Geller JL, Vasiliauskas EA et al. Treatment with infliximab is associated with increased markers of bone formation in patients with Crohn's disease. *J Clin Gastroenterol*, 40(1), 55-63 (2006).

[39] Bernstein CN, Leslie WD. The pathophysiology of bone disease in gastrointestinal disease. *European journal of gastroenterology & hepatology*, 15(8), 857-864 (2003).

[40] Hessov I, Mosekilde L, Melsen F et al. Osteopenia with normal vitamin D metabolites after small-bowel resection for Crohn's disease. *Scandinavian journal of gastroenterology*, 19(5), 691-696 (1984).

[41] Croucher PI, Vedi S, Motley RJ, Garrahan NJ, Stanton MR, Compston JE. Reduced bone formation in patients with osteoporosis associated with inflammatory bowel disease. *Osteoporosis international : a journal established as result of cooperation between the European Foundation for Osteoporosis and the National Osteoporosis Foundation of the USA*, 3(5), 236-241 (1993).

[42] Ishige T. Growth failure in pediatric onset inflammatory bowel disease: mechanisms, epidemiology, and management. *Transl Pediatr*, 8(1), 16-22 (2019).

[43] Heuschkel R, Salvestrini C, Beattie RM, Hildebrand H, Walters T, Griffiths A. Guidelines for the management of growth failure in childhood inflammatory bowel disease. *Inflamm Bowel Dis*, 14(6), 839-849 (2008).

[44] Hildebrand H, Karlberg J, Kristiansson B. Longitudinal growth in children and adolescents with inflammatory bowel disease. *J Pediatr Gastroenterol Nutr*, 18(2), 165-173 (1994).

[45] Levine A, Griffiths A, Markowitz J et al. Pediatric modification of the Montreal classification for inflammatory bowel disease: the Paris classification. *Inflamm Bowel Dis*, 17(6), 1314-1321 (2011).

[46] Ampuero J, Rojas-Feria M, Castro-Fernandez M, Cano C, Romero-Gomez M. Predictive factors for erythema nodosum and pyoderma gangrenosum in inflammatory bowel disease. *J Gastroenterol Hepatol*, 29(2), 291-295 (2014).

[47] Weizman A, Huang B, Berel D et al. Clinical, serologic, and genetic factors associated with pyoderma gangrenosum and erythema nodosum in inflammatory bowel disease patients. *Inflamm Bowel Dis*, 20(3), 525-533 (2014).

[48] Pellicer Z, Santiago JM, Rodriguez A, Alonso V, Anton R, Bosca MM. Management of cutaneous disorders related to inflammatory bowel disease. *Annals of gastroenterology : quarterly publication of the Hellenic Society of Gastroenterology*, 25(1), 21-26 (2012).

[49] Requena L, Sanchez Yus E. Erythema nodosum. *Seminars in cutaneous medicine and surgery*, 26(2), 114-125 (2007).

[50] van der Velden JJ, van Marion AM, Kremer B, Straetmans JM, Henquet CJ, Frank J. Erythema nodosum as an early sign of Crohn's disease. *International journal of dermatology*, 46 Suppl 3, 27-29 (2007).

[51] Farhi D, Cosnes J, Zizi N et al. Significance of erythema nodosum and pyoderma gangrenosum in inflammatory bowel diseases: a cohort study of 2402 patients. *Medicine (Baltimore)*, 87(5), 281-293 (2008).

[52] Chowaniec M, Starba A, Wiland P. Erythema nodosum - review of the literature. *Reumatologia*, 54(2), 79-82 (2016).

[53] Schwartz RA, Nervi SJ. Erythema nodosum: a sign of systemic disease. *Am Fam Physician*, 75(5), 695-700 (2007).

[54] Blake T, Manahan M, Rodins K. Erythema nodosum - a review of an uncommon panniculitis. *Dermatol Online J*, 20(4), 22376 (2014).

[55] Acosta KA, Haver MC, Kelly B. Etiology and therapeutic management of erythema nodosum during pregnancy: an update. *Am J Clin Dermatol*, 14(3), 215-222 (2013).

[56] Gregory B, Ho VC. Cutaneous manifestations of gastrointestinal disorders. Part II. *Journal of the American Academy of Dermatology*, 26(3 Pt 2), 371-383 (1992).

[57] Timani S, Mutasim DF. Skin manifestations of inflammatory bowel disease. *Clinics in dermatology*, 26(3), 265-273 (2008).

[58] Agrawal D, Rukkannagari S, Kethu S. Pathogenesis and clinical approach to extraintestinal manifestations of inflammatory bowel disease. *Minerva gastroenterologica e dietologica*, 53(3), 233-248 (2007).

[59] Cohen PR. Neutrophilic dermatoses: a review of current treatment options. *American journal of clinical dermatology*, 10(5), 301-312 (2009).

[60] Van Assche G, Dignass A, Reinisch W et al. The second European evidence-based Consensus on the diagnosis and management of Crohn's disease: Special situations. *Journal of Crohn's & colitis*, 4(1), 63-101 (2010).

[61] Poritz LS, Lebo MA, Bobb AD, Ardell CM, Koltun WA. Management of peristomal pyoderma gangrenosum. *J Am Coll Surg*, 206(2), 311-315 (2008).

[62] Bender-Heine A, Grantham JT, Zaslau S, Jansen R. Metastatic Crohn disease: a review of dermatologic manifestations and treatment. *Cutis*, 99(6), E33-E40 (2017).

[63] Palamaras I, El-Jabbour J, Pietropaolo N et al. Metastatic Crohn's disease: a review. *J Eur Acad Dermatol Venereol*, 22(9), 1033-1043 (2008).

[64] Aberumand B, Howard J, Howard J. Metastatic Crohn's Disease: An Approach to an Uncommon but Important Cutaneous Disorder. *Biomed Res Int*, 2017, 8192150 (2017).

[65] Siroy A, Wasman J. Metastatic Crohn disease: a rare cutaneous entity. *Arch Pathol Lab Med*, 136(3), 329-332 (2012).

[66] Ickrath F, Stoevesandt J, Schulmeyer L, Glatzel C, Goebeler M, Kerstan A. Metastatic Crohn's disease: an underestimated entity. *J Dtsch Dermatol Ges*, 19(7), 973-982 (2021).

[67] Goyal A, Mansel RE, Young HL, Douglas-Jones A. Metastatic cutaneous Crohn's disease of the nipple: report of a case. *Diseases of the colon and rectum*, 49(1), 132-134 (2006).

[68] Veloso FT, Carvalho J, Magro F. Immune-related systemic manifestations of inflammatory bowel disease. A prospective study of 792 patients. *Journal of clinical gastroenterology*, 23(1), 29-34 (1996).

[69] Lankarani KB, Sivandzadeh GR, Hassanpour S. Oral manifestation in inflammatory bowel disease: a review. *World journal of gastroenterology : WJG*, 19(46), 8571-8579 (2013).

[70] Greer RO, Jr., Lindenmuth JE, Juarez T, Khandwala A. A double-blind study of topically applied 5% amlexanox in the treatment of aphthous ulcers. *Journal of oral and maxillofacial surgery : official journal of the American Association of Oral and Maxillofacial Surgeons*, 51(3), 243-248; discussion 248-249 (1993).

[71] Rodriguez M, Rubio JA, Sanchez R. Effectiveness of two oral pastes for the treatment of recurrent aphthous stomatitis. *Oral diseases*, 13(5), 490-494 (2007).

[72] Cohen PR. Sweet's syndrome--a comprehensive review of an acute febrile neutrophilic dermatosis. *Orphanet journal of rare diseases*, 2, 34 (2007).

[73] Maalouf D, Battistella M, Bouaziz JD. Neutrophilic dermatosis: disease mechanism and treatment. *Current opinion in hematology*, 22(1), 23-29 (2015).

[74] Stoevesandt J, Keita DU, Goebeler M. Disease-related burden and long-term outcome in orofacial granulomatosis: observations from a large single-centre cohort. *Clin Exp Dermatol*, 47(6), 1169-1173 (2022).

[75] Gavioli CFB, Florezi GP, Dabronzo MLD, Jimenez MR, Nico MMS, Lourenco SV. Orofacial Granulomatosis and Crohn Disease: Coincidence or Pattern? A Systematic Review. *Dermatology*, 237(4), 635-640 (2021).

[76] Bogenrieder T, Rogler G, Vogt T, Landthaler M, Stolz W. Orofacial granulomatosis as the initial presentation of Crohn's disease in an adolescent. *Dermatology*, 206(3), 273-278 (2003).

[77] Haaramo A, Kolho KL, Pitkaranta A, Kanerva M. A 30-year follow-up study of patients with Melkersson-Rosenthal syndrome shows an association to inflammatory bowel disease. *Annals of medicine*, 51(2), 149-155 (2019).

[78] Zbar AP, Ben-Horin S, Beer-Gabel M, Eliakim R. Oral Crohn's disease: is it a separable disease from orofacial granulomatosis? A review. *Journal of Crohn's & colitis*, 6(2), 135-142 (2012).

[79] Phillips F, Verstockt B, Sladek M et al. Orofacial Granulomatosis Associated with Crohn's Disease: a Multicentre Case Series. *Journal of Crohn's & colitis*, 16(3), 430-435 (2022).

[80] Shah J, Shah A, Hassman L, Gutierrez A. Ocular Manifestations of Inflammatory Bowel Disease. *Inflammatory bowel diseases*, 27(11), 1832-1838 (2021).

[81] Harbord M, Annese V, Vavricka SR et al. The First European Evidence-based Consensus on Extra-intestinal Manifestations in Inflammatory Bowel Disease. *Journal of Crohn's & colitis*, 10(3), 239-254 (2016).

[82] Isene R, Bernklev T, Hoie O et al. Extraintestinal manifestations in Crohn's disease and ulcerative colitis: results from a prospective, population-based European inception cohort. *Scandinavian journal of gastroenterology*, 50(3), 300-305 (2015).

[83] Mintz R, Feller ER, Bahr RL, Shah SA. Ocular manifestations of inflammatory bowel disease. *Inflammatory bowel diseases*, 10(2), 135-139 (2004).

[84] Troncoso LL, Biancardi AL, de Moraes HV, Jr., Zaltman C. Ophthalmic manifestations in patients with inflammatory bowel disease: A review. *World journal of gastroenterology : WJG*, 23(32), 5836-5848 (2017).

[85] Mady R, Grover W, Butrus S. Ocular complications of inflammatory bowel disease. *ScientificWorldJournal*, 2015, 438402 (2015).

[86] Sainz de la Maza M, Molina N, Gonzalez-Gonzalez LA, Doctor PP, Tauber J, Foster CS. Clinical characteristics of a large cohort of patients with scleritis and episcleritis. *Ophthalmology*, 119(1), 43-50 (2012).

[87] Rossi RE, Conte D, Massironi S. Primary sclerosing cholangitis associated with inflammatory bowel disease: an update. *European journal of gastroenterology & hepatology*, 28(2), 123-131 (2016).

[88] Gizard E, Ford AC, Bronowicki JP, Peyrin-Biroulet L. Systematic review: The epidemiology of the hepatobiliary manifestations in patients with inflammatory bowel disease. *Alimentary pharmacology & therapeutics*, 40(1), 3-15 (2014).

[89] Mertz A, Nguyen NA, Katsanos KH, Kwok RM. Primary sclerosing cholangitis and inflammatory bowel disease comorbidity: an update of the evidence. *Annals of gastroenterology : quarterly publication of the Hellenic Society of Gastroenterology*, 32(2), 124-133 (2019).

[90] de Vries AB, Janse M, Blokzijl H, Weersma RK. Distinctive inflammatory bowel disease phenotype in primary sclerosing cholangitis. *World journal of gastroenterology : WJG*, 21(6), 1956-1971 (2015).

[91] Rasmussen HH, Fallingborg JF, Mortensen PB, Vyberg M, Tage-Jensen U, Rasmussen SN. Hepatobiliary dysfunction and primary sclerosing cholangitis in patients with Crohn's disease. *Scandinavian journal of gastroenterology*, 32(6), 604-610 (1997).

[92] Pardi DS, Loftus EV, Jr., Kremers WK, Keach J, Lindor KD. Ursodeoxycholic acid as a chemopreventive agent in patients with ulcerative colitis and primary sclerosing cholangitis. *Gastroenterology*, 124(4), 889-893 (2003).

[93] Christensen B, Micic D, Gibson PR et al. Vedolizumab in patients with concurrent primary sclerosing cholangitis and inflammatory bowel disease does not improve liver biochemistry but is safe and effective for the bowel disease. *Alimentary pharmacology & therapeutics*, 47(6), 753-762 (2018).

[94] Lindor KD, Kowdley KV, Harrison ME, American College of G. ACG Clinical Guideline: Primary Sclerosing Cholangitis. *Am J Gastroenterol*, 110(5), 646-659; quiz 660 (2015).

[95] European Association for the Study of the L. EASL Clinical Practice Guidelines: management of cholestatic liver diseases. *J Hepatol*, 51(2), 237-267 (2009).

[96] Antonini F, Pezzilli R, Angelelli L, Macarri G. Pancreatic disorders in inflammatory bowel disease. *World J Gastrointest Pathophysiol*, 7(3), 276-282 (2016).

[97] Weber P, Seibold F, Jenss H. Acute pancreatitis in Crohn's disease. *Journal of clinical gastroenterology*, 17(4), 286-291 (1993).

[98] Barthet M, Hastier P, Bernard JP et al. Chronic pancreatitis and inflammatory bowel disease: true or coincidental association? *The American journal of gastroenterology*, 94(8), 2141-2148 (1999).

[99] Joossens S, Vermeire S, Van Steen K et al. Pancreatic autoantibodies in inflammatory bowel disease. *Inflammatory bowel diseases*, 10(6), 771-777 (2004).

[100] Gaspar R, Branco CC, Macedo G. Liver manifestations and complications in inflammatory bowel disease: A review. *World J Hepatol*, 13(12), 1956-1967 (2021).

[101] European Association for the Study of the L. EASL Clinical Practice Guidelines: Autoimmune hepatitis. *J Hepatol*, 63(4), 971-1004 (2015).

[102] Saubermann LJ, Deneau M, Falcone RA et al. Hepatic Issues and Complications Associated With Inflammatory Bowel Disease: A Clinical Report From the NASPGHAN Inflammatory Bowel Disease and Hepatology Committees. *J Pediatr Gastroenterol Nutr*, 64(4), 639-652 (2017).

[103] DeFilippis EM, Kumar S. Clinical Presentation and Outcomes of Autoimmune Hepatitis in Inflammatory Bowel Disease. *Dig Dis Sci*, 60(10), 2873-2880 (2015).

[104] Reddy KR, Beavers KL, Hammond SP, Lim JK, Falck-Ytter YT, American Gastroenterological Association I. American Gastroenterological Association Institute guideline on the prevention and treatment of hepatitis B virus reactivation during immunosuppressive drug therapy. *Gastroenterology*, 148(1), 215-219; quiz e216-217 (2015).

[105] Dehghani T, Gholizadeh O, Daneshvar M et al. Association Between Inflammatory Bowel Disease and Viral Infections. *Curr Microbiol*, 80(6), 195 (2023).

[106] Sinh P, Cross RK. Cardiovascular Comorbidities and Inflammatory Bowel Disease: Causes and Consequences. *Gastroenterol Hepatol (N Y)*, 20(4), 204-215 (2024).

[107] Murthy SK, Robertson McCurdy AB, Carrier M, McCurdy JD. Venous thromboembolic events in inflammatory bowel diseases: A review of current evidence and guidance on risk in the post-hospitalization setting. *Thromb Res*, 194, 26-32 (2020).

[108] Biondi RB, Salmazo PS, Bazan SGZ, Hueb JC, de Paiva SAR, Sassaki LY. Cardiovascular Risk in Individuals with Inflammatory Bowel Disease. *Clin Exp Gastroenterol*, 13, 107-113 (2020).

[109] Chen B, Collen LV, Mowat C et al. Inflammatory Bowel Disease and Cardiovascular Diseases. *The American Journal of Medicine*, 135(12), 1453-1460 (2022).

[110] Cainzos-Achirica M, Glassner K, Zawahir HS et al. Inflammatory Bowel Disease and Atherosclerotic Cardiovascular Disease: JACC Review Topic of the Week. *J Am Coll Cardiol*, 76(24), 2895-2905 (2020).

[111] Bernstein CN, Blanchard JF, Houston DS, Wajda A. The incidence of deep venous thrombosis and pulmonary embolism among patients with inflammatory bowel disease: a population-based cohort study. *Thrombosis and haemostasis*, 85(3), 430-434 (2001).

[112] Yuhara H, Steinmaus C, Corley D et al. Meta-analysis: the risk of venous thromboembolism in patients with inflammatory bowel disease. *Alimentary pharmacology & therapeutics*, 37(10), 953-962 (2013).

[113] Nguyen GC, Sam J. Rising prevalence of venous thromboembolism and its impact on mortality among hospitalized inflammatory bowel disease patients. *The American journal of gastroenterology*, 103(9), 2272-2280 (2008).

[114] Sinagra E, Aragona E, Romano C et al. The role of portal vein thrombosis in the clinical course of inflammatory bowel diseases: report on three cases and review of the literature. *Gastroenterol Res Pract*, 2012, 916428 (2012).

[115] Maconi G, Bolzacchini E, Dell'Era A, Russo U, Ardizzone S, de Franchis R. Portal vein thrombosis in inflammatory bowel diseases: a single-center case series. *Journal of Crohn's & colitis*, 6(3), 362-367 (2012).

[116] Naymagon L, Tremblay D, Zubizarreta N et al. The Natural History, Treatments, and Outcomes of Portal Vein Thrombosis in Patients With Inflammatory Bowel Disease. *Inflammatory bowel diseases*, 27(2), 215-223 (2021).

[117] Elkrief L, Hernandez-Gea V, Senzolo M et al. Portal vein thrombosis: diagnosis, management, and endpoints for future clinical studies. *Lancet Gastroenterol Hepatol*, 9(9), 859-883 (2024).

[118] Mansour M, Doumet G, Kadan A et al. Early diagnosis and treatment of perianal Crohn's disease in a 1-year-old infant: Case report and review of literature. *Clin Case Rep*, 12(6), e8963 (2024).

[119] Singh B, Mc CMNJ, Jewell DP, George B. Perianal Crohn's disease. *Br J Surg*, 91(7), 801-814 (2004).

[120] Spinelli A, Yanai H, Girardi P et al. The Impact of Crohn's Perianal Fistula on Quality of Life: Results of an International Patient Survey. *Crohns Colitis 360*, 5(3), otad036 (2023).

[121] Pogacnik JS, Salgado G. Perianal Crohn's Disease. *Clin Colon Rectal Surg*, 32(5), 377-385 (2019).

[122] Bonheur JL, Braunstein J, Korelitz BI, Panagopoulos G. Anal skin tags in inflammatory bowel disease: new observations and a clinical review. *Inflammatory bowel diseases*, 14(9), 1236-1239 (2008).

[123] Safar B, Sands D. Perianal Crohn's disease. *Clin Colon Rectal Surg*, 20(4), 282-293 (2007).

[124] Schwartz DA, Ghazi LJ, Regueiro M et al. Guidelines for the multidisciplinary management of Crohn's perianal fistulas: summary statement. *Inflammatory bowel diseases*, 21(4), 723-730 (2015).

[125] Sato S, Sasaki I, Naito H et al. Management of urinary complications in Crohn's disease. *Surgery today*, 29(8), 713-717 (1999).

[126] Pardi DS, Tremaine WJ, Sandborn WJ, McCarthy JT. Renal and urologic complications of inflammatory bowel disease. *The American journal of gastroenterology*, 93(4), 504-514 (1998).

[127] Pak CY, Sakhaee K, Fuller C. Successful management of uric acid nephrolithiasis with potassium citrate. *Kidney international*, 30(3), 422-428 (1986).

[128] Kazi AM, Hashmi MF. Glomerulonephritis. In: *StatPearls.* (Treasure Island (FL), 2024)

[129] Corica D, Romano C. Renal Involvement in Inflammatory Bowel Diseases. *Journal of Crohn's & colitis*, 10(2), 226-235 (2016).

[130] Ambruzs JM, Walker PD, Larsen CP. The histopathologic spectrum of kidney biopsies in patients with inflammatory bowel disease. *Clin J Am Soc Nephrol*, 9(2), 265-270 (2014).

[131] Kiryluk K, Li Y, Scolari F et al. Discovery of new risk loci for IgA nephropathy implicates genes involved in immunity against intestinal pathogens. *Nat Genet*, 46(11), 1187-1196 (2014).

[132] Wang J, Anders RA, Wu Q et al. Dysregulated LIGHT expression on T cells mediates intestinal inflammation and contributes to IgA nephropathy. *J Clin Invest*, 113(6), 826-835 (2004).

[133] Forshaw MJ, Guirguis O, Hennigan TW. IgA nephropathy in association with Crohn's disease. *Int J Colorectal Dis*, 20(5), 463-465 (2005).

[134] Ben-Ami H, Ginesin Y, Behar DM, Fischer D, Edoute Y, Lavy A. Diagnosis and treatment of urinary tract complications in Crohn's disease: an experience over 15 years. *Can J Gastroenterol*, 16(4), 225-229 (2002).

[135] Jansen R, Zaslau S. Hydronephrosis and Ureteral Obstruction in Crohn's Disease. *Open Journal of Urology*, 3(5), 219-221 (2013).

[136] Angelberger S, Fink KG, Schima W et al. Complications in Crohn's disease: right-sided ureteric stenosis and hydronephrosis. *Inflammatory bowel diseases*, 13(8), 1056-1057 (2007).

[137] Vagianos C, Malgarinos G, Spyropoulos C, Triantafillidis JK. Entero-vesical fistulas in CROHN'S disease: A case series report and review of the literature. *Int J Surg Case Rep*, 41, 477-480 (2017).

[138] Wade G, Zaslau S, Jansen R. A review of urinary fistulae in Crohn's disease. *Can J Urol*, 21(2), 7179-7184 (2014).

[139] Hsu MW, Chen WC, Wei TN, Huang CP. Management of Enterovesical Fistula in a Patient with Crohn's Disease: A Case Report and Literature Review. *Diagnostics (Basel)*, 13(9) (2023).

[140] Levy C, Tremaine WJ. Management of internal fistulas in Crohn's disease. *Inflammatory bowel diseases*, 8(2), 106-111 (2002).

[141] Manganiotis AN, Banner MP, Malkowicz SB. Urologic complications of Crohn's disease. *Surg Clin North Am*, 81(1), 197-215, x (2001).

[142] Gruner JS, Sehon JK, Johnson LW. Diagnosis and management of enterovesical fistulas in patients with Crohn's disease. *Am Surg*, 68(8), 714-719 (2002).

[143] Zhu YF, Tao GQ, Zhou N, Xiang C. Current treatment of rectovaginal fistula in Crohn's disease. *World journal of gastroenterology : WJG*, 17(8), 963-967 (2011).

[144] Casadesus D, Villasana L, Sanchez IM, Diaz H, Chavez M, Diaz A. Treatment of rectovaginal fistula: a 5-year review. *Aust N Z J Obstet Gynaecol*, 46(1), 49-51 (2006).

[145] Willis S, Rau M, Schumpelick V. Chirurgische Therapie hoher anorectaler und rectovaginaler Fisteln mittels transanaler endorectaler Verschiebelappenplastik. *Der Chirurg*, 71(7), 836-840 (2000).

[146] Li Destri G, Scilletta B, Tomaselli TG, Zarbo G. Rectovaginal fistula: a new approach by stapled transanal rectal resection. *J Gastrointest Surg*, 12(3), 601-603 (2008).

[147] Ji XQ, Wang LX, Lu DG. Pulmonary manifestations of inflammatory bowel disease. *World journal of gastroenterology : WJG*, 20(37), 13501-13511 (2014).

[148] Rothfuss KS, Stange EF, Herrlinger KR. Extraintestinal manifestations and complications in inflammatory bowel diseases. *World journal of gastroenterology : WJG*, 12(30), 4819-4831 (2006).

[149] Songur N, Songur Y, Tuzun M et al. Pulmonary function tests and high-resolution CT in the detection of pulmonary involvement in inflammatory bowel disease. *Journal of clinical gastroenterology*, 37(4), 292-298 (2003).

[150] Raj AA, Birring SS, Green R, Grant A, de Caestecker J, Pavord ID. Prevalence of inflammatory bowel disease in patients with airways disease. *Respir Med*, 102(5), 780-785 (2008).

[151] Vasishta S, Wood JB, McGinty F. Ulcerative tracheobronchitis years after colectomy for ulcerative colitis. *Chest*, 106(4), 1279-1281 (1994).

[152] Spira A, Grossman R, Balter M. Large airway disease associated with inflammatory bowel disease. *Chest*, 113(6), 1723-1726 (1998).

[153] Zeitz J, Ak M, Muller-Mottet S et al. Pain in IBD Patients: Very Frequent and Frequently Insufficiently Taken into Account. *PLoS One*, 11(6), e0156666 (2016).

[154] Borren NZ, van der Woude CJ, Ananthakrishnan AN. Fatigue in IBD: epidemiology, pathophysiology and management. *Nat Rev Gastroenterol Hepatol*, 16(4), 247-259 (2019).

[155] Canakis A, Qazi T. Sleep and Fatigue in IBD: an Unrecognized but Important Extra-intestinal Manifestation. *Current gastroenterology reports*, 22(2), 8 (2020).

[156] Grygiel-Gorniak B, Puszczewicz M. Fatigue and interleukin-6 - a multi-faceted relationship. *Reumatologia*, 53(4), 207-212 (2015).

[157] Szigethy E, Craig AE, Iobst EA et al. Profile of depression in adolescents with inflammatory bowel disease: implications for treatment. *Inflammatory bowel diseases*, 15(1), 69-74 (2009).

[158] McGing JJ, Radford SJ, Francis ST, Serres S, Greenhaff PL, Moran GW. Review article: The aetiology of fatigue in inflammatory bowel disease and potential therapeutic management strategies. *Alimentary pharmacology & therapeutics*, 54(4), 368-387 (2021).

[159] Schirbel A, Reichert A, Roll S et al. Impact of pain on health-related quality of life in patients with inflammatory bowel disease. *World journal of gastroenterology : WJG*, 16(25), 3168-3177 (2010).

Section II. Surgery

Chapter 7

Preoperative Optimization

John J. Kessler II[1], MD
and Hugo Bonatti[2,*], MD
[1]University of Maryland Medical Center, Baltimore, Maryland, USA
[2]University of Maryland School of Medicine, Baltimore, Maryland, USA

Abstract

Patients with Crohn's disease (CD) are known to have high rates of post-surgical complications. These complications have been linked to various preoperative conditions common in this patient population. Clinicians must take steps preoperatively to decrease the rate of complications and improve patient outcomes. The goal of preoperative patient optimization is to identify and correct specific factors known to increase adverse outcomes. Some of the critical aspects to the preoperative tune-up are corticosteroid use, nutrition, current smoking, cross sectional imaging, infection, and venous thromboembolism. To decrease postoperative complications, corticosteroids should ideally be weaned six weeks prior to surgery. Caloric and micronutrient deficiency should be identified and treated. Nutritional optimization can be done through a combination of surgical delay (if possible), enteral nutrition, parenteral nutrition, and micronutrient supplementation. Smoking cessation for eight weeks prior to surgery is ideal, however, any reduction in smoking decreases adverse outcomes. Cross sectional imaging is required for surgical planning and identification of abdominal and pelvic infections. Preoperative treatment of abdominal and pelvic abscesses with antibiotics and percutaneous drainage improves postoperative outcomes. Lastly, patients with CD are more likely to develop deep vein thromboses, therefore venous thromboembolism prophylaxis may be indicated while hospitalized.

Introduction

Surgical management of Crohn's disease (CD) has remained an important part of a multidisciplinary approach to a patient's treatment. Between 50-85% of patients will undergo abdominal surgery for their Crohn's disease and over half of those receiving one operation will undergo reoperation [1, 2]. Patients with CD are at an increased risk of postoperative complications compared to the general population due to the nature of their disease and treatment course [3]. The rates of postoperative complications after surgery for CD is more than double the complication rate in the general population [4, 5]. The goal of patient optimization

* Corresponding Author's Email: hbonatti@som.umaryland.edu

In: Surgery for Crohn's Disease. Second Edition
Editors: Stephen M. Kavic, Rebecca Brown and Kerri Lopez
ISBN: 979-8-89530-676-5

is to modify specific risk factors for postoperative complications including surgical site infection (SSI), anastomotic, leak, intraabdominal sepsis, and reoperation. During the preoperative phase, surgeons should evaluate patients for these known risk factors and take action to improve patient outcomes through steroid management, nutritional optimization, smoking cessation, preoperative treatment of infection, and prophylaxis for venous thromboembolism.

Corticosteroids

Corticosteroids are frequently used in the medical management of active CD, and as a result, a substantial portion of patients will have exposure to corticosteroids [6]. There is some disagreement regarding corticosteroid use resulting in increased postoperative complications. Brewer found no association between corticosteroid exposure and infectious complications [7]. Other studies have demonstrated a distinct dose dependent relationship between preoperative steroid use and rates of postoperative complications. At doses of prednisone <10mg/day there was no increased risk of SSI, while doses >10mg/day increased the risk of SSI [8]. At higher doses of prednisone, >20mg/day prednisone equivalent for at least six weeks, the rates of all surgical complications were increased including superficial SSI, deep SSI, anastomotic leak, and delayed wound healing [9, 10]. Lastly, at doses of prednisone >40 mg/day, the rates of both surgical and non-surgical complications were increased [11].

Because of the increased risk of complication, the European Crohn's and Colitis Organization (ECCO) recommends tapering off steroids at least six weeks prior to elective surgery for CD [12]. In cases where completely stopping steroids is not feasible, a reduction to <20mg/day prednisone is recommended. In the setting of emergency surgery where time for steroid taper is not possible, a postoperative steroid taper decreases the rates of surgical complications [13]. Additionally, if high dose steroids are unable to be weaned, due to either the need for emergency surgery or inability to tolerate cessation, surgeons should consider staged surgery, as temporary stoma creation for fecal diversion decreases the risk of anastomotic leak in this patient population [14, 15].

Another consideration of high dose steroid exposure during the perioperative period is adrenal insufficiency due to corticosteroid suppression of the hypothalamus/pituitary axis [16]. CD patients treated with either high dose stress steroids, low dose stress steroids, or no stress dosing have shown no difference in hemodynamic stability postoperatively if they had been completely weaned off steroids prior to surgery [17, 18]. As a result, perioperative steroid stress dose is not recommended in patients weaned from steroids [18]. Additionally, CD patients are on maintenance corticosteroids that could not be weaned further, should be kept on their maintenance dose in leu of stress dosing [19].

Biologic Therapy

Biologic agents, also known as disease modifiers, are monoclonal antibodies including anti-tumor necrosis factor alfa (anti-TNF) agents, vedolizumab (VDZ), and Ustekinumab (UST). These drugs have shown remarkable success in inducing remission for patients with moderate to severe CD, however, their effect on the immune system has raised concern for post operative complications [6, 15].

Data on the anti-TNF agents, infliximab, adalimumab, certolizumab pegol, and natalizumab are conflicting. Several meta-analyses have shown preoperative exposure to anti-TNF therapy increases the rates of overall complications including SSI, anastomotic leak, and reoperation [20-24]. Other larger meta-analyses have shown no such findings, with no increase in rates of any postoperative complication [25, 26]. One study also demonstrated no difference in postoperative complications when comparing 4-, 8-, and 12-week anti-TNF dosing to surgery intervals [27]. Additionally, the use of serum levels of anti-TNF agents, nor time from last dose influenced the rates of SSI or anastomotic complications [28]. Current ECCO guidelines do not recommend termination of anti-TNF agents prior to elective surgery in patients with CD; and recommend against delay of surgery due to recent anti-TNF agent exposure [15].

VDZ is a monoclonal antibody that targets integrin, selectively inhibiting leukocyte migration into the gastrointestinal tract [29]. Similarly to anti-TNF agents, there are also conflicting results regarding preoperative VDZ exposure and surgical complications. Two studies have shown increased SSI, readmission, and reoperation rates in those exposed to VDZ compared to patients exposed to anti-TNF and biologic therapy naive patients [30, 31]. Conversely, other meta-analyses have shown no increase in postoperative complications when comparing patients exposed to VDZ, patients exposed to anti-TNF, and biologic therapy naive patients [23, 32, 33]. VDZ is considered safe in the surgical setting and current ECCO guidelines do not require the termination of VDZ agents prior to elective surgery in patients with CD, or a delay of surgery due to recent VDZ exposure [15].

UST, the newest FDA approved monoclonal antibody used in the management of CD, inhibits interleukin 12/23 p40 [29]. Fewer patients have been exposed to UST compared to older biologic agents. Several studies have shown no difference in postoperative complications including SSI, anastomotic leak, and intraabdominal sepsis when comparing patients exposed to UST or anti-TNF agents [34-36]. Conversely, one single centered series showed high rates of intraabdominal sepsis in patients exposed to UST compared to patients free of biologic therapy for at least 12 weeks prior to major abdominal surgery [37]. Because the overall rates of postoperative complications in patients on UST therapy are similar to rates of postoperative complications in patients on anti-TNF therapy, the use of UST is safe in the perioperative setting [36].

When evaluating the use of biologic agents, ECCO guidelines state preoperative anti-TNF therapy, VDZ, and UST do not increase the risk of postoperative complications in CD patients undergoing major abdominal surgery [15]. Even though these guidelines do not advocate for delay of surgery due to recent biologic agent therapy, the contradicting data regarding biologic agent therapy and possibly increased rates of postoperative complications has caused some institutions to adjust the timing of elective surgery to allow for a longer preoperative drug free interval [29]. Patel advocates for the scheduling of elective surgery at the halfway point between biologic agent dosses. This timing maximizes both preoperative washout and postoperative healing before the next dose [14].

Other Immunomodulators

Purine analogues or thiopurines (i.e., azathioprine and 6-mercaptopurine) are frequently used in addition to other agents to reduce steroid doses and the need for surgical intervention [38]. Multiple studies have shown preoperative use of purine analogues does not increase the rates of surgical complication including infections [9, 39, 40]. Current ECCO guidelines indicate thiopurines can be continued perioperatively [12]. The recommendation is to hold thiopurines on the day of surgery and resume as early as post op day 1 when oral medications are resumed [41].

Methotrexate (MTX) is also used in Crohn's disease to reduce corticosteroids and induce and maintain remission [42]. Most studies concerning MTX in the perioperative setting have observed patients with rheumatoid arthritis undergoing orthopedic procedures. These studies have shown preoperative MTX use does not increase postoperative complications including would healing and infectious complications [43-45]. One small study of fifteen patients with irritable bowel disease (14 with CD) who continued MTX in the preoperative period, showed no increase in early postoperative complications after major abdominal surgery [46]. There are no official guidelines regarding MTX use in the preoperative setting for CD available; however, published data show perioperative methotrexate may not increase adverse effects and could be continued until the day of surgery [47].

Nutrition

Malnutrition is an independent risk factor for postoperative complications. Approximately 70% of CD patients meet the clinical criteria for malnutrition [48]. The prevalence of malnutrition increases to 80% of patients with active disease, while 40% of patients in remission meet criteria [49]. There are several factors inherent to the disease process of CD that increase the rates of caloric and micronutrient malnutrition including decreased nutrient intake, decreased absorption, and increased nutritional requirements. Decreased intake is due to the symptoms of CD including bowel obstruction, abdominal pain, bloating, and drug side effects. Decreased nutrient absorption of the intestines is attributed to inflammation, drug nutrient interactions, changes to gut flora, decreased area of absorption post resection, and nutrient loss in diarrhea [50-52]. Lastly, the hyper metabolic state observed in systemic inflammation increases the nutritional requirements [51].

Postoperative complications associated with preoperative malnutrition in patients with CD, include abscess formation, anastomotic leak, intraabdominal sepsis, SSI (superficial, deep, and organ space), delayed wound healing, and wound dehiscence [25, 53-55]. To reduce the rates of these complications, appropriate evaluation and treatment of malnutrition must occur in the preoperative setting.

All CD patients should undergo evaluation for malnutrition preoperatively. The European Society for Clinical Nutrition and Metabolism (ESPEN) states severe malnutrition is present if at least one of the following criteria is met [56].

1) Weight loss of >10-15% within the last six months
2) BMI <18.5 kg/m^2

3) Nutritional Risk Screening (NRS-2002) >5
4) Serum Albumin <30g/L (with no evidence of Hepatic or renal dysfunction)

Of note, albumin is a negative acute phase reactant and more closely represents disease severity rather than nutritional status [57]. However, its strong association with postoperative complications and nutritional supplementation directly corrects hypoalbuminemia, serum albumin is an effective tool in the evaluation of malnutrition. During the history and physical, in addition to BMI calculation and blood work, the patient should be asked about any weight loss in the last six months and complete the NRS-2002. Meeting ESPEN criteria for malnutrition has been associated with increased risk of postoperative complications, of which SSIs are most likely [56]. In patients meeting the criteria for malnutrition, initiation of nutritional optimization should occur in the preoperative phase for improved surgical outcomes [58].

Preoperative interventions for malnutrition include both supplemental nutrition and delay of operation. The benefit of correction of malnutrition includes deceased rates of both infectious and noninfectious surgical complications as well as non-surgical complications [59-61]. ESPEN guidelines suggest delay of surgery for 7-14 days to allow for correction of malnutrition [56]. In cases of severe disease, longer periods of nutrition lasting 3-6 months can correlate with decreased risks of complications [62]. There are no definitive guidelines for length of nutritional optimization or endpoint goals, but some institutions have used serum albumin >30g/L as the marker for successful improvement of nutritional status and have shown decreased rates of complications when achieved [14].

When initiating supplemental nutrition, the aim is for patients to meet 100% of their caloric need and consume 1.2-1.5 g/kg total body weight of protein [58]. In CD patients especially those in active disease, caloric expenditure of Calories/kg body weight can be up to 24% higher compared to the general population [63]. Enteral nutrition (EN) is preferred over parenteral nutrition (PN) but there is disagreement over natural nutrition with oral nutritional supplements (ONS) verses starting enteral nutrition via nasogastric or nasojejunal (NJ) feeding tube when malnutrition has been identified. Patel has seen decreased rates of complications when initiating EN as a first step in nutritional optimization over natural nutrition with ONS [14]. The average increase from ONS is about 600 kcal/day, therefore clinical judgement should be used to evaluate if a patient is likely to succeed with ONS alone or EN should be initiated [63]. If a patient has been unable to meet caloric need with ONS alone, EN should be added via NG or NJ tube [56]. When selecting a formula for EN, ideal formulas are low in long-chain triglycerides, low in monounsaturated fatty acids, high in medium- chain triglycerides and high omega-6 to omega-3 ratios [64].

When a patient has no oral intake and EN is used for 100% of nutritional requirements, it is classified as exclusive enteral nutrition (EEN). EEN has shown multiple benefits in the preoperative phase of CD management. Multiple studies have shown decreased markers of inflammation and proinflammatory cytokines after EEN [65-67]. Heerasing et. al. demonstrated EEN to be as effective as steroids in inducing remission [68]. EEN has been shown to promote mucosal healing [69]. There are also decreased rates of sepsis and postoperative infections, and recurrence in patients receiving EEN [66, 70]. Lastly, EEN has been shown to decrease operative times, decrease the length of resected bowel, and decrease the need for surgery. After EEN preoperatively, up to 25% of patients may no longer require the originally planned operation [66, 70]. One downside to EEN is poor patient compliance [68].

Parenteral nutrition is added to a patient's nutritional regimen when EN fails to provide adequate nutrition. ESPEN guidelines indicate adding PN with a patients EN meets <60% of their caloric need [56]. Total parenteral nutrition (TPN) is only utilized when EN is contraindicated [58]. Contraindications for EN include bowel obstruction, high output enterocutaneous fistula, short remaining bowel after prior resection [52, 69].

A poorly studied issue is best management of obese/morbidly obese CD patients. It should be considered that even if CD patients have a high BMI, they still may be protein depleted. Nevertheless, due to the well-known negative effects of obesity in surgical patients, weight management preoperatively seems beneficial even if good study data are not available. The best approach seems dietary counseling with reduction of intake of fat and carbohydrates and an increase in protein intake. Ideally, a body mass index <30kg/m2 should be achieved and this may delay surgery significantly. This is feasible in stable patients but one should consider patient compliance and the discomfort during the wait time as well as the development of an acute bout of the disease.

Micronutrients are an often-overlooked portion of the preoperative evaluation CD patients. Over 60% of patients present with a deficiency in at least one micronutrient [71]. The micronutrients most commonly deficient in this patient population are iron, B12, folate, vitamin D, vitamin A, vitamin K, vitamin C, selenium, zinc, B6, and B1. Like caloric deficiency, the rates of micronutrient deficiencies increase in states of active disease [71, 72]. These deficiencies are relevant in the preoperative phase because many have been linked to increased rates of surgical complications. Although no clear guidelines exist, testing levels of various Vitamins, zinc and selenium may be advisable. If patients are deficient, supplementation should be started prior to surgery.

Anemia is present in over 50% of CD patients in active disease and iron deficiency anemia is the most common cause of anemia in CD [72, 73]. Preoperative iron deficiency is known to increase rates of post operative complications [73]. There have been mixed results from preoperative iron supplementation studies. Some studies of CD patients have shown decreased rates of post operative blood transfusion and decreased rates of adverse surgical outcomes while other studies have shown no difference between those receiving iron supplementation preoperatively and those given placebo [72, 74, 75]. International consensus conference on Anema Management in Surgical patients recommends iron supplementation preoperatively with oral or intravenous iron in patients with iron deficiency anemia [75]. Vitamin D deficiency also increased rates of surgical complications including infection and poor wound healing [76]. Deficiencies in zinc, vitamin A, and vitamin C also increase rates of poor wound healing, while deficiencies in folate, B6, and B12 increase rates of venous thrombosis [74]. There is minimal data regarding individual micronutrient supplementation effects on surgical outcomes for Crohn's patients and there are no definitive guidelines for preoperative micronutrient supplementation.

Cannabis

Cannabis has been used as an additional resource in the management of multiple chronic illnesses. Approximately 20% of CD patients actively use cannabis for treatment of their disease [77]. Even with this rate of use, cannabis in CD remains controversial, however, cannabinoids have been shown to cause some symptomatic relief. Patients have experienced increased appetite and decreased rates of GI symptoms including pain, nausea, and vomiting, but cannabis did not alter rates or remission or need for surgery [78]. In one study cannabis has been shown to increase appetite but no weight gain or increased in nutritional status was achieved [79].

Smoking

Smoking is another well-known risk factor for postoperative complications in patients without CD, but smoking does have additional impacts in this patient population. Because 30-40% of CD patients undergoing surgery are current smokers, preoperative evaluation should include investigating current smoking status [80]. Active smoking increased the likelihood of SSI by over 50% and in CD patients is associated with an increased risk for intraabdominal sepsis as well as overall morbidity [81, 82]. Due to these increased risks, any current smoker should be counseled on smoking cessation and referred to a smoking cessation clinic with the goal of stopping smoking at least 8 weeks preoperatively. The benefits of smoking cessation are significant in this patient population. There is a four-fold reduction in the rate of endoscopic CD recurrence with cessation [83]. Additionally, ex-smokers have the same rates of endoscopic recurrence and disease relapse as nonsmokers [62]. Even if full cessation is not possible there are benefits to smoking reduction. A smoking reduction of >50% for 6-8 weeks prior to surgery resulted in decreased rates of postoperative complications including wound complications, cardiovascular complications, and need for reoperation [84]. Lastly, even abstinence of smoking only day of surgery proves to be beneficial with a reduction of surgical complications [82]. Ideally, smoking is stopped two months prior to elective surgery but if that is not possible any amount of time will improve patient outcomes.

Imaging

Imaging is a critical portion of presurgical evaluation and preoperative optimization of patients with CD [12]. Imaging allows for the identification of the current anatomic locations of disease and the extent of disease activity. Imaging also identifies areas of stricture, fistulae, abscesses, and phlegmon [85]. This information provides the opportunity for not only surgical planning but allows for targeted presurgical interventions that can improve patient outcomes [36]. Areas of active infection can be addressed with pre surgical interventions and delineating areas of fibrosis, which are most successfully treated with surgery, from areas of inflammation, which may require additional medical management, can improve surgical outcomes [14, 86].

The three modes of imaging for the evaluation of Crohn's disease in the preoperative setting are ultrasonography (US), magnetic resonance imaging (MRI), and computed tomography (CT). All three have equivalent overall sensitivity in detection of disease, however, each modality has distinct advantages and disadvantages [87, 88]. The benefits of US include low cost, noninvasive, widespread, and does not expose the patient to radiation. This modality is particularly useful in the identification of superficial fistulas and abscesses. The downsides of US include a decreased accuracy in deep and pelvic spaces. Additionally, US is highly technician-dependent where the skill of the operator can have a great impact on the usefulness of the imaging [89].

MRI and CT are the two most used imaging modalities in the preoperative setting. Compared to US, they have improved sensitivity for deep spaces [87]. MRI is preferred in the elective preoperative setting for two reasons. First, MRI does not expose the patient to any radiation. Many patients with CD are at risk for increased radiation exposure over the course of their disease; therefore, no added radiation is beneficial to patients [14]. Second, MRI has the highest level of sensitivity in detecting and assessing abscesses, fistulas, areas of stenosis, and perforation [85, 90]. The downsides of MRI include higher cost, lesser availability, and takes longer to perform.

CT imaging is the modality of choice in the emergent and acute setting. It is widely available, faster to complete, and more accurate in detecting free perforation, a rare complication of Crohn's disease, in comparison to MRI [91, 92]. The major downside to CT imaging is the added radiation exposure, however, low dose CT has improved the amount of radiation to which patients are exposed [91]. CT- enterography is a specialized modality with improved ability to detect scattered areas of CD involvement within the intestinal tract. In the preoperative setting, clinical judgment should be used in selection of imaging modality. They can be done alone or in combination and factors that should be considered include patient age, radiation exposure history, clinical status, and modality availability.

Colonoscopy is an additional tool for anatomic evaluation in the presurgical setting and is useful for evaluation of the disease severity and extent, specifically in the colon. Biopsies from colonoscopies can be taken which gives essential information on disease activity. It is not required prior to all surgeries for CD but can be useful when employed intentionally. In preparation for a partial colectomy, colonoscopy is used for evaluation of planned anastomotic sites to ensure the target location for both proximal and distal anastomosis are disease free. In patients where the operative plan is limited to the small bowel (i.e., resection and stricturoplasty) a colonoscopy is not necessarily required [14]. It should also be noted that presurgical imaging and colonoscopy are not foolproof. As a result, intraoperatively surgeons should always search for possible additional lesions that could dictate a change to the surgical plan. Between 9-26% of patients have unexpected intraoperative findings leading to deviation from the planned procedure [93, 94]. With this rate of modification, patients should also be made aware of the possibility of modifications to their operation.

Infection

Abscesses and phlegmon occur in 10-30% of patients throughout their disease course and are suggestive of penetrating Crohn's disease [95, 96]. In the event preoperative imaging identifies an abscess, steps can be taken to reduce the morbidity of these infections. Untreated, these preoperative abscesses result in higher rates of surgical and non-surgical complications as well as overall postoperative mortality [9, 97, 98]. Appropriate presurgical intervention and treatment of abdominal and pelvic abscesses can reduce the rates of intraabdominal septic complications, anastomotic leak, and unplanned stoma creation [97, 99, 100]. Additionally, preoperative treatment of these abscesses increased the likelihood of successful laparoscopic surgical intervention and decreased the length of resected bowel, days hospitalized, and costs

[99-101]. Percutaneous drainage and antibiotics as a delay to surgery are not possible in all patients. Those who are unstable may require surgical drainage.

Percutaneous drains (PD) and antibiotics are the non-surgical options to treat abdominal and pelvic abscess. Broad spectrum antibiotics are initiated, and the abscess is evaluated for feasibility of drain placement. PD are placed under visualization using either CT or US and multiple drains are common in patients with multiple abscesses [86]. Abscesses that are well defined and unilocular are more likely to be successfully targeted and treated with PD [102]. Deeper abscesses, particularly pelvic abscesses, are less likely to be accessible for PD placement [100]. Culturing abscess drainage and susceptibility testing dictates narrowing of a patient's antibiotic treatment [99]. In addition, multidrug resistant bacteria can now be identified rapidly through advanced microbiologic testing allowing for early initiation of appropriate directed treatment and isolation measures. After PD placement and antibiotic initiation, clinical improvement is usually seen within 24-72 hours. Drainage is expected to stop within one week of treatment. In the event PD continues to have high output after one week the drain should be assessed for misplacement and fistula formation using CT or MRI [86].

In this setting percutaneous drainage and antibiotics are a temporizing measure that functions as a bridge to surgery. This window of time can allow for optimization of infection as well as the other aspects of preoperative care. The rate of successful drainage is 74-100% and up to 29% may no longer need their originally planned operation [103-104]. Patients are more likely to no longer need surgery if they do not have active luminal inflammation, are free from active perianal disease and fistulization, and are naive to medical management [86, 100, 105, 106]. Due to the chronicity of CD, drains may have to remain in place for a prolonged time.

Venous Thromboembolism

Patients with Crohn's disease are twice as likely to develop deep venous thrombosis (DVT), and venous thromboembolism (VTE)when compared to the general population [107, 108]. This increased risk is attributed to active disease, systemic inflammation, regular steroid exposure, malnutrition, chronic anemia, thrombocytosis, prolonged hospitalization, decreased mobility, and emergency surgery [107-109]. In hospitalized patients prior to surgery VTE prophylaxis is indicated and can reduce the rates of VTE complications [12]. VTE prophylaxis should be given according to the American College of Chest Physicians Evidence-Based Clinical Practice Guidelines [110, 111].

Conclusion

The goal of preoperative patient optimization is to identify and correct specific factors known to increase adverse postoperative outcomes. The most important targets of the preoperative tune-up are corticosteroids, nutrition, current smoking, cross sectional imaging, infection, and VTEs. Corticosteroids should ideally be weaned six weeks prior to surgery. Caloric and micronutrient deficiency should be identified and treated. Nutritional optimization can be done with a combination of surgical delay (if possible), enteral nutrition, parenteral nutrition, and micronutrient supplementation. Smoking cessation for eight weeks prior to surgery is ideal, however, any reduction in smoking decreases adverse outcomes. Cross sectional imaging is required for surgical planning and identification of infections. Preoperative treatment of abdominal and pelvic abscesses with antibiotics and percutaneous drainage improves postoperative outcomes. Lastly, patients with CD are more likely to develop DVTs, therefore VTE prophylaxis may be indicated.

References

[1] Aras, Oguz AZ, Apar S. Patel, Emma K. Satchell, Nicholas J. Serniak, Raphael M. Byrne, and Burt Cagir. 2024. "Comparison of Outcomes in Small Bowel Surgery for Crohn's Disease: A Retrospective NSQIP Review." *International Journal of Colorectal Disease* 39 (1): 119.

[2] Yamamoto, T., R. N. Allan, and M. R. B. Keighley. 2000. "Risk Factors for Intra-Abdominal Sepsis After Surgery in Crohn's Disease." *Diseases of the Colon & Rectum* 43 (8): 1141–1145.

[3] Papay, Pavlov, Walter Reinisch, Elien Ho, Cornelia Gratzer, Donata Lissner, Harald Herkner, Stefan Riss, et al. 2010. "The Impact of Thiopurines on the Risk of Surgical Recurrence in Patients with Crohn's Disease After First Intestinal Surgery." *American Journal of Gastroenterology* 105 (5): 1158–1164.

[4] Luglio, G., L. Pellegrini, A. Rispo, F. P. Tropeano, N. Imperatore, G. Pagano, A. Amendola, A. Testa, G. D. De Palma, and F. Castiglione. 2022. "Post-Operative Morbidity in Crohn's Disease: What is the Impact of Patient-, Disease- and Surgery-Related Factors?" *International Journal of Colorectal Disease* 37 (2): 411–419.

[5] Tolstrup, Mai-Britt, Sara Kehlet Watt, and Ismail Gögenur. 2017. "Morbidity and Mortality Rates After Emergency Abdominal Surgery: An Analysis of 4346 Patients Scheduled for Emergency Laparotomy Or Laparoscopy." *Langenbeck's Archives of Surgery* 402 (4): 615–623.

[6] Torres, Joana, Stefanos Bonovas, Glen Doherty, Torsten Kucharzik, Javier P. Gisbert, Tim Raine, Michel Adamina, et al. 2020. "ECCO Guidelines on Therapeutics in Crohn's Disease: Medical Treatment." *Journal of Crohn's and Colitis* 14 (1): 4–22.

[7] Bruewer, Matthias, Markus Utech, Emile J. M. Rijcken, Christoph Anthoni, Mike G. Laukoetter, Sabine Kersting, Norbert Senninger, and Christian F. Krieglstein. 2003. "Preoperative Steroid Administration: Effect on Morbidity among Patients Undergoing Intestinal Bowel Resection for Crohn's Disease." *World Journal of Surgery* 27 (12): 1306–1310.

[8] Stuck, Andreas E., Christoph E. Minder, and Felix J. Frey. 1989. "Risk of Infectious Complications in Patients Taking Glucocorticosteroids." *Clinical Infectious Diseases* 11 (6): 954–963.

[9] Aberra, Faten N., James D. Lewis, David Hass, John L. Rombeau, Benjamin Osborne, and Gary R. Lichtenstein. 2003. "Corticosteroids and Immunomodulators: Postoperative Infectious Complication Risk in Inflammatory Bowel Disease Patients." *Gastroenterology* 125 (2): 320–327.

[10] Rizzo, Gianluca, Alessandro Armuzzi, Daniela Pugliese, Alessandro Verbo, Alfredo Papa, Claudio Mattana, Gian Lodovico Rapaccini, Luisa Guidi, and Claudio Coco. 2011. "Anti-TNF-Alpha Therapies do Not Increase Early Postoperative Complications in Patients with Inflammatory Bowel Disease. an Italian Single-Center Experience." *International Journal of Colorectal Disease* 26 (11): 1435–1444.

[11] Subramanian, Venkataraman, Sonia Saxena, Jin-Yong KANG, and Richard C. G. POLLOK. 2008. "Preoperative Steroid use and Risk of Postoperative Complications in Patients with Inflammatory Bowel Disease Undergoing Abdominal Surgery." *The American Journal of Gastroenterology* 103 (9): 2373–2381.

[12] Bemelman, Willem A., Janindra Warusavitarne, Gianluca M. Sampietro, Zuzana Serclova, Oded Zmora, Gaetano Luglio, Anthony de Buck van Overstraeten, et al. 2018. "ECCO-ESCP Consensus on Surgery for Crohn's Disease." *Journal of Crohn's and Colitis* 12 (1): 1–16.

[13] Alomari, Mohammad, Pravallika Chadalavada, Sadaf Afraz, Mu'ed AlGhadir-AlKhalaileh, Zoilo K. Suarez, Alec Swartz, Mamoon Rashid, Shrouq Khazaaleh, Benjamin L. Cohen, and Asad Ur Rahman. 2024. "Post-Hospitalization Short Versus Long Steroid Taper Strategies in Patients with Acute Severe Ulcerative Colitis: A Comparison of Clinical Outcomes." *Crohn's & Colitis 360* 6 (2): 25.

[14] Patel, Kamal V., Amir A. Darakhshan, Nyree Griffin, Andrew B. Williams, Jeremy D. Sanderson, and Peter M. Irving. 2016. "Patient Optimization for Surgery Relating to Crohn's Disease." *Nature Reviews Gastroenterology & Hepatology* 13 (12): 707–719.

[15] Adamina, Michel, Stefanos Bonovas, Tim Raine, Antonino Spinelli, Janindra Warusavitarne, Alessandro Armuzzi, Oliver Bachmann, et al. 2020. "ECCO Guidelines on Therapeutics in Crohn's Disease: Surgical Treatment." *Journal of Crohn's and Colitis* 14 (2): 155–168.

[16] Fraser, Charles G., Fred S. Preuss, and Walter D. Bigford. 1952. "Adrenal Atrophy and Irreversible Shock Associated with Cortisone Therapy." *JAMA : The Journal of the American Medical Association* 149 (17): 1542–1543.

[17] Zaghiyan, Karen N., M. D, Zuri Murrell M. D, Gil Y. Melmed M. D, and Phillip R. Fleshner M. D. 2012. "High-Dose Perioperative Corticosteroids in Steroid-Treated Patients Undergoing Major Colorectal Surgery: Necessary Or Overkill?" *The American Journal of Surgery* 204 (4): 481–486.

[18] Zaghiyan, Karen, Gil Melmed, Zuri Murrell, and Phillip Fleshner. Oct 1, 2011. "Are High-Dose Perioperative Steroids Necessary in Patients Undergoing Colorectal Surgery Treated with Steroid Therapy within the Past 12 Months?" *The American Surgeon* 77 (10): 1295-1299.

[19] Marik, Paul E. and Joseph Varon. 2008. "Requirement of Perioperative Stress Doses of Corticosteroids: A Systematic Review of the Literature." *Archives of Surgery (Chicago. 1960)* 143 (12): 1222–1226.

[20] Hmed Ali, Usama, Sean T. Martin, Abhishek D. Rao, and Ravi P. Kiran. 2014. "Impact of Preoperative Immunosuppressive Agents on Postoperative Outcomes in Crohn's Disease." *Diseases of the Colon & Rectum* 57 (5): 663–674.

[21] Billioud, Vincent, Alexander C. Ford, Emilie Del Tedesco, Jean-Frédéric Colombel, Xavier Roblin, and Laurent Peyrin-Biroulet. 2013. "Preoperative use of anti-TNF Therapy and Postoperative Complications in Inflammatory Bowel Diseases: A Meta-analysis." *Journal of Crohn's and Colitis* 7 (11): 853–867.

[22] Kopylov, Uri, Shomron Ben-Horin, Oded Zmora, Rami Eliakim, and Lior H. Katz. 2012. "Anti-tumor Necrosis Factor and Postoperative Complications in Crohn's Disease: Systematic Review and Meta-analysis." *Inflammatory Bowel Diseases* 18 (12): 2404–2413.

[23] Law, Cindy CY, Conor Bell, Deborah Koh, Yueyang Bao, Vipul Jairath, and Neeraj Narula. 2020. "Risk of Postoperative Infectious Complications from Medical Therapies in Inflammatory Bowel Disease." *Cochrane Database of Systematic Reviews* 2021 (12): 13256.

[24] Lin, Yang-Sheng, Sheng-Wei Cheng, Yuan-Hung Wang, Kee-Hsin Chen, Ching-Ju Fang, and Chiehfeng Chen. 2019. "Systematic Review with Meta-analysis: Risk of Post-operative Complications Associated with Pre-operative Exposure to Anti-tumour Necrosis Factor Agents for Crohn's Disease." *Alimentary Pharmacology & Therapeutics* 49 (8): 966–977.

[25] Huang, Wenpeng, Yanbo Tang, Legen Nong, and Yifan Sun. 2015. "Risk Factors for Postoperative Intra-Abdominal Septic Complications After Surgery in Crohn's Disease: A Meta-Analysis of Observational Studies." *Journal of Crohn's and Colitis* 9 (3): 293–301.

[26] Xu, YanYan, LiSheng Yang, Ping An, Bing Zhou, and Gang Liu. 2019. "Meta-Analysis: The Influence of Preoperative Infliximab use on Postoperative Complications of Crohn's Disease." *Inflammatory Bowel Diseases* 25 (2): 261–269.

[27] Qiu, YuJie, ZiCheng Zheng, Gang Liu, XinYu Zhao, and AnQi He. 2019. "Effects of Preoperative Anti-Tumour Necrosis Factor Alpha Infusion Timing on Postoperative Surgical Site Infection in Inflammatory Bowel Disease: A Systematic Review and Meta-Analysis." *United European Gastroenterology Journal* 7 (9): 1198–1214.

[28] Fumery, Mathurin, Philippe Seksik, Claire Auzolle, Nicolas Munoz-Bongrand, Jean-Marc Gornet, Gilles Boschetti, Eddy Cotte, et al. 2017. "Postoperative Complications After Ileocecal Resection in Crohn's Disease: A Prospective Study from the REMIND Group." *American Journal of Gastroenterology* 112 (2): 337–345.

[29] Baumgart, Daniel C. and Catherine Le Berre. 2021. "Newer Biologic and Small-Molecule Therapies for Inflammatory Bowel Disease." *The New England Journal of Medicine* 385 (14): 1302–1315.

[30] Lightner, Amy L., Kellie L. Mathis, Chung Sang Tse, John H. Pemberton, Bo Shen, Gursimran Kochhar, Amandeep Singh, et al. 2018. "Postoperative Outcomes in Vedolizumab-Treated Patients Undergoing Major Abdominal Operations for Inflammatory Bowel Disease: Retrospective Multicenter Cohort Study." *Inflammatory Bowel Diseases* 24 (4): 871–876.

[31] Guo, Daxin, Ke Jiang, Jiaze Hong, Mengting Zhang, Yetan Shi, and Bin Zhou. 2021. "Association between Vedolizumab and Postoperative Complications in IBD: A Systematic Review and Meta-Analysis." *International Journal of Colorectal Disease* 36 (10): 2081–2092.

[32] Yamada, Akihiro, Yuga Komaki, Nayan Patel, Fukiko Komaki, Arthur S. Aelvoet, Anthony L. Tran, Joel Pekow, et al. 2017. "Risk of Postoperative Complications among Inflammatory Bowel Disease Patients Treated Preoperatively with Vedolizumab." *The American Journal of Gastroenterology* 112 (9): 1423–1429.

[33] Yung, Diana E., Nir Horesh, Amy L. Lightner, Shomron Ben-Horin, Rami Eliakim, Anastasios Koulaouzidis, and Uri Kopylov. 2018. "Systematic Review and Meta-Analysis: Vedolizumab and Postoperative Complications in Inflammatory Bowel Disease." *Inflammatory Bowel Diseases* 24 (11): 2327–2338.

[34] Shim, Hang Hock, Christopher Ma, Paulo G. Kotze, Cynthia H. Seow, Heba Al-Farhan, Ahmed K. Al-Darmaki, Jack X. Q. Pang, et al. 2018. "Preoperative Ustekinumab Treatment is Not Associated with Increased Postoperative Complications in Crohn's Disease: A Canadian Multi-Centre Observational Cohort Study." *Journal of the Canadian Association of Gastroenterology* 1 (3): 115–123.

[35] Lightner, Amy L., Nicholas P. McKenna, Chung Sang Tse, Neil Hyman, Radhika Smith, Gayane Ovsepyan, Phillip Fleshner, et al. 2018. "Postoperative Outcomes in Ustekinumab-Treated Patients Undergoing Abdominal Operations for Crohn's Disease." *Journal of Crohn's and Colitis* 12 (4): 402–407.

[36] Garg, Rajat, Babu P. Mohan, Suresh Ponnada, Miguel Regueiro, Amy L. Lightner, and Benjamin Click. 2021. "Postoperative Outcomes After Preoperative Ustekinumab Exposure in Patients with Crohn's Disease: A Systematic Review and Meta-Analysis." *Annals of Gastroenterology* 34 (5): 691–698.

[37] Lightner, Amy L., Fabian Grass, Ahmad Alsughayer, Molly M. Petersen, Laura E. Raffals, and Edward V. Loftus. 2019. "Postoperative Outcomes in Ustekinumab-Treated Patients Undergoing Abdominal Operations for Crohn's Disease: Single-Center Series." *Crohn's & Colitis 360* 1 (2).

[38] Szamosi, Tamas, Janos Banai, Laszlo Lakatos, Zsofia Czegledi, Gyula David, Ferenc Zsigmond, Tunde Pandur, et al. 2010. "Early Azathioprine/Biological Therapy is Associated with Decreased Risk for First Surgery and Delays Time to Surgery but Not Reoperation in both Smokers and Nonsmokers with Crohn's Disease, while Smoking Decreases the Risk of Colectomy in Ulcerative Colitis." *European Journal of Gastroenterology & Hepatology* 22 (7): 872–879.

[39] Colombel, Jean Frédéric, Edward V. Loftus, William J. Tremaine, John H. Pemberton, Bruce G. Wolff, Tonia Young-Fadok, William S. Harmsen, Cathy D. Schleck, and William J. Sandborn. 2004. "Early Postoperative Complications are Not Increased in Patients with Crohn's Disease Treated Perioperatively with Infliximab Or Immunosuppressive Therapy." *The American Journal of Gastroenterology* 99 (5): 878–883.

[40] Papay, pavlov, Walter Reinisch, Elien Ho, Cornelia Gratzer, Donata Lissner, Harald Herkner, Stefan Riss, et al. 2010. "The Impact of Thiopurines on the Risk of Surgical Recurrence in Patients with Crohn's Disease After First Intestinal Surgery." *American Journal of Gastroenterology* 105 (5): 1158–1164.

[41] Lightner, Amy L. and Bo Shen. 2017. "Perioperative use of Immunosuppressive Medications in Patients with Crohn's Disease in the New "Biological Era."" *Gastroenterology Report* 5 (3): 165–177.

[42] Feagan, B. G., J. Rochon, R. N. Fedorak, E. J. Irvine, G. Wild, L. Sutherland, A. H. Steinhart, G. R. Greenberg, R. Gillies, and M. Hopkins. 1995. "Methotrexate for the Treatment of Crohn's Disease. the North American Crohn's Study Group Investigators." *The New England Journal of Medicine* 332 (5): 292–297.

[43] Heldmann, F. and J. Braun. 2010. "Perioperative use of Methotrexate." *Clinical and Experimental Rheumatology* 28 (5 Suppl 61): S110–S113.

[44] Murata, Koichi, Tadashi Yasuda, Hiromu Ito, Makoto Yoshida, Makoto Shimizu, and Takashi Nakamura. 2006. "Lack of Increase in Postoperative Complications with Low-Dose Methotrexate Therapy in Patients with Rheumatoid Arthritis Undergoing Elective Orthopedic Surgery." *Modern Rheumatology* 16 (1): 14–19.

[45] Sreekumar, Ramankutty, Julie Gray, Peter Kay, and David Michael Grennan. 2011. "Methotrexate and Post Operative Complications in Patients with Rheumatoid Arthritis Undergoing Elective Orthopaedic Surgery--a Ten Year Follow-Up." *Acta Orthopaedica Belgica* 77 (6): 823–826.

[46] Afzali, Anita, Christopher J. Park, Kehao Zhu, Jie Kate Hu, Prachi Sharma, Mika N. Sinanan, and Scott D. Lee. 2016. "Preoperative use of Methotrexate and the Risk of Early Postoperative Complications in Patients with Inflammatory Bowel Disease." *Inflammatory Bowel Diseases* 22 (8): 1887–1895.

[47] Lightner, Amy L. and Bo Shen. 2017. "Perioperative use of Immunosuppressive Medications in Patients with Crohn's Disease in the New "Biological Era."" *Gastroenterology Report* 5 (3): 165–177.

[48] Dragana D. Mijač, Goran L.J. Janković, Jagoda Jorga, and Miodrag N. Krstić. 2010. "Nutritional Status in Patients with Active Inflammatory Bowel Disease: Prevalence of Malnutrition and Methods for Routine Nutritional Assessment." *European Journal of Internal Medicine* 21 (4): 315–319.

[49] Sökülmez, Pınar, Ali Eba Demirbağ, Perihan Arslan, and Selçuk Dişibeyaz. 2014. "Effects of Enteral Nutritional Support on Malnourished Patients with Inflammatory Bowel Disease by Subjective Global Assessment." *The Turkish Journal of Gastroenterology* 25 (5): 493–507.

[50] Balestrieri, Paola, Mentore Ribolsi, Michele Pier Luca Guarino, Sara Emerenziani, Annamaria Altomare, and Michele Cicala. 2020. "Nutritional Aspects in Inflammatory Bowel Diseases." *Nutrients* 12 (2): 372.

[51] Schwartz, Emily. 2016. "Perioperative Parenteral Nutrition in Adults with Inflammatory Bowel Disease." *Nutrition in Clinical Practice* 31 (2): 159–170.

[52] Wędrychowicz, Andrzej, Andrzej Zając, and Przemysław Tomasik. 2016. "Advances in Nutritional Therapy in Inflammatory Bowel Diseases: Review." *World Journal of Gastroenterology : WJG* 22 (3): 1045–1066.

[53] Alves, Arnaud, Yves Panis, Yoram Bouhnik, Marc Pocard, Eric Vicaut, and Patrice Valleur. 2007. "Risk Factors for Intra-Abdominal Septic Complications After a First Ileocecal Resection for Crohn's Disease: A Multivariate Analysis in 161 Consecutive Patients." *Diseases of the Colon & Rectum* 50 (3): 331–336.

[54] Kiyoshi Maeda, Hisashi Nagahara, Masatsune Shibutani, Hiroshi Otani, Katsunobu Sakurai, Takahiro Toyokawa, Hiroaki Tanaka, et al. 2014. "A Preoperative Low Nutritional Prognostic Index Correlates with the Incidence of Incisional Surgical Site Infections After Bowel Resection in Patients with Crohn's Disease." *Surgery Today* 45 (11): 1366–1372.

[55] Yamamoto, T., R. N. Allan, and M. R. B. Keighley. 2000. "Risk Factors for Intra-Abdominal Sepsis After Surgery in Crohn's Disease." *Diseases of the Colon & Rectum* 43 (8): 1141–1145.

[56] Bischoff, Stephan C., Palle Bager, Johanna Escher, Alastair Forbes, Xavier Hébuterne, Christian Lodberg Hvas, Francisca Joly, et al. 2023. "ESPEN Guideline on Clinical Nutrition in Inflammatory Bowel Disease." *Clinical Nutrition (Edinburgh, Scotland)* 42 (3): 352–379.

[57] Wagner, I. Janelle, MD and John L. Rombeau MD. 2011. "Nutritional Support of Surgical Patients with Inflammatory Bowel Disease." *The Surgical Clinics of North America* 91 (4): 787–803.

[58] Stephan C. Bischoff, Johanna Escher, Xavier Hébuterne, Stanisław Kłęk, Zeljko Krznaric, Stéphane Schneider, Raanan Shamir, et al. 2020. "ESPEN Practical Guideline: Clinical Nutrition in Inflammatory Bowel Disease." *Clinical Nutrition* 39 (3): 632–653.

[59] Ayoub, Fares, Amir Y. Kamel, Ahmed Ouni, Naueen Chaudhry, Yan Ader, Sanda Tan, Atif Iqbal, Ellen M. Zimmermann, and Sarah C. Glover. 2019. "Pre-Operative Total Parenteral Nutrition Improves Post-Operative Outcomes in a Subset of Crohn's Disease Patients Undergoing Major Abdominal Surgery." *Gastroenterology Report* 7 (2): 107–114.

[60] Brennan, Gregory T., Iris Ha, Christopher Hogan, Emily Nguyen, M. M. Jamal, Matthew L. Bechtold, and Douglas L. Nguyen. 2018. "Does Preoperative Enteral Or Parenteral Nutrition Reduce Postoperative Complications in Crohn's Disease Patients: A Meta-Analysis." *European Journal of Gastroenterology & Hepatology* 30 (9): 997–1002.

[61] Meade, Susanna, Kamal V. Patel, Raphael P. Luber, Dearbhaile O'Hanlon, Andra Caracostea, Polychronis Pavlidis, Sailish Honap, et al. 2022. "A Retrospective Cohort Study: Pre-operative Oral Enteral Nutritional Optimisation for Crohn's Disease in a UK Tertiary IBD Centre." *Alimentary Pharmacology & Therapeutics* 56 (4): 646–663.

[62] Ayoub, Fares, Amir Y. Kamel, Ahmed Ouni, Naueen Chaudhry, Yan Ader, Sanda Tan, Atif Iqbal, Ellen M. Zimmermann, and Sarah C. Glover. 2019. "Pre-Operative Total Parenteral Nutrition Improves Post-Operative Outcomes in a Subset of Crohn's Disease Patients Undergoing Major Abdominal Surgery." *Gastroenterology Report* 7 (2): 107–114.

[63] Harries, A. D., L. A. Jones, V. Danis, R. Fifield, R. V. Heatley, R. G. Newcombe, and J. Rhodes. 1983. "Controlled Trial of Supplemented Oral Nutrition in Crohn's Disease." *The Lancet (British Edition)* 1 (8330): 887–890.

[64] Ajabnoor, Sarah M. and Alastair Forbes. 2019. "Effect of Fat Composition in Enteral Nutrition for Crohn's Disease in Adults: A Systematic Review." *Clinical Nutrition (Edinburgh, Scotland)* 38 (1): 90–99.

[65] Heerasing, N., B. Thompson, P. Hendy, G. A. Heap, G. Walker, R. Bethune, S. Mansfield, et al. 2017. "Exclusive Enteral Nutrition Provides an Effective Bridge to Safer Interval Elective Surgery for Adults with Crohn's Disease." *Alimentary Pharmacology & Therapeutics* 45 (5): 660–669.

[66] Honggang Wang, Lugen Zuo, Jie Zhao, Jianning Dong, Yi Li, Lili Gu, Jianfeng Gong, Qinghong Liu, and Weiming Zhu. 2016. "Impact of Preoperative Exclusive Enteral Nutrition on Postoperative Complications and Recurrence After Bowel Resection in Patients with Active Crohn's Disease." *World Journal of Surgery* 40 (8): 1993–2000.

[67] Nguyen, Douglas L., Berkeley Limketkai, Valentina Medici, Mardeli Saire Mendoza, Lena Palmer, and Matthew Bechtold. 2016. "Nutritional Strategies in the Management of Adult Patients with Inflammatory Bowel Disease: Dietary Considerations from Active Disease to Disease Remission." *Current Gastroenterology Reports* 18 (10): 55.

[68] MacLellan, Amber, Jessica Moore-Connors, Shannan Grant, Leah Cahill, Morgan G. I. Langille, and Johan Van Limbergen. 2017. "The Impact of Exclusive Enteral Nutrition (EEN) on the Gut Microbiome in Crohn's Disease: A Review." *Nutrients* 9 (5): 0447.

[69] Grass, Fabian, Basile Pache, David Martin, Dieter Hahnloser, Nicolas Demartines, and Martin Hübner. 2017. "Preoperative Nutritional Conditioning of Crohn's Patients-Systematic Review of Current Evidence and Practice." *Nutrients* 9 (6): 562.

[70] Li, G., J. Ren, G. Wang, D. Hu, G. Gu, S. Liu, H. Ren, X. Wu, and J. Li. 2014. "Preoperative Exclusive Enteral Nutrition Reduces the Postoperative Septic Complications of Fistulizing Crohn's Disease." *European Journal of Clinical Nutrition* 68 (4): 441–446.

[71] Scaldaferri, F., M. Pizzoferrato, L. R. Lopetuso, T. Musca, F. Ingravalle, L. L. Sicignano, M. Mentella, et al. 2017. "Nutrition and IBD: Malnutrition and/Or Sarcopenia? A Practical Guide." *Gastroenterology Research and Practice* 2017: 1.

[72] Weisshof, Roni and Irit Chermesh. 2015. "Micronutrient Deficiencies in Inflammatory Bowel Disease." *Current Opinion in Clinical Nutrition and Metabolic Care* 18 (6): 576–581.

[73] Baron, D.M., H. Hochrieser, M. Posch, B. Metnitz, A. Rhodes, R.P. Moreno, R.M. Pearse, and P. Metnitz. 2014. "Preoperative Anaemia is Associated with Poor Clinical Outcome in Non-Cardiac Surgery Patients." *British Journal of Anaesthesia* 113 (3): 416–423.

[74] Hwang, Caroline, Viveca Ross, and Uma Mahadevan. 2012. "Micronutrient Deficiencies in Inflammatory Bowel Disease: From A to Zinc." *Inflammatory Bowel Diseases* 18 (10): 1961–1981.

[75] Shander, Aryeh, Howard L. Corwin, Jens Meier, Michael Auerbach, Elvira Bisbe, Jeanna Blitz, Jochen Erhard, et al. 2023. "Recommendations from the International Consensus Conference on Anemia Management in Surgical Patients (ICCAMS)." *Annals of Surgery* 277 (4): 581–590.

[76] Iglar, Paul J. and Kirk J. Hogan. 2015. "Vitamin D Status and Surgical Outcomes: A Systematic Review." *Patient Safety in Surgery* 9 (1): 14.

[77] Lal, Simon, Neeraj Prasad, Manijeh Ryan, Sabrena Tangri, Mark S. Silverberg, Allan Gordon, and Hillary Steinhart. 2011. "Cannabis use Amongst Patients with Inflammatory Bowel Disease." *European Journal of Gastroenterology & Hepatology* 23 (10): 891–896.

[78] Kafil, Tahir S., Tran M. Nguyen, John K. MacDonald, and Nilesh Chande. 2020. "Cannabis for the Treatment of Crohn's Disease and Ulcerative Colitis: Evidence from Cochrane Reviews." *Inflammatory Bowel Diseases* 26 (4): 502–509.

[79] Fliss Isakov, Naomi, Chen Seidenberg, David Meiri, Michal Yackobovitch-Gavan, Nitsan Maharshak, and Ayal Hirsch. 2023. "Medical Cannabis Increases Appetite but Not Body Weight in Patients with Inflammatory Bowel Diseases." *Nutrients* 16 (1): 78.

[80] Reese, George E., Theodore Nanidis, Catherine Borysiewicz, Takayuki Yamamoto, Timothy Orchard, and Paris P. Tekkis. 2008. "The Effect of Smoking After Surgery for Crohn's Disease: A Meta-Analysis of Observational Studies." *International Journal of Colorectal Disease* 23 (12): 1213–1221.

[81] Morar, Pritesh S., Jonathan D. Hodgkinson, Samantha Thalayasingam, Kanyada Koysombat, Martha Purcell, Ailsa L. Hart, Janindra Warusavitarne, and Omar Faiz. 2015. "Determining Predictors for Intra-Abdominal Septic Complications Following Ileocolonic Resection for Crohn's Disease—Considerations in Pre-Operative and Peri-Operative Optimisation Techniques to Improve Outcome." *Journal of Crohn's and Colitis* 9 (6): 483–491.

[82] Nolan, Margaret B., David P. Martin, Rodney Thompson, Darrell R. Schroeder, Andrew C. Hanson, and David O. Warner. 2017. "Association between Smoking Status, Preoperative Exhaled Carbon Monoxide Levels, and Postoperative Surgical Site Infection in Patients Undergoing Elective Surgery." *JAMA Surgery* 152 (5): 476–483.

[83] Bolckmans, Roel, Thordis Kalman, Sandeep Singh, Keshara C. Ratnatunga, Pär Myrelid, Simon Travis, and Bruce D. George. 2020. "Does Smoking Cessation Reduce Surgical Recurrence After Primary Ileocolic Resection for Crohn's Disease?" *Diseases of the Colon & Rectum* 63 (2): 200–206.

[84] Møller, Ann M., Nete Villebro, Tom Pedersen, and Hanne Tønnesen. 2002. "Effect of Preoperative Smoking Intervention on Postoperative Complications: A Randomised Clinical Trial." *The Lancet (British Edition)* 359 (9301): 114–117.

[85] Rimola, Jordi, Núria Planell, Sonia Rodríguez, Salvadora Delgado, Ingrid Ordás, Anna Ramírez-Morros, Carmen Ayuso, et al. 2015. "Characterization of Inflammation and Fibrosis in Crohn's Disease Lesions by Magnetic Resonance Imaging." *The American Journal of Gastroenterology* 110 (3): 432–440.

[86] Feagins, Linda A., Stefan D. Holubar, Sunanda V. Kane, and Stuart J. Spechler. 2011. "Current Strategies in the Management of Intra-Abdominal Abscesses in Crohn's Disease." *Clinical Gastroenterology and Hepatology* 9 (10): 842–850.

[87] Qiu, Y., R. Mao, B. -L Chen, X. -H Li, Y. He, Z. -R Zeng, Z. -P Li, and M. -H Chen. 2014. "Systematic Review with Meta-analysis: Magnetic Resonance Enterography Vs. Computed Tomography Enterography for Evaluating Disease Activity in Small Bowel Crohn's Disease." *Alimentary Pharmacology & Therapeutics* 40 (2): 134–146.

[88] Horsthuis, Karin, Shandra Bipat, Roelof J. Bennink, and Jaap Stoker. 2008. "Inflammatory Bowel Disease Diagnosed with US, MR, Scintigraphy, and CT: Meta-Analysis of Prospective Studies." *Radiology* 247 (1): 64–79.

[89] Parente, Fabrizio, Salvatore Greco, Mirko Molteni, Andrea Anderloni, Giovanni Maconi, and Gabriele Bianchi Porro. 2004. "Modern Imaging of Crohn's Disease using Bowel Ultrasound." *Inflammatory Bowel Diseases* 10 (4): 452–461.

[90] Lee, Seung Soo, Ah Young Kim, Suk-Kyun Yang, Jun-Won Chung, So Yeon Kim, Seong Ho Park, and Hyun Kwon Ha. 2009. "Crohn Disease of the Small Bowel: Comparison of CT Enterography, MR Enterography, and Small-Bowel Follow-through as Diagnostic Techniques." *Radiology* 251 (3): 751–761.

[91] Panes, J., Y. Bouhnik, W. Reinisch, J. Stoker, S. A. Taylor, D. C. Baumgart, S. Danese, et al. 2013. "Imaging Techniques for Assessment of Inflammatory Bowel Disease: Joint ECCO and ESGAR Evidence-Based Consensus Guidelines." *Journal of Crohn's and Colitis* 7 (7): 556–585.

[92] Zissin, R., A. Osadchy, and G. Gayer. 2009. "Abdominal CT Findings in Small Bowel Perforation." *British Journal of Radiology* 82 (974): 162–171.

[93] Seastedt, Kenneth P., Koiana Trencheva, Fabrizio Michelassi, Doaa Alsaleh, Jeffrey W. Milsom, Toyooki Sonoda, Sang W. Lee, and Govind Nandakumar. 2014. "Accuracy of CT Enterography and

Magnetic Resonance Enterography Imaging to Detect Lesions Preoperatively in Patients Undergoing Surgery for Crohn's Disease." *Diseases of the Colon & Rectum* 57 (12): 1364–1370.

[94] Spinelli, Antonino, Gionata Fiorino, Piero Bazzi, Matteo Sacchi, Cristiana Bonifacio, Sarah De Bastiani, Alberto Malesci, et al. 2014. "Preoperative Magnetic Resonance Enterography in Predicting Findings and Optimizing Surgical Approach in Crohn's Disease." *Journal of Gastrointestinal Surgery* 18 (1): 83–91.

[95] Peyrin-Biroulet, Laurent, Edward V. Loftus, Jean-Frederic Colombel, and William J. Sandborn. 2010. "The Natural History of Adult Crohn's Disease in Population-Based Cohorts." *American Journal of Gastroenterology* 105 (2): 289–297.

[96] Van Assche, Gert, Axel Dignass, Julian Panes, Laurent Beaugerie, John Karagiannis, Mathieu Allez, Thomas Ochsenkühn, et al. 2010. "The Second European Evidence-Based Consensus on the Diagnosis and Management of Crohn's Disease: Definitions and Diagnosis." *Journal of Crohn's & Colitis* 4 (1): 7–27.

[97] Tzivanakis, A., J. C. Singh, R. J. Guy, S. P. L. Travis, N. J. Mortensen, and B. D. George. 2012. "Influence of Risk Factors on the Safety of Ileocolic Anastomosis in Crohn's Disease Surgery." *Diseases of the Colon & Rectum* 55 (5): 558–562.

[98] Zerbib, P., D. Koriche, S. Truant, A. F. Bouras, G. Vernier-Massouille, D. Seguy, F. R. Pruvot, A. Cortot, and J. F. Colombel. 2010. "Pre-operative Management is Associated with Low Rate of Post-operative Morbidity in Penetrating Crohn's Disease." *Alimentary Pharmacology & Therapeutics* 32 (3): 459–465.

[99] Lobatón, T., J. Guardiola, F. Rodriguez-Moranta, M. Millán-Scheiding, M. Peñalva, J. De Oca, and S. Biondo. 2013. "Comparison of the Long-Term Outcome of Two Therapeutic Strategies for the Management of Abdominal Abscess Complicating Crohn's Disease: Percutaneous Drainage Or Immediate Surgical Treatment." *Colorectal Disease* 15 (10): 1267–1272.

[100] Nguyen, Douglas L., William J. Sandborn, Edward V. Loftus, David W. Larson, Joel G. Fletcher, Brenda Becker, Jay Mandrekar, William S. Harmsen, and David H. Bruining. 2012. "Similar Outcomes of Surgical and Medical Treatment of Intra-Abdominal Abscesses in Patients with Crohn's Disease." *Clinical Gastroenterology and Hepatology* 10 (4): 400–404.

[101] Sahai, A., M. Belair, D. Gianfelice, S. Cote, J. Gratton, and R. Lahaie. 1997. "Percutaneous Drainage of Intra-Abdominal Abscesses in Crohn's Disease: Short and Long Term Outcome." *The American Journal of Gastroenterology* 92 (2): 275–278.

[102] Gervais, Debra A., Peter F. Hahn, Mary J. O'neill, and Peter R. Mueller. 2002. "Percutaneous Abscess Drainage in Crohn Disease: Technical Success and Short- and Long-Term Outcomes during 14 Years." *Radiology* 222 (3): 645–651.

[103] Clancy, Cillian, Therese Boland, Joseph Deasy, Deborah McNamara, and John P. Burke. 2016. "A Meta-analysis of Percutaneous Drainage Versus Surgery as the Initial Treatment of Crohn's Disease-related Intra-abdominal Abscess." *Journal of Crohn's and Colitis* 10 (2): 202–208.

[104] de Groof, E. Joline, Frank Carbonnel, Christianne J. Buskens, and Willem A. Bemelman. 2014. "Abdominal Abscess in Crohn's Disease: Multidisciplinary Management." *Digestive Diseases (Basel)* 32 (1): 103–109.

[105] Bermejo, Fernando, Elena Garrido, Maria Chaparro, Jordi Gordillo, Míriam Mañosa, Alicia Algaba, Antonio López-San Román, et al. 2011. "Efficacy of Different Therapeutic Options for Spontaneous Intraabdominal Abscesses in Crohn's Disease." *Gastroenterology* 140 (5): S–437.

[106] Nguyen, Douglas L., Emily T. Nguyen, and Matthew L. Bechtold. 2015. "Outcomes of Initial Medical Compared with Surgical Strategies in the Management of Intra-Abdominal Abscesses in Patients with Crohn's Disease: A Meta-Analysis." *European Journal of Gastroenterology & Hepatology* 27 (3): 235–241.

[107] Bryant, Robert V., Vipul Jairath, Nicola Curry, and Simon P. L. Travis. 2014. "Thrombosis in Inflammatory Bowel Disease: Are we Tailoring Prophylaxis to those most at Risk?" *Journal of Crohn's and Colitis* 8 (2): 166–171.

[108] Irving, Peter M., K. John Pasi, and David S. Rampton. 2005. "Thrombosis and Inflammatory Bowel Disease." *Clinical Gastroenterology and Hepatology* 3 (7): 617–628.

[109] Wallaert, Jessica B., Randall R. De Martino, Priscilla S. Marsicovetere, Philip P. Goodney, Sam R. G. Finlayson, John J. Murray, and Stefan D. Holubar. 2012. "Venous Thromboembolism After Surgery for Inflammatory Bowel Disease: Are there Modifiable Risk Factors? Data from ACS NSQIP." *Diseases of the Colon & Rectum* 55 (11): 1138–1144.

[110] Spinelli, A., M. Allocca, M. Jovani, and S. Danese. 2014. "Review Article: Optimal Preparation for Surgery in Crohn's Disease." *Alimentary Pharmacology & Therapeutics* 40 (9): 1009–1022.

[111] Geerts, William H., David Bergqvist, Graham F. Pineo, John A. Heit, Charles M. Samama, Michael R. Lassen, and Clifford W. Colwell. 2008. "Prevention of Venous Thromboembolism: American College of Chest Physicians Evidence-Based Clinical Practice Guidelines (8th Edition)." *Chest* 133 (6 Suppl): 381S–453S.

Chapter 8

Crohn's Disease of the Foregut

Hossam Abdou[1], MD
Joseph Edwards[1], MD
and Stephen M. Kavic[2,*], MD, MSHPE
[1]Surgery, University of Maryland Medical Center, Baltimore, Maryland, USA
[2]University of Maryland School of Medicine, Baltimore, Maryland, USA

Abstract

Crohn's disease results in transmural inflammation involving any portion of the gastrointestinal tract from the mouth to the anus. However, Crohn's disease most commonly affects the lower gastrointestinal tract, often sparing the proximal portions. Here, we review the presentation and management of Crohn's disease of the esophagus, stomach, and duodenum. Like all forms of Crohn's disease, the initial management is typically medical. Unlike the remainder of the GI tract, however, bypass techniques are preferred to resection or strictureplasty techniques, given the morbidity associated with resection. Surgeons that often encounter Crohn's disease will inevitably face the patient with Crohn's of the foregut, either in isolation, or more commonly, in conjunction with ileal or colonic disease. The purpose of this overview is to assist clinicians in evaluating and managing Crohn's Disease of the foregut.

Prevalence

The prevalence of symptomatic Crohn's disease (CD) involving the esophagus, stomach, and/or duodenum has been reported to be between 0.5 and 4% [1-7]. With more liberal use of esophagogastroduodenoscopy (EGD), however, recent studies suggest that occult findings in the upper gastrointestinal tract are far more frequent, ranging from 16 to 51% [8-10, 11]. In adolescents and children, EGD is recommended at initial evaluation, per the 2020 European Society for Pediatric Gastroenterology, Hepatology, and Nutrition [Levine]. This may explain why the rate of upper GI involvement is higher in children and adolescents, with rates reported up to 28% [12-14].

Presently, upper endoscopic evaluation is recommended for use only in CD patients with upper GI symptoms, in accordance with the American College of Gastroenterology's most recent guidelines [15]. However, given that there are frequent endoscopic findings, some argue

* Corresponding Author's Email: skavic@som.umaryland.edu

In: Surgery for Crohn's Disease. Second Edition
Editors: Stephen M. Kavic, Rebecca Brown and Kerri Lopez
ISBN: 979-8-89530-676-5

that EGD should be included as part of the routine diagnostic work-up [9, 10], In a retrospective review, published in 2014, endoscopic and pathologic changes of the upper GI tract in 138 patients with CD were examined [8]. Seventy of 138 patients (51%) demonstrated macroscopic disease-specific findings. The definition of disease-specific findings involving the upper GI tract and results of this study are detailed in Figure 8.1. Additionally, in a prospective analysis published in 2012, 119 patients with CD underwent histologic and endoscopic examination before and after medical therapy [10]. All symptomatic patients showed relief of symptoms following treatment, and while 63% of patients were asymptomatic at presentation, nearly half of these patients (47%) demonstrated mucosal healing on post-treatment biopsy.

The prevalence of CD involving the foregut does not seem to vary significantly with age. In children with CD, histologic evidence by endoscopy of the upper GI tract is also frequently documented (30-80%) [16-18]. Nonetheless, symptomatic disease in this region is uncommon.

Location	Any findings (%)	CD specific findings* (%)	Granuloma detection (%)
Esophagus	14	7	0
Stomach: upper to mid	51	48	6
Stomach: lower	60	25	25
Duodenum: bulb	42	32	11
Duodenum: 2nd portion	19	18	0
Total	75	51	11

* Crohn's disease (CD) specific findings included: aphthae, longitudinal/irregular erosions and ulcers, Bamboo joint appearances, protruded or notch like appearances in the duodenum and fistula or stricture irrespective of location. Esophageal lesions were considered non-CD related when relation with reflux esophagitis was suspected. Gastroduodenal lesions were considered non-CD related when relation with H. pylori or NSAIDs was suspected.

Figure 8.1. Frequency of identification of characteristic findings and granulomas on EGD, based on a review of 138 patients.

Clinical Manifestations

Isolated involvement of the esophagus, stomach or duodenum is exceptionally rare. While Crohn's gastritis is the most common site of upper-GI involvement, it is often continuous with duodenal inflammation, and thus often termed, "gastroduodenal CD." Overall, however, patients are more commonly diagnosed with disease in the terminal ileum, and symptomatic involvement of the foregut is identified secondarily. Patients with Crohn's of the foregut, often present with the signs and symptoms of CD outlined earlier.

In a study by Nugent and Roy, which examined 89 patients with gastroduodenal CD, 46 of 89 patients (52%) had documented distal disease before the development of upper GI symptoms [4]. At a follow-up interval of 12 years, distal disease had developed in 82 of 89 patients (92%); 53 of 89 patients (60%) had contiguous gastroduodenal involvement, and two of 36 patients with duodenal disease also had involvement in the proximal jejunum.

Importantly, symptoms of CD involving the foregut can be difficult to differentiate from other more common ailments of the upper gastrointestinal tract, such as gastroesophageal reflux and peptic ulcer disease. According to a retrospective analysis performed at Mayo Clinic over a 15-year period, 83% of patients with endoscopically/pathologically diagnosed esophageal involvement had symptoms, with 54% reporting dysphagia, 33% reporting odynophagia, 25% with GERD, and 13% reporting chest pain [19]. Some patients with involvement of the esophagus may also present with oral aphthous ulceration [20].

Symptom	Nugent and Roy [4]	Worsey [15]	Farmer [16]	Poggioli [17]
Postprandial pain	79	71	100	100
Weight loss	64	65	72	55
Nausea and vomiting	61	32	72	55
Bloating	NR	68	NR	NR
Bleeding and anemia	17	NR	9	33

NR = not recorded.

Figure 8.2. Presenting symptoms of gastroduodenal Crohn's disease.

The presenting symptoms of patients with gastroduodenal CD from several series are outlined in Figure 8.2 [1, 4, 21-23]. The most common symptoms of gastroduodenal involvement included postprandial pain, nausea, vomiting, and weight loss. Notably, the pain associated with gastroduodenal CD was relieved by antacids or acid suppressive therapy, as is seen in peptic ulcer disease.

Much like CD that involves any region of the gastrointestinal tract, advanced manifestations of CD in the foregut include stricture, obstruction, fistulization, or bleeding. Of these complications in esophageal CD, stricture presents most frequently. In Decker's review, the clinical course and outcome in twenty patients with symptoms of esophageal CD is described well. Four of twenty patients (20%) presented with esophageal stricture [20]. The overwhelming majority presented with dysphagia and were found to have esophageal ulceration and/or erosion (90%) without complication. Obstruction is the most common presenting symptom in gastroduodenal CD, and remains the most common indication for surgery in CD involving the foregut, ranging from 70-90% [4, 7, 24]. Bleeding and perforation are rarely associated with CD and are more likely due to another disease processes such as peptic ulcer disease [25].

Fistulization of the esophagus in CD can also occur, involving communication with the proximal and/or distal airway, however this is much more rare. Fistulas involving the stomach and/or duodenum are also infrequent, and if they arise, are more often attributed to primary colonic or distal small bowel disease. Fistulization to the pancreatic gland, although vanishingly rare, has also been described in gastroduodenal CD [26-30]. Likewise, granulomatous involvement of the gallbladder and common bile duct obstruction have been reported [29-32].

Studies examining surgical patients who present with complications of CD involving the esophagus, stomach or duodenum, suggest that the patient population should be considered high risk. CD of the upper gastrointestinal tract has been associated with increased recurrence, need for surgery and length of hospitalization [33, 34]. Interestingly, in a recent cross-sectional query of the National Institute of Diabetes and Digestive and Kidney Diseases Inflammatory Bowel Disease Genetics Consortium (IBDGC), published by Lazarev in 2014, 175 of 1,759 patients (10%) with CD involving the esophagus, stomach or duodenum were compared to patients with isolated jejunal disease, 115 of 1,759 patients (7%) [35]. In this study, while patients with upper tract involvement seemed to present at an earlier age, they were less likely to have stricturing and undergo multiple surgeries. Instead, independent predictors of structuring behavior and multiple abdominal surgeries included ileal involvement, longer duration of disease and isolated jejunal disease. Current classification schemes do not reflect a difference between CD of the duodenum and jejunum.

Diagnosis and Classification

A diagnosis of subtle disease involving the esophagus, stomach or duodenum can be done endoscopically, and reported prevalence varies dramatically based on clinical presentation. This variance is further complicated by non-specific gross and/or histologic findings identified on endoscopy, as universal criteria for CD involving the upper gastrointestinal tract have yet to be defined. While findings of macroscopic ulceration or aphthous lesions are frequently seen in CD of the upper GI tract, erythema, edema and other inflammatory changes cannot exclusively be attributed to CD.

The histology of gastric CD in particular is difficult to interpret. The occurrence of epithelioid granulomas is considered a histological hallmark of the disease, however this finding is detected infrequently [1, 8, 9]. A list of commonly accepted CD-specific findings in the upper GI tract is included in Figure 8-1.

Upper GI studies with contrast are best utilized to characterize fistulas or obstructive lesions. Although these findings are uncommon, they have been well described in the literature. The shape of the distended stomach and a rigid stenotic antrum and duodenum has been described as the "ram's horn deformity," seen in gastroduodenal CD [36]. Similarly, a tube-like appearance of the antrum, pylorus and duodenum has been termed, the "pseudo-Billroth I," characterizing CD which involves the stomach and duodenum as similar in appearance to a surgical end-to-end gastro-duodenostomy [37].

Current systems used to classify CD include the Vienna and Montreal classifications. The Montreal classification system is the most recently updated version (see Figure 8.2) [38]. Note that this classification scheme may be revised to further subclassify L4 disease into two categories, esophageal-gastric-duodenal, and jejunal, reflecting increasing evidence that supports clinically distinct differences between the two [35].

Medical Treatment

The current therapeutic approach to CD accounts for the broad spectrum of disease involvement. The medical management is reviewed in detail in an earlier chapter. Most clinicians, however, assume that the entire GI tract is at risk for the subsequent manifestation of CD. As a result, patients with CD of the foregut are treated with standard therapy, including 5-aminosalicylic acid and steroids. The efficacy of more recent immunosuppressive treatments has not been specifically evaluated in CD of the upper GI tract, but has been reported to be successful [39, 40]. Other modalities that have been used, but have not been widely adopted, include endoscopic dilation and local steroid injection for obstructive lesions [20, 41-43].

The optimal non-steroid management regimen for gastroduodenal disease is currently unknown and are typically utilized in addition to other medications if there is endoscopic/histopathlogic evidence of gastroduodenal CD [44]. Regimens that include steroids combined with acid-blocking therapy, as well as immunomodulators such as 6-MP and azothioprine have shown success in treating non-obstructing disease, with at least one study showing that steroids could be successfully weaned after achieving some level of acute disease control [45-47]. While there is a paucity of quality studies to direct the optimal medical treatment of esophageal CD, it is likely that the same regimens used for GD CD can be utilized.

Intuitively, a step-up approach from medical management to endoscopic management should guide treatment before surgery is performed as inflammation becomes chronic and these other therapies become ineffective.

More recent studies have assessed the role of biologics in treating UGI-CD. For example, one study showed that 5 of 18 patients with esophageal CD were successfully treated with infliximab only, while 2 of 18 patients were treated with induction steroid therapy followed by maintenance infliximab. None of these patients had recurrence of disease after successful treatment. There is even one case report of the successful treatment of pyloric stenosis in a patient treated with adalimumab treatment, without the use of steroids. Although these studies are not prospective studies, they show the potential efficacy of using anti-TNF therapy to treat UGI-CD without the need for steroids.

Endoscopic management is also a potential treatment option for patients who experience strictures as sequelae of their UGI CD. A recent single-center prospective randomized controlled study examined the role of endoscopic balloon dilation in patients with duodenal strictures, ultimately including 45 patients treated, and compared the efficacy of serial dilation (dilations performed every 2-4 weeks for 3 dilations on average) vs intermittent dilation (dilations performed when obstructive symptoms arose). While both methods were deemed to be safe and effective, serial dilations showed greater recurrence-free survival from last EBD (815 days vs. 291 days), as well as greater mean diameter of the duodenal diameter when compared to the intermittent dilation group [48].

Surgical Management

Esophageal Crohn's Disease

In general, an anastomosis to the esophagus within the chest has a significant risk of complications. This risk is amplified in patients with CD, making resection with anastomosis particularly unappealing. Therefore, CD of the esophagus, when presenting with severe complications, requires esophagectomy.

Fortunately, esophageal disease is infrequent. Unfortunately, the consequence for surgeons is that there is a paucity of quality literature to guide management. Early case reports, from the 1960's to the 1980's, often documented very poor outcomes [49, 50]. More recent literature on the topic has focused on endoscopic and medical therapies for strictures and obstruction, as alternatives to esophagectomy [20, 41-43]. The most common endoluminal therapies include dilation, steroid injection, and topical application of other immunosuppressive regimens.

Despite modern advancements in surgical technique and post-operative care, which have likely improved associated morbidity and mortality, the use of esophagectomy for surgical management of esophageal CD should be reserved for severe cases. It is worrisome to replace the native esophagus with intestinal conduit, as a replacement with colon may lead to recurrent disease within the chest if Crohn's develops within the colon. Given the morbidity of both medical immunosuppression as well as surgical complications, it is also essential to consider first and eliminate the more common causes of chronic esophageal inflammation, such as gastroesophageal reflux.

Gastroduodenal Crohn's Disease

The most common indications for surgery in gastroduodenal CD include obstruction and refractory painful ulceration. Isolated gastric disease is extremely rare [51, 52]. Options for surgical management of complicated gastroduodenal CD include bypass, resection, or strictureplasty. Unlike the management of CD involving the distal small bowel and colon, bypass is more commonly used than resection, as resection in this region is associated with significant morbidity [53]. Bypass techniques most frequently used include gastro-jejunostomy, gastro-duodenostomy, and Roux-en-Y gastro-jejunostomy.

In one of the largest and most recent studies performed on surgical management of patients with gastroduodenal CD, Shapiro retrospectively examined 30 patients who underwent surgical intervention between 1995 and 2006 at Mount Sinai Medical Center [24]. Eleven patients underwent open bypass, thirteen had laparoscopic bypass, two underwent strictureplasty, and four had fistula takedown. The average length of follow-up was 58 months, 27% (n = 7) experienced major complications, including five patients in the open bypass group and one patient in the laparoscopic bypass group, and there was one death. The authors concluded that surgery is a viable and safe option for patients with intractable gastroduodenal CD. Furthermore, in the era of widespread use of proton pump inhibitors, vagotomy is no longer considered necessary to prevent marginal ulceration post-operatively. Results of this study in comparison to other published series are listed in Figure 8.3. These studies report significant complication rates, yet serious morbidity (such as anastomotic leak and sepsis) is uncommon, and mortality rates are also very low.

A comparison between bypass and strictureplasty has not been prospectively evaluated in CD of the upper GI tract. Initial analysis in the early 1990s, suggested that strictureplasty may be associated with a significant complication rate. In one analysis, 9 of 13 patients (69%) required reoperation for complication and/or recurrent disease. However, a more recent report from the same surgical group published a surgical recurrence rate of only 25% (2 of 8 patients) in this patient population [7, 54, 55]. Another recent study corroborates this data noting only 1 of 10 patients with surgical recurrence [56]. Although these results represent small sample sizes, they suggest that refinements in technique can result in improved outcomes. Currently, strictureplasty remains an acceptable alternative to bypass for CD involving the duodenum and is used according to surgeon preference and clinical situation [57].

Study (Sample Size)	Open Bypass	Laparoscopic Bypass	Strictureplasty	Vagotomy	Morbidity	Mortality
Worsey [15] (n = 34)	21	0	15	21	6 (18%)*	NR
Nugent and Roy [4] (n = 33)	32	0	0	18	8 (24%)*	NR
Yamamoto [7] (n = 23)	13	0	10	4	13 (57%)	NR
Shapiro [19] (n = 30)	11	13	2	1	14 (47%)	1 (3%)

*Morbidity in these series was recorded as recurrence requiring surgical revision.

Figure 8.3. Surgical management and outcomes in patients with Crohn's disease of the foregut.

Current recommendations include strictureplasty for short segment disease within a segment of small bowel when the segment is surgically accessible and the procedure may be accomplished with minimal risk to adjacent structures. Therefore, patients with stricturing disease in the second and fourth portions of the duodenum may be better served by bypass techniques (gastro-duodenal or gastro-jejunal). Disease in the first portion or third portion may be amenable to Heineke-Mikulicz strictureplasty.

Cancer Risk and Management

Small-intestinal adenocarcinoma associated with preexisting CD has been rarely reported and requires complete oncologic resection [58-65]. Cancer of the small intestine, arising in CD patients, has been associated with younger age at presentation and has a male predilection. There is a poor prognosis due to delay in diagnosis, often attributed to difficulty in differentiating underlying CD and early signs of invasive carcinoma. These cases emphasize the need to perform a careful and thorough endoscopic evaluation, with the use of biopsy of any concerning lesions, to rule out malignancy in patients with CD.

Conclusion

Crohn's disease isolated to the foregut is a rare condition, which more commonly manifests in association with contiguous involvement in the distal gastrointestinal tract. Crohn's disease-specific lesions are increasingly being identified with the use of upper endoscopy, and practitioners still debate when best to perform an endoscopic exam. Medical therapy continues to be the mainstay of management in the majority of patients who present with Crohn's disease involving the stomach, esophagus and/or duodenum; however surgeons still have a vital role. Surgical intervention for Crohn's disease of the foregut can be performed safely and with good outcomes, yet should be reserved for patients with severe complications and/or disease that is refractory to medical treatment.

References

[1] Reynolds HL, Stellato TA. Crohn's disease of the foregut. *Surg Clin N Am* 2001;81:117-135.

[2] Farmer RG, Whelan G, Fazio VW. Long-term follow-up of patients with Crohn's disease: relationship between the clinical pattern and prognosis. *Gastroenterology* 1985;88:1818-1825.

[3] Legge DA, Carlson HC, Judd ES. Roentgenologic features of regional enteritis of the upper gastrointestinal tract. *Am J Roentgenol* 1970;110:355-360.

[4] Nugent FW, Roy MA. Duodenal Crohn's disease: an analysis of 89 cases. *Am J Gastroenterol* 1989;84:861-862.

[5] Sandler RS, Golden AL. Epidemiology of Crohn's disease. *J Clin Gastroenterol* 1986;8:160-165.

[6] Tootla F, Lucas RJ, Bernacki EG, et al. Gastroduodenal Crohn's disease. *Arch Surg* 1980;111:855-857.

[7] Yamamoto T, Bain IM, Connolly AB, et al. Outcome of strictureplasty for duodenal Crohn's disease. *Br J Surg* 1999;86:259-262.

[8] Sakuraba A, Iwao Y, Matsuoka K, Naganuma M, Ogata H, Kanai T, Hibi T. Endoscopic and pathologic changes of the upper gastrointestinal tract in Crohn's disease. *BioMed Res Int* 2014;1-6.

[9] Turner D, Griffiths AM. Esophageal, gastric, and duodenal manifestations of IBD and the role of upper endoscopy in IBD diagnosis. *Curr Gastroenterol Rep* 2007;9:475-478.

[10] Annunziata ML, Caviglia R, Papparella LG, Cicala M. Upper gastrointestinal involvement of Crohn's disease: a prospective study on the role of upper endoscopy in the diagnostic work-up. *Dig Dis Sci* 2012;57:1618-1623.

[11] Horjus Talabur Horje CS, Meijer J, Rovers L, van Lochem EG, Groenen MJM, Wahab PJ. Prevalence of upper gastrointestinal lesions at primary diagnosis in adults with inflammatory bowel disease. *Inflamm Bowel Dis* 2016;22(08):1896–1901.

[12] Goodhand J, Dawson R, Hefferon M, et al. Inflammatory bowel disease in young people: the case for transitional clinics. *Inflamm Bowel Dis* 2010;16(06):947–952.

[13] Ammoury RF, Pfefferkorn MD. Significance of esophageal Crohn disease in children. *J Pediatr Gastroenterol Nutr* 2011;52(03): 291–294.

[14] Renault M, Goodier A, Subramony C, Hood B, Bishop P, Nowicki M. Age-related differences in granulomatous gastritis: a retrospective, clinicopathological analysis. *J Clin Pathol* 2010;63(04): 347–350.

[15] Lichtenstein, Gary R; Loftus, Edward V; Isaacs, Kim L; Regueiro, Miguel D; Gerson, Lauren B; Sands, Bruce E. ACG Clinical Guideline: Management of Crohn's Disease in Adults. *Am J Gastroenterol* 113(4):p 481-517, April 2018. | doi: 10.1038/ajg.2018.27.

[16] Dolgin SE. Surgical management of upper gastrointestinal and small bowel Crohn's disease. *Sem Ped Surg* 2007;16:172-177.

[17] Ruushka T, Vaajalahti P, Arajarvi P, et al. Prospective evaluation of upper gastrointestinal mucosal lesions in children with ulcerative colitis and Crohn's disease. *J Pediatr Gastrointest Nutr* 1994;19:181-186.

[18] Lenaerts C, Roy CC, Vaillancourt M, et al. High incidence of upper gastrointestinal tract involvement in children with Crohn disease. *Pediatrics* 1989;83:777-781.

[19] DeFelice KM, Katzka DA and Raffals LE. Crohn's disease of the esophagus: clinical features and treatment outcomes in the biological era. *Inflamm Bowel Dis*. 2015; 21: 2106-2113.

[20] Anton G, Decker G, Loftus EV, Pasha TM, Tremaine WJ, Sandborn WJ. Crohn's disease of the esophagus: clinical features and outcomes. *Inflamm Bowel Dis* 2001;7:113-119.

[21] Worsey MJ, Hull T, Ryland L, et al. Strictureplasty is an effective option in the operative management of duodenal Crohn's disease. Dis Colon Rectum 1999;42:596-600.

[22] Farmer RG, Hawk WA, Turnbull RB. Crohn's disease of the duodenum (transmural duodenitits): clinical manifestations, report of 11 cases. *Am J Dig Dis* 1972;17:191-198.

[23] Poggioli G, Stocchi L, Laureti S, et al. Duodenal involvement of Crohn's disease: three different clinicopathologic patterns. *Dis Colon Rectum* 1997;40:179-183.

[24] Shapiro M, Greenstein AJ, Bryn J, Corona J, Greenstein AJ, Salky B, Harris MT, Divino CM. Surgical management and outcomes of patients with duodenal Crohn's disease. *J Am Coll Surg* 2008;207:36-42.

[25] Podugu A, Tandon K, Castro FJ. Crohn's disease presenting as acute gastrointestinal hemorrhage. *World J Gastroenterol* 2016; 22(16):4073–4078.

[26] Jacobson IM, Schapiro RH, Warshaw AL. Gastric and duodenal fistulas in Crohn's disease. *Gastroenterology* 1985;89:1347-1352.

[27] Gschwantler M, Kogelbauer G, Klose W, et al. The pancreas as a site of granulomatous inflammation in Crohn's disease. *Gastroenterology* 1995;108:1246-1249.

[28] Omata F, Arakawa S, Takahashi H, et al. Crohn's disease associated with pancreatitis of unknown etiology: a case report. *Gastroenterol Jpn* 1993;28:420-423.

[29] Spiess SE, Braun M, Vogelzang RL, et al. Crohn's disease of the duodenum complicated by pancreatitis and common bile duct obstruction. *Am J Gastroenterol* 1992;87:1033-1036.

[30] Guellouz S, Pariente B, Benet C, Baudry C, Lourenco N, Kraemer A, Allez M, Gornet JM. Cephalic duodenopancreatectomy for hyperalgic duodenal Crohn's disease fistulized in the pancreatic gland. *Case Rep Gastroenterol* 2014;8:72-76.

[31] Foutch PG, Ferguson DR. Duodenal Crohn's disease complicated by common bile duct obstruction: report of a case and review of the literature. *Am J Gastroenterol* 1984;79:520-524.

[32] Post AB, van Stolk R, Broughan TA, et al. Crohn's disease of the gallbladder. *J Clin Gastroenterol* 1993;139-142.

[33] Wolters FL, Russel MG, Sijbrandij J, et al. Phenotype at diagnosis predicts recurrence rates in Crohn's disease. *Gut* 2006;55:1124-1130.

[34] Chow DK, Sung J, Yu JC, et al. Upper gastrointestinal tract phenotype of Crohn's disease is associated with early surgery and further hospitalization. *Inflamm Bowel Dis* 2009;15:551-557.

[35] Lazarev M, Huang C, Bitton A, Cho JH, Duerr RH, McGovern DP, Proctor DD, Regueiro M, Rioux JD, Schumm PP, Taylor KD, Silverberg MS, Steinhart AH, Hutfless S, Brant SR. Relationship between proximal Crohn's disease location and disease behavior and surgery: a cross-sectional study of the IBD genetics consortium. *Am J Gastroenterol* 2013;108:106-112.

[36] Farman J, Faegenburg D, Dallemand S, et al. Crohn's disease of the stomach: the "ram's horn" sign. *Am J Roentgenol* 1975;123:242-251.

[37] Thompson WM, Cockrill H, Rice RP. Regional enteritis of the duodenum. *Am J Roentgenol* 1975;123:252-261.

[38] Silverberg MS, Satsangi J, Ahmad T, et al. Toward an integrated clinical, molecular and serological classification of inflammatory bowel disease: report of a working party of the 2005 Montreal World Congress of Gastroenterology. *Can J Gastroenterol* 2005;19:5-36.

[39] Odashima M, Otaka M, Jin M, Horikawa Y, Matsuhashi T, Ohba R, Koizumi S, Kinoshita N, Takahashi T, Watanabe S. Successful treatment of refractory duodenal Crohn's disease with infliximab. *Dig Dis Sci* 2007;52:31-32.

[40] Karaoglu AO, Yukselen V. Obstructing Crohn's disease of the duodenum: is surgery always mandatory? *Int J Clin Pract* 2004;58:221-223.

[41] Anderson JM. Treatment of espophageal strictures with intralesional steroids. *Gastrointest Endosc* 1995;41:333.

[42] 42.Tamboer C, Verhamme M, Dhondt E, et al. Endoscopic treatment of stenosis in recurrent Crohn's disease with balloon dilation combined with local corticosteroid injection. *Gastrointest Endosc* 1995;42:252-255.

[43] Rupp T, Earle D, Dick P, et al. Randomized trial of dilation plus intralesional steroids vs dilation alone for benign gastroesophageal strictures. *Gastrointest Endosc* 1993;39:287.

[44] Korelitz BI, Adler DJ, Mendelsohn RA, Sacknoff AL. Long-term experience with 6-mercaptopurine in the treatment of Crohn's disease. *Am J Gastroenterol* 1993;88(08):1198–1205.

[45] Griffiths AM, Alemayehu E, Sherman P. Clinical features of gastroduodenal Crohn's disease in adolescents. *J Pediatr Gastroenterol Nutr* 1989;8(02):166–171.

[46] Nugent FW, Richmond M, Park SK. Crohn's disease of the duodenum. *Gut* 1977;18(02):115–120.

[47] Miehsler W, Püspök A, Oberhuber T, Vogelsang H. Impact of different therapeutic regimens on the outcome of patients with Crohn's disease of the upper gastrointestinal tract. *Inflamm Bowel Dis* 2001;7(02):99–105.

[48] Zhang, J., Qian, X., Zhu, L. et al. Clinical outcomes of serial endoscopic balloon dilation for duodenal Crohn's disease-associated strictures. *Surg Endosc* 38, 4512–4520 (2024). https://doi.org/10.1007/s00464-024-10992-8.

[49] Howden FM, Mills LR, Rubin J. Crohn's disease of the esophagus. *Am Surg* 1994;60:656-660.

[50] Dyer NH, Cook PL, Harper RA. Oesophageal stricture associated with Crohn's disease. *Gut* 1969;10:549-554.

[51] Ingle SB, Pujari GP, Patle YG, Nagoba BS. An unusual case of Crohn's disease with isolated gastric involvement. *J Crohn's Colitis* 2011;5:69-70.

[52] Ingle SB, Hinge CR, Dakhure S, Bhosale SS. Isolated gastric Crohn's disease. *World J Clin Cases* 2013;1:71-73.

[53] Ghahremani GG, Gore RM, Breuer RI, et al. Esophageal manifestations of Crohn's disease. *Gastrointest Radiol* 1982;7:199-203.

[54] Yamamamoto T. The role of strictureplasty in the surgical management of duodenal Crohn's disease. *J Crohn's Colitis* 2013;7:237.

[55] Yamamoto T, Fazio VW, Tekkis PP. Safety and efficacy of strictureplasty for Crohn's disease: a systematic review and meta-analysis. *Dis Colon Rectum* 2007;50:1968-1986.

[56] Moon JS, Lee JL, Yu CS, et al. Clinical Characteristics and Postoperative Outcomes of Patients Presenting With Upper Gastrointestinal Tract Crohn Disease. *Ann Coloproctol* 2020;36(4):243-248.

[57] Yang L, Wu G, Wu Q, et al. Surgical Management of Duodenal Crohn's Disease. *World J Gastrointest Surg* 2023;15(6):1159-1168.

[58] Collier PE, Turowski P, Diamond DL. Small intestinal adenocarcinoma complicating regional enteritis. *Cancer* 1985;55:516-521.

[59] Fresko D, Lazarus S, Dotan J, et al. Early presentation of carcinoma of the small bowel in Crohn's disease: case reports and review of the literature. *Gastroenterology* 1982;7:199-203.
[60] Greenstein AJ, Sachar DB, Smith H, et al. A comparison of cancer risk in Crohn's disease and ulcerative colitis. *Cancer* 1980;46:403-407.
[61] Greenstein AJ, Sachar DB, Smith H, et al. A comparison of cancer risk in Crohn's disease and ulcerative colitis. *Cancer* 1981;48:2742-2745.
[62] Guye SN, Prior P, McCartney JL, et al. Malignancy in Crohn's disease. *Gut* 1980;21:1024-1029.
[63] Hawker PC, Guge SN, Thompson H, et al. Adenocarcinoma of the small intestine complicating Crohn's disease. *Gut* 1982;23:188-193.
[64] Meiselman MS, Ghahremani GG, Kaufman MW. Crohn's disease of the duodenum complicated by adenocarcinoma. *Gastrointest Radiol* 1987;12:333-336.
[65] Traube J, Simpson S, Riddel RH, et al. Crohn's disease and adenocarcinoma of the bowel. *Dig Dis Sci* 1980;25:939-944.

Chapter 9

Small Bowel Surgery

Brady A. Campbell[1], MD, MPH
Stephen M. Kavic[2], MD, MSHPE
and Rebecca F. Brown[2,*], MD
[1]University of Maryland Medical Center, Baltimore, Maryland, USA
[2]University of Maryland School of Medicine, Baltimore, Maryland, USA

Abstract

While the terminal ileum is the most frequently involved portion of the intestine in patients with Crohn's disease, it is more difficult to discern the relative frequency of isolated small bowel involvement in this disease. Stricturing disease is commonly encountered, and we review both the pathophysiology as well as the major techniques of resection and strictureplasty. An algorithm for penetrating disease is also presented, including strategies for the operative management of fistulizing disease. As with other portions of the GI tract, multi-disciplinary care is paramount to optimal outcomes. However, the surgeon plays a central role in the management of complicated small bowel disease, especially in cases of obstruction, perforation, and fistulization.

Introduction

An estimated 75% of Crohn's patients ultimately require surgery, with as many as 50% of patients needing operative intervention within ten years of their diagnosis [1]. Many patients present with small bowel involvement, where the terminal ileum is the most common site of disease. Resection of the terminal ileum necessarily involves the cecum, and there is some overlap between colectomy and small intestinal resection that increases the difficulty of interpreting the literature. In this chapter, we will examine the disease patterns that may necessitate small bowel surgery in Crohn's disease (CD), discuss major surgical approaches to management of stricturing and penetrating presentations, and discuss preoperative and postoperative considerations for management of this complicated patient population.

* Corresponding Author's Email: rfbrown@som.umaryland.edu

In: Surgery for Crohn's Disease. Second Edition
Editors: Stephen M. Kavic, Rebecca Brown and Kerri Lopez
ISBN: 979-8-89530-676-5

Location

Approximately one third of patients with a diagnosis of CD have isolated small bowel involvement, while another one third will have ileocolonic or terminal ileal disease [2]. The remaining third typically present with colitis, which is discussed in another chapter in this text. Terminal ileal predominance accounts for the classical presentation of Crohn's obstruction requiring surgery, secondary to stricturing disease at the terminal ileum [3].

Duodenal involvement is the least common small bowel location, found in fewer than 5% of patients. Duodenal disease generally manifests with gastric outlet obstruction. Unlike terminal ileal disease, which often requires resection, the primary treatment remains immunosuppression into the late stages of disease [4]. Once the symptoms can no longer be controlled, a bypass of the diseased segment (gastro-jejunostomy or duodeno-jejunostomy) should be considered.

Isolated jejunal disease is also extremely rare, with estimates ranging from 1% of isolated jejunal disease [5], to 10% for jejunal-ileal disease [6, 7] Jejunal disease is notably difficult to diagnose as well, due to the inaccessibility of endoscopy. In the largest series of jejunal CD, Tonelli found combined resection and strictureplasty was the most common treatment required [8].

Preoperative Considerations

Prior to an elective operation for CD, the first consideration is the determination of medical management of the patient. Medical management should be initiated and/or optimized to determine if symptomatic control without surgical intervention is possible. However, some patients will desire or require a surgical reset – like those with fibrostenotic disease would have little to no improvement with anti-inflammatory medications or systemic therapies. However, the optimal management of Crohn's disease is multi-disciplinary, and the surgeon should not hesitate to be integrally involved in the consideration of early surgical intervention as part of the multi-faceted approach to management for these patients.

Once the decision to operate has been made, each patient should be optimized for surgery. Patients will require general anesthesia, and guidelines for cardiac workup before invasive procedures have been well established [9]. Routine assessment includes basic laboratory studies (CBC, CMP, and coagulation studies), chest radiograph and electrocardiogram (EKG) in most patients. It is our practice to type and screen all patients undergoing intestinal resection.

Most patients with CD have a thorough history of localizing studies, of which a CT scans are the most useful to assist in localization and the diagnosis of complex CD [9] It is mandatory that the surgeon review the preoperative imaging, and to repeat studies if there has been a substantial interval between imaging and operation.

Perhaps the most important perioperative factor to consider, specific to Crohn's patients, is overall nutrition status. Often, patients with CD are significantly malnourished, due to poor oral intake, malabsorption, systemic inflammation, and medication side effects. Optimizing preoperative nutrition is critical for postoperative wound healing, particularly if a primary bowel anastomosis is constructed. It has been demonstrated in elective colorectal resections that anastomotic dehiscence is associated with hypoalbuminemia (<3.5 g/dL) [10, 11]. Enteral nutritional support is preferred to optimize preoperative nutrition.

Though CD patients may have a broad spectrum of nutritional deficiencies, components including an elemental diet and omega-3 fatty acids have been advocated by some to promote ease of digestion and prevent proinflammatory leukotriene and prostaglandin generation, respectively [10, 12-14]. A course of total parenteral nutrition prior to surgery of at least 2-4 weeks is also recommended by some for nutritional repletion prior to elective surgery, though the risk/benefit ratio of this intervention has not been demonstrated [15, 16].

Preoperative management of immunosuppressive agents is constantly evolving. Generally, biologic regimens can be safely continued or stopped just prior to surgery [17], while chronic steroid use necessitates continued perioperative use. The concept of stress dose steroids to prevent adrenal insufficiency remains highly debated. This has also not been studied specifically in the Crohn's population, so individual assessments should be made for each patient. Historically, stress dose steroids have been implemented when patients are treated with ≥ 10mg per day of prednisone (or an equivalent) for 3 months. For large intestinal surgery, a regimen of the patient's pre-operative dose, plus 25 mg of hydrocortisone at induction, and 100 mg of hydrocortisone/day for 2-3 days is utilized [3, 18]. In the elective setting, a standard preoperative antibiotic regimen determined by an institutional antibiogram, should be administered. In the setting of an emergent operation, generally for perforating disease, a broader regimen should be considered perioperatively.

In small bowel surgery for CD, a bowel preparation regimen is not recommended. There is no evidence to suggest a bowel preparation mitigates postoperative complications. However, if there is suspected terminal ileal disease and a colonic anastomosis is expected, surgeons should consider a bowel prep on an individualized basis.

Disease Patterns

Fibrostenotic Disease of the Small Bowel

The most frequent indication for surgery in CD patients is obstructing disease, which includes fibrostenotic pathology [19]. Obstructing disease in Crohn's patients is thought to develop from the progressive wall thickening subsequent to recurrent bouts of inflammation. Once progressed to a fibrostenotic level and the luminal diameter is narrowed, it does not respond well to medical management as the benefits of minimizing inflammation dwindle (Figure 9.1). Additionally, medically refractory obstruction may arise from neoplasms or other inflammatory masses such as a phlegmon or abscess [20].

Duodenal Obstruction

Duodenal involvement in CD is relatively rare, occurring in less than 5% of patients [21]. The proximal duodenum is the most common location for duodenal CD, followed by the descending portion [22]. Obstruction due to stricturing is the most common presentation, with symptoms typical of proximal obstruction - abdominal pain, nausea, vomiting, and early satiety [23].

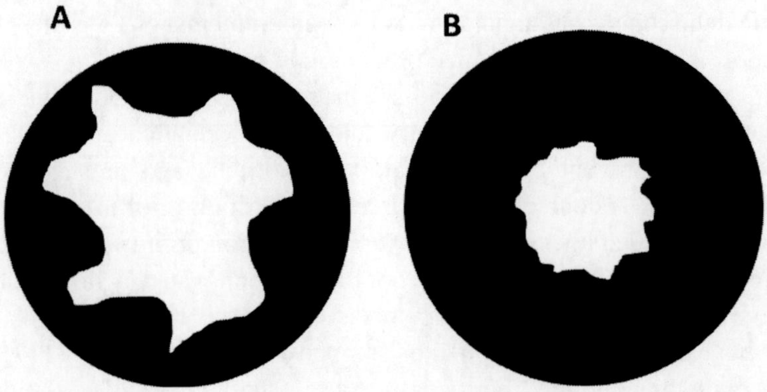

Figure 9.1. Inflammation of the intestine, in cross-section. A: Normal wall, moderate inflammation. In this setting, anti-inflammatory management will restore the luminal diameter of the intestine. B: Thickened wall, minimal inflammation. In the advanced state, medical management will have minimal effect on the lumen, and the patient will require surgical intervention for clinical relief.

Diagnosis of small bowel disease is typically made by upper gastrointestinal series or esophagogastroduodenoscopy (EGD). Early stenotic disease may show thickening and blunting of mucosal folds, cobblestoning, or erosions. Progression of stenotic disease may lead to scarring and fibrosis of the bowel segment. More characteristically, deep linear ulcerations with opposing wall sacculations are seen [24-26]. Often time, duodenal involvement is suggested with CT findings, which may include signs of gastric outlet obstruction, duodenal mural thickening, hyperemia of the mucosa, soft tissue stranding as well as sites of extra-duodenal inflammation, which is later confirmed on EGD [25].

Although initial management should include multidisciplinary care and early optimization of medical therapy, including antacid and anti-inflammatory medications such as steroids and biologic agents [21], surgical intervention is eventually required in up to 90% of these patients [22]. In the face of duodenal obstruction, the surgeon is faced with two options: bypass or strictureplasty. Duodenal resection is typically avoided due to high morbidity and mortality, although partial duodenectomy or formal pancreaticoduodenectomy may be required in special cases [26].

Surgical options for duodenal bypass include gastrojejunostomy, gastroduodenostomy, and Roux-en-Y-gastrojejunostomy. Strictureplasty, on the other hand, allows for restoration of the constricted lumen throughout the affected portion of bowel. The operative technique for stricureplasty is based on the length of strictured segment and is described in detail later in this chapter. However, duodenal strictureplasty is often quite difficult, as the mobilization required to perform appropriate stricureplasty is often difficult to extensive inflammation inherent to CD. The complexity is further increased due to the retroperitoneal location and proximity to sensitive vascular and pancreaticobiliary structures[26]. Currently, there is no high-level evidence supporting one technique over the other.

Jejunoileal Obstruction

Up to 10% of CD patients are affected by diffuse jejunoileal disease, with obstruction being the most common indication for surgical intervention. Generally, several strictures develop, and the series of strictures leads to chronic, high-grade obstruction that presents as postprandial cramping, nausea and vomiting [6]. This condition can progress to complete obstruction, for which surgery is mandatory. In jejunoileal obstruction, multiple tight strictures are often present, transforming the bowel into alternating saccular segments and tight strictures. This pathology does not simply cause classic obstructive symptoms - the stagnation that occurs in these saccular segments can also lead to bacterial overgrowth, leading to diarrhea, malabsorption, and nutrient deficiency as well [6].

Surgical intervention is warranted when medical management fails, when the obstruction becomes complete, or when acute sepsis develops. Treatment selection has varied over time, but a recent systematic review and meta-analysis favors bowel resection over strictureplasty in fibrostenotic CD [27]. Importantly, if short bowel syndrome is a concern, strictureplasty should remain the operation of choice. The surgical approach to strictureplasty is discussed in detail later in this chapter.

Terminal Ileal Obstruction

Chronic obstruction in the terminal ileal and ileocecal region is the most common indication for operative intervention in CD [28]. Traditionally, ileocecectomy with ileal-ascending colon anastomosis was performed for this condition. The terminal ileum is often the most aggressive site of CD, with inflamed bowel walls, friable hemorrhagic mucosa, and deep ulcerations [29]. As such, there has been a hesitancy to preserve the ileocecal region in these patients. In addition, the ileocecal valve itself may be involved in the inflammatory process, complicating local repair options.

However, strictureplasty of the terminal ileal and ileocecal region is possible. Strictureplasty, primarily of the Finney type (see section on Strictureplasty), has demonstrated no difference relative to ileocecectomy in ten-year outcomes and clinical relapse of terminal ileitis [29]. Terminal ileal strictureplasty remains a viable alternative to segmental resection.

For bowel resection, the primary considerations are the margin resection and anastomotic technique. In ileocecal resection for CD, randomized controlled data have demonstrated no benefit with respect to recurrence rates between a limited resection (2cm margins from macroscopic disease) and an extended resection (12cm margins from macroscopic disease), several years postoperatively [30]. Therefore, radical resection is currently not recommended, particularly as bowel conservation is a fundamental component of surgical intervention in patients with small bowel disease [21].

There is limited quality data comparing stapled vs. hand-sewn, and end-to-end or side-to-side anastomosis after ileocecectomy in CD [31]. Reports from the late 1990s retrospectively examined whether there was a difference in outcomes in stapled vs. sutured end-to-end anastomoses. These studies suggested that a stapled technique was associated with fewer complications and less recurrent disease at the anastomotic site [32, 33]. A 2004 study suggested that recurrent disease was less frequent in patients with stapled and hand-sewn side-to-side anastomoses relative to those constructed using stapled end-to-side technique [34]. McLeod, in 2009, published the first multicenter randomized controlled data assessing the influence of anastomotic type on recurrence of disease. It was found that disease recurrence rates were similar between end-to-end and side-to-side ileocolic anastomoses in patients who underwent ileocecectomy for CD [35]. Overall, the literature appears to favor stapling anastomoses over hand-sewing [36]. However, until high-level, validated evidence emerges, ileocolic anastomosis is recommended in a way that the surgeon is most comfortable.

Penetrating Disease of the Small Bowel

Penetrating CD, typically due to full thickness inflammation, can broadly be broken into fistulous or perforating disease. Notably, perforating disease typically includes abscess formation. A fistula is an abnormal epithelialized connection between two organs and is one of the most common complications of penetrating CD, occurring in 30-40% of patients. The interested reader is directed to an excellent review on the process of fistula formation in CD, reported by Scharl and Rogler in 2014 [37]. In active CD, full thickness inflammation promotes the creation of pathologic fistulae either to nearby intestine and contained completely within the alimentary tract (around 25%) [38], or between a portion of the alimentary tract and a nearby organ such as the skin (around 6%) [39], bladder (up to 8%) or vagina [40]. Fistulae often develop at sites of active disease, however, one-fourth of fistulae in Crohn's patients form at anastomotic sites from previous bowel resection [38]. Internal fistulae, those that form between two internal organs, can often remain subclinical. External fistulae, in which there is a fistulous tract with the skin, are easier to identify.

Internal Fistulae

In CD, a segment of the small bowel, upon becoming inflamed, can form an inflammatory adhesion and ultimately fistulize with another segment of bowel. The ileum is the most common site of active inflammation in the small bowel, and it is therefore by far the most common segment of small bowel involved in internal fistulae formation. Most frequently and likely due to proximity, the target organ for fistulization is the sigmoid colon, however, ileocecal fistulae and ileoenteric fistulae are common as well. Small bowel fistula formation can occur without ileal involvement, although this is rare. Gastrocolic and duodenocolic fistulae have been reported in small case series [41].

An inflamed portion of small bowel, the ileum in 64% of cases [40, 41], fistulizes with an additional segment of small bowel, is also common. Entero-enteric was the most frequent type of fistula observed in a cohort of Japanese CD patients [42]. In addition, the small bowel can internally fistulize with a solid organ outside of the alimentary tract. In up to 8% of CD patients, fistulae between bowel and the urinary system (ureter and bladder) can form spontaneously. With involvement in 64% of cases, the ileum is the most common segment of bowel involved in these fistulae [40, 41].

Diagnosis of Small Bowel Fistula

Since they are often subclinical, internal fistulae of the small bowel can develop and progress without overt signs and symptoms. Typically, it is only recognized late in the process when septic or obstructive symptoms necessitate diagnostic imaging [43]. The most common presenting symptoms for internal fistulae involving the small bowel are abdominal pain and diarrhea, although fever from abscess formation is seen as well. In one classic series of patients, up to 25% of CD patients with fistula are diagnosed intraoperatively, or on pathologic examination of the resected specimen [44]. Cross-sectional imaging (CT or MRI) or contrast studies will illustrate a fistula. In practice, the severe inflammation present often masks the small aperture of the fistula, and it may only be diagnosed intraoperatively.

Enterovesical fistulae in CD are almost always ileovesical. Both urinary and gastrointestinal symptoms may bring attention to the diagnosis, perhaps even as the first clinical manifestation of the patient's CD. Reported in over half of patients with enterovesical fistulae, pneumaturia is the most common presenting symptom. Although pneumaturia may be an uncommon clinical sign, it is pathognomonic for this disorder.

Dysuria, fecaluria, suprapubic pain and recurrent urinary tract infections (UTI), generally due to *Escherichia coli*, are common symptoms as well. When suspected, diagnostic confirmation of the fistula is necessary, particularly for surgical planning. Imaging techniques used in the case of a suspected enterovesical fistula. These include cystoscopy, colonoscopy, the "poppy seed" test, transabdominal ultrasonography, computerized tomography, magnetic resonance imaging, barium enema, and a cystogram. In the poppy seed test, a few grams of poppy seeds are ingested orally. If there is a significant fistula, then the seeds pass through and are visible in the urine.

Although each modality has its own advantages and disadvantages, Golabek proposed an optimized diagnostic imaging algorithm after a best evidence examination of the literature. Once clinically suspected, both transabdominal ultrasound and the "Poppy seed" test are performed. If these tests are negative, but fistula is still suspected, CT/MRI imaging and cystoscopy with biopsy are undertaken[45]. Sigmoidoscopy may demonstrate the enteral side of the fistula; cystoscopy can show the bladder side.

Management of Small Bowel Fistula

Enterocutaneous Fistulae

Enterocutaneous fistulae (ECF) in CD can be a significant management challenge. These fistulae generally develop after a previous bowel resection and are classically ileocutaneous. In the early postoperative setting, ECF can present 7-10 days postoperatively due to anastomotic breakdown. If an ECF presents in a delayed fashion, typically after two weeks postoperatively, it may be attributed to a previously contained anastomotic leak [43]. They are initially managed with skin care, as well as nutritional support. Sepsis is the most common cause of mortality from ECF.

A fistula is considered high-output if its output is greater than 500 milliliters (mL) per 24 hours, and in these cases, supplemental parenteral nutrition is often needed to avoid malnutrition. Multiple methods may be used to reduce fistula output, including restriction of hypo-osmolar fluids, consumption of electrolytes with high concentrations of glucose and sodium, anti-secretory agents (e.g., proton pump inhibitors, octreotide) and anti-motility agents (e.g., loperamide) [38]. ECF may close spontaneously or with the assistance of anti-secretory medications, however, if medical management has not promoted fistula closure after two months, surgical treatment with ECF resection is often required.

Prior to surgical treatment of ECF, it is imperative that the patient is nutritionally optimized, managed with skin care, and has intestinal anatomy defined. Cross sectional imaging, most commonly CT imaging, is useful to help delineate anatomy, but an upper GI contrast study with small bowel follow-through or magnetic resonance enterography are both appropriate choices as well.

While not a complication of CD *per se*, peri-ileostomy cutaneous fistulae can form after the initial resection. Early postoperative peri-stomal fistulae develop due to excess tension placed on sutures between the abdominal fascia and bowel serosa, leading to bowel injury and subsequent fistulization with the skin. This complication begets another operation in which the ileostomy must be further exteriorized, and a second stoma allowed to mature [43]. However, fistulizing CD may also develop in the stoma, which likely represents disease relapse rather than a technical misadventure.

Enteroenteric Fistula

An internal fistula involving the ileum or other small bowel region does not represent an indication for surgery; rather, deleterious sequela from the fistula must be present. Malabsorption, diarrhea, malnutrition, and bacterial overgrowth can occur if the fistulous tract that forms between two segments of bowel creates an intestinal bypass [39]. Internal fistula can also exteriorize, becoming enterocutaneous in nature. As previously discussed, ECF is associated with a high risk of malnutrition and septic complications and is an indication for eventual surgical treatment [43]. Finally, the presence of an abscess related to an intra-abdominal fistula is associated with a high-risk for progression to sepsis or obstruction, often necessitating surgical intervention after initial control of the inflammatory process.

While surgical management is often eventually indicated due to persistent symptoms of infectious complications, medical therapy is the first line treatment of non-acute small bowel fistulous CD [39]. While isolated enteroenteric fistulae can generally be managed medically, 40% of patients will require surgery by one year, and an additional 33% will undergo surgical intervention within 9 years [3]. In surgical repair of internal fistulae involving the small bowel, the inflamed segment (usually ileal) is excised with either diversion or primary anastomosis. When the small bowel segment fistulizes with the sigmoid, it is often the practice of surgeons to primarily close the fistulous opening in the "innocent bystander" sigmoid, rather than resecting it, assuring there is minimal inflammation of the colon. It is worth paying scrupulous attention to the character of the sigmoid colon, as suturing inflamed bowel may lead to a high rate of failure with subsequent leak, abscess, or sepsis.

Enterovesical Fistula

Enterovesical fistulae due to CD require prompt evaluation and management, due to the potential development of recurrent urinary tract infection (UTI) and resultant urosepsis. Once recognized, the first line of management is often medical. Consistent with general management of CD, initial medical management with sulfasalazine, corticosteroids, 6-mercaptopurine and antibiotics such as metronidazole is often used [3, 46]. In addition, bowel rest with total parenteral nutrition and urethral catheter drainage is recommended for conservative management.

The role of TNF-alpha monoclonal antibodies in fistulizing small bowel disease is not clear, with some studies showing superior fistula closure rates [47], while others reserve it for second line therapy after surgery [45]. The goal of medical therapy is to reduce inflammation while preventing recurrent UTIs, allowing for the fistula tract to heal spontaneously. However, a majority of patients (up to 80%) will have persistent or recurrent symptoms, necessitating a surgical repair of the enterovesical fistula [47].

The goal of operative management of enterovesical fistulae is to resect the involved small bowel segment and close the resultant cystostomy. The small bowel is typically re-anastomosed. The bladder repair may be endoscopic, open, or laparoscopic.

Laparoscopic repair of ileovesical fistula is currently the most frequent approach. In the majority of cases, the resection can be done with a primary re-anastomosis of bowel segments. The bowel is bluntly dissected off the bladder wall. The bladder is then infused with a methylene blue solution via a Foley catheter if the hole is not clearly visible. Once identified, the vesicular injury is then oversewn in one or two layers. Although some cystotomies have been left to heal spontaneously once divided from the fistula, it is our practice to attempt primary closure [45]. Some authors have advocated interposing an omental flap between the bladder and bowel, as the high vascularity may promote healing, however, high-level evidence for this technique still lacks [45, 48].

In turning the attention to the bowel, the fistulous segment should be resected. If deemed feasible, primary re-anastomosis should be attempted. A two-stage procedure is recommended in cases where the pathology or operation led to gross contamination of the abdomen with bowel contents, or a large abdominopelvic abscess is noted [45]. A temporary diverting ileostomy can be constructed, with closure of the colon (Hartmann's pouch), and re-anastomosis can be done in delayed fashion. While definitive surgical management of enterovesical fistulae is often quite successful, there is a risk of recurrence, in addition to other postoperative complications including abscess formation, enterocutaneous fistula development at the anastomotic site, and anastomotic failure.

Anti-TNF Alpha Biologic Therapy in Fistulous Disease

An integral component of the medical treatment of fistulizing CD is the use of chimeric monoclonal antibodies, or human monoclonal antibodies against tumor necrosis factor alpha (TNF-alpha). The best known in this class are infliximab or adalimumab. Briefly, TNF-alpha is a proinflammatory cytokine implicated in the pathogenesis of CD. In 2002, the ACCENT I trial demonstrated that intermittent infliximab infusion therapy helped maintain remission of CD for the duration of the study (54 weeks) and allowed patients to discontinue corticosteroid use [49]. In 2004, the ACCENT II trial showed that infliximab infusion promoted and maintained closure of externally draining fistulae in CD, with an acceptable safety profile [50]. This led to FDA approval of infliximab for the treatment of fistulizing CD, and its clinical use has since been extended to treat various other manifestations.

While there has been a small amount of literature suggesting superior fistula closure rates in small bowel fistulae with anti-TNF therapy [47], surgery remains the first line treatment once a patient becomes symptomatic. Anti-TNF use as a maintenance agent after a bowel resection is not clear either. In the case of enterovesical fistulae, there is no consensus on the use of anti-TNF therapy currently.

Small Bowel Perforation

CD associated small bowel perforations are often sequelae of bowel microperforations due to chronic inflammation inherent to CD and can present as abscesses or free perforation. When perforations are present with penetrating disease, it has been shown to portend more frequent future abdominal operations, faster clinical symptomatic recurrence, and a higher immunosuppression requirement [51]. Small bowel perforations due to CD lead to more complex procedures, longer inpatient hospital stays, and increased likelihood of needing temporary fecal diversion with ileostomy [52].

Crohn's Related Abscess

Abscesses occur in 10-30% of CD patients and are most common between the ages of 20-30 [53, 54]. Often, abscesses in CD are formed at sites of prior bowel anastomoses. However, as many as half of abscesses in Crohn's patients are spontaneous and form due to microperforations in diseased segments of bowel, usually in the ileocecal region [53].

Several mechanisms have been proposed for abscess development. The first, and most common, involves transmural inflammation with fistulization to contiguous tissues, allowing for the direct spread of pathogenic bacteria. Second, diseased bowel can disseminate bacteria hematogenously, leading to intra-abdominal seeding. Finally, at the time of operation, peritoneal contamination with bowel contents can lead to a postoperative abscess [55]. The complex interactions between the bacteria and host lead to accumulation of neutrophils and the fibrin encasement of the abscess. The abscesses are generally polymicrobial, with *Escherichia coli* and *Enterococcus* as the most common aerobes, and *Bacteroidis fragilis* and *Peptostreptococcus* as the most common anaerobes [56].

Diagnosis of Intra-Abdominal Abscess

The diagnosis of abscess is generally suspected in a patient with CD who presents with fever or a new abdominal mass. CD associated complications such as fistulae and stricture are often present and can be assessed by using an enterography protocol with imaging. When prospectively compared, MR and CT enterography showed no difference in sensitivity, however, image quality was higher with CT [57]. Nonetheless, approximately 10% of abscesses remain clinically unsuspected, and are diagnosed intraoperatively for refractory disease [54].

Management of Crohn's Related Abscesses

Classically, Crohn's related abscesses required surgical drainage, however, trends in management have shifted toward percutaneous drainage and/or the use of medical management [56, 58]. Immunosuppressive therapy management in the face of septic complications presents a challenge. The clinician wants to pursue mutually exclusive goals: to preserve immune function to deal with infection, but also suppress the immune response to minimize intestinal inflammation. Usually, in the acute setting, the management of infection trumps the management of inflammation.

Initial management of a spontaneous abscess, regardless of size, location, immunosuppression regimen or associated fistula, involves treatment with a broad-spectrum antibiotic regimen. Appropriate regimens include ticarcillin-clavulanate, ertapenem or moxifloxacin as monotherapy, or dual therapy with metronidazole and a fluoroquinolone (ciprofloxacin or levofloxacin) or an appropriate cephalosporin (i.e., cefazolin, ceftriaxone or cefuroxime). As indicated in Figure 9.2, after initiation of treatment with antibiotics, an abscess <3 cm can be observed for a short course, with a recommended repeat imaging study 4-6 weeks after initial diagnosis assuming no clinical deterioration. For those with abscesses >3 cm, an associated fistula, or on steroids, percutaneous drainage under radiologic guidance is indicated. If the abscess persists, a resection of the offending bowel region is indicated. If the abscess resolves, immunosuppression therapy can be safely resumed [56]. The duration and severity of symptoms typically give some indication of the success of purely medical management.

Percutaneous drainage has become much more common, with a 2007 report of 3,296 hospitalizations for intraabdominal abscesses in patients with CD finding that approximately 39% were treated medically, 29% with percutaneous drainage, and 32% with surgery, representing a greater than fourfold increase in the use of percutaneous drainage since 1998 [58]. Percutaneous abscess drainage is typically performed by interventional radiologists, and can be done under ultrasonographic, CT or fluoroscopic guidance. Typically, catheters are between 8 and 16 French, and require daily flushing with saline to maintain patency. In clinically improving patients, catheters can be removed when drainage is between 10-20 mL/d, however, if there are persistent signs and symptoms of infection, reimaging may be indicated to assess the placement of the catheter while looking for another potential focus of infection. Conversely, persistently high-output (>50 mL/day) from a percutaneous drain may indicate a contrast study through the catheter. Upon injection of contrast, the small bowel can then be assessed for fistulization using X-ray [59].

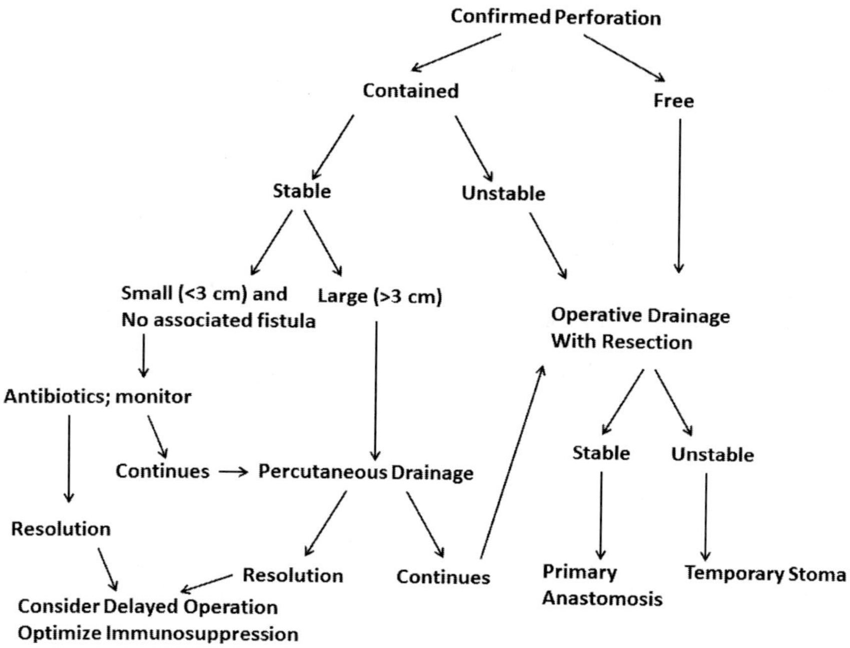

Figure 9.2. A suggested management algorithm for perforation of the small bowel, adapted in part from Feagins LA, et al., (2011) Clinical gastroenterology and hepatology: the official clinical practice journal of the American Gastroenterological Association 9:842-850.

Percutaneous drainage has a very high success rate, particularly when there is not an associated fistula. Although delayed interval resection of the diseased segment is often required, an initial percutaneous approach is more successful in allowing for a primary re-anastomosis at the time of surgery, rather than temporary diversion [10, 56]. Repeated studies have demonstrated that an interval resection following percutaneous drainage allows for an easier operation, with increased likelihood of primary re-anastomosis [60, 61]. Furthermore, one study demonstrated that two-thirds of abscesses treated percutaneously may not require surgery for at least one year [55]. For recurrent abscesses, repeated percutaneous drainage is often attempted, however, ultimately, they may need to be drained surgically. This operation involves thorough irrigation and debridement of the abscess cavity, followed by an en-bloc bowel resection [56]. Notably, studies assessing optimal management of recurrent spontaneous abscess in CD are lacking.

Free Perforation

The most morbid presentation of penetrating disease results from a free perforation into the abdominal cavity. Spontaneous free perforations of the small intestine can be caused by many conditions, including trauma, infections, neoplasms, drugs, vascular disease or, as with CD, immune-mediated or inflammatory conditions [62]. Unlike an abscess, which is walled off or contained due to a retroperitoneal location or a closed space, a free perforation usually presents with generalized peritonitis and requires emergent surgical intervention. Fortunately, in CD, free perforation is quite rare, estimated to be less than 2%, though higher in Asian populations [62, 63]. The most common location for free perforation is in the ileum, though jejunal and duodenal perforations are also seen. Importantly, they may herald the presence of a CD-induced neoplasm such as an adenocarcinoma or lymphoma [62].

Diagnosis of Free Perforation

In a stable patient with suspected free perforation, obtaining a plain film of the abdomen is performed concomitantly with resuscitation and initiation of broad-spectrum antibiosis. However, the lack of pneumoperitoneum on plain film should not exclude free perforation. Free air is only present in 20% of perforations in CD patients, and this percentage may be even lower in ileal disease [64]. If the patient is unstable, or free air is present, the patient is then promptly taken to the operating room for emergent exploration. After thorough examination of the small bowel, resection is performed in almost all cases of perforated jejunoileal disease, followed by primary re-anastomosis or construction of a temporary ileostomy, and thorough irrigation of the abdomen [62, 65]. In the rarer case of a gastroduodenal perforation, debridement and primary repair is recommended [64].

Management of Free Perforation

The choice of diversion, in the form of an ileostomy, has traditionally been a function of the location of perforation, the hemodynamic stability of the patient, and the length of time since presentation. In extreme cases, resection without anastomosis, leaving the GI tract in discontinuity with temporary abdominal closure, may be prudent. In these cases, return to the operating room for definitive anastomosis or stoma formation should follow the index operation within 48 hours. All patients should prudently be started on antibiotic therapy as well, with initial broad-spectrum coverage, until more definitive source control is obtained.

Ultimately initial decisions for management of Crohn's related perforations are dictated by the clinical presentation, with a good clinical algorithm located in Figure 9.2.

Operative Considerations and Technique

General Considerations

In any operation for CD, the full length of the small bowel should be examined and described in the operative note. As it is a transmural process, the extent of CD is defined by visual inspection of the bowel. Palpation of the mesenteric margin of the bowel wall is another key indicator of the extent of disease, and once the mesenteric border of the intestine is easily palpable, normal intestine has been reached [3].

The majority of patients (70-90%) with small bowel CD will require an operation at some point in their clinical course [66]. Patients with acute perforation, or those with short segmental disease, are typically appropriate candidates for segmental resection. Generally, resection of up to half of the small bowel length is well tolerated, unless the ileocecal valve is not left intact

[67]. Normally, enough small bowel length can be maintained, however, those with medically refractory disease, or those with poor compliance, are at risk for short gut syndrome.

Short gut syndrome is a functional entity, and there is no specific length of bowel that serves as a reliable threshold to predict the need for supplemental parenteral nutrition. However, it typically occurs in adults with fewer than 200 cm of intestine and can be a significant problem in the Crohn's population [68]. When there is inadequate small bowel, malabsorption of both micronutrients and macronutrients can result. Ileal resection can rapidly lead to large fluid losses, and inability to absorb certain nutrients such as vitamin B_{12}. Jejunal resections, while generally better tolerated, can also lead to nutrient deficiencies [67].

Additionally, extensive loss of small bowel length can cause a hormonal imbalance. Notably, the negative feedback mechanism for gastrin generation is removed leading to hypergastrinemic peptic ulcer disease and gastroesophageal reflux [69]. Short gut syndrome, therefore, necessitates close monitoring of nutritional status, frequent supplementation and carries the potential for harmful systemic sequelae, including a decreased life expectancy [70]. It becomes a surgical dictum that minimization of small bowel resection is advantageous. The strictureplasty is such a surgical technique, one in which one or multiple small bowel strictures are surgically opened, rather than resected, presenting an alternative, bowel-preserving operation for patients with a history of segmental resection [71].

Resection

The first step to resection is to identify the extent and location(s) of disease based on pre-operative radiographic data as well as intraoperative visual and tactile guidance. The small intestine should be examined visually and/or manually in its entirety (from ligament of treitz to ileocecal valve) to identify all areas of disease, especially if pre-operative imaging is unavailable or inconsistent. Resection margins should then be identified. It is unnecessary to remove bowel to negative microscopic margins. Finally, because of the recurrent nature of the disease, the surgeon should measure and document the extent of small intestine resected in addition to the amount of bowel remaining.

Management of the Mesentery

The mesenteric pathology in CD may be more challenging to the surgeon than the intestine itself. Changes can include mesenteric fat growth ("creeping fat," which can encompass the circumference of the bowel), diffuse inflammation with enlarged lymph nodes, and friable tissue. Energy devices often have difficulty forming a proper seal in this setting. Vessels may fracture while the energy dissipates into the surrounding fatty coat.

Caution must also be taken when clamping the inflamed mesentery of CD patients. The surgeon should always be aware of the "corkscrew" vessels that penetrate near the bowel wall, as well as the presence of excess adipose tissue and pathologically enlarged lymph nodes, which still maintain their relationship to the underlying vasculature[3]. Mesentery can be managed by obtaining proximal control with atraumatic clamps, followed by ligation and control of remaining areas of bleeding [31]. Alternatively, serial, overlapping clamps can be used with a particular goal to prevent hematoma formation [3].

Anastomotic Configuration

Many anastomotic configurations for CD have been studied, including end-to-side, side-to-side, end-to-end, and the Kono-S. It is an active field of research, without one clearly superior anastomosis currently. Previous data suggests that stapled anastomoses have a slightly lower recurrence rate than a hand-sewn approach [36]. Recent data from He et al. supports this approach as well, and advocates for a side-to-side anastomosis based on results from their meta-analysis [72], given that the side-to-side anastomosis results in greater luminal width of the bowel.

A more recent innovation in anastomotic configuration was by Kono and colleagues, who proposed a novel technique for primary re-anastomosis after resection for CD, known as the Kono-S anastomosis [6], which initial results have found to be safe and effective [73]. To attempt to reduce anastomotic recurrence of CD after resection, a functional end-to-end handsewn anastomosis has been proposed. Once the bowel to be resected has been identified, that segment is divided transversely with a GIA stapler device, dividing the associated mesentery close to the bowel. Then, the corners of the staple lines are sutured together, and the staple lines are re-approximated in an interrupted fashion, to exclude the mesentery. On both sides of the newly re-apposed suture line, an anti-mesenteric longitudinal enterotomy is made. These two enterotomies are then re-approximated in two layers, allowing a large transverse lumen of 7-8 cm [74, 75]. Prospective data regarding recurrence rates of obstruction and active disease at the anastomotic site have not been established, however, two recent studies have found similar safety and efficacy profiles of Kono-S and conventional side-to-side anastomoses [76, 77].

Fecal Diversion

Pre-operative conditions preclude some patients with small bowel Crohn's disease from being candidates for primary anastomosis. As many as 20% of patients will require a temporary ileostomy following resection due to poor nutritional status, chronic steroid therapy, sepsis, and the presence of an enterocutaneous fistula. There is no literature to suggest any benefit to choosing either a loop or end ileostomy in these cases; however recent data suggests that anastomotic complications can be reduced by performance of a split-stoma in these "high-risk" patients that have at least two of the aforementioned factors [78]. A split-stoma involves exteriorization of both free ends of bowel after resection, with delayed re-anastomosis. Diversion is beneficial because it allows time for treatment of the underlying deficiency or heightened state of inflammation. Additionally, there is a growing body of evidence to suggest that fecal diversion, in and of itself, is associated with a lower risk of recurrence [35]. The mechanism is not entirely understood, but is thought to be related to the poor integrity of the intestinal mucosa, as well as decreasing fecal stasis due to a narrow anastomosis [35, 79-81].

Strictureplasty

The strictureplasty was first described by Katariya in 1977, in which a small case series of nine patients with obstructing tubercular strictures was described [82]. Within the next several years, the procedure was adapted to patients with CD, and early results were promising. The first use of strictureplasty for CD of the small bowel, reported by Lee, examined nine patients with chronic intestinal obstruction, as diagnosed by barium enema or enteroclysis. Using strictureplasty as one of three methods of relief of obstruction (minimal resections and short-segment bypasses were also used), no major complications were observed, yet a lasting benefit was realized in terms of weight gain up to three years postoperatively [83]. Suddenly, the strictureplasty for small bowel CD gained favor as a safe and effective alternative to resection for obstructing small bowel lesions. While resection is more common than strictureplasty, except in those cases where short gut syndrome is a concern [27], strictureplasty remains an important surgical tool in the management of CD. Due to varying lengths of strictures, there are multiple techniques, including the Heineke-Mikulicz, Finney, Jaboulay and Michelassi, which will be described further.

Indications for Strictureplasty

There are several current indications for small bowel strictureplasty in CD. Primarily, it should be used in patients with a history of prior bowel resections over >100 cm, or in patients with or at risk for short gut syndrome. This often presents as multiple long stricutred segments, especially in patients with previous resections. In addition, patients with rapid recurrence of disease with obstruction, or strictures at previous anastomotic sites, particularly ileorectal or ileocolic, are also candidates for strictureplasty [84, 85]. Currently, evidence supports the use of strictureplasty primarily in the jejunal and ileal regions, as treatment of duodenal strictures has yet to be sufficiently investigated to recommend strictureplasty over bypass or resection, primarily due to the low prevalence of duodenal stricturing disease [22, 29, 85, 86]. Biologic medications do not appear to alter the role of strictureplasty, as rates have remained the same over time, with similar surgical outcomes [87].

Contraindications to Strictureplasty

Preoperative malnutrition is a contraindication to strictureplasty, as it is with any procedure involving intestinal anastomoses due to risk of post-operative leak. A pre-operative serum albumin level <2.0 g/dL is reported as a cutoff for prohibitive malnutrition [84]. Additionally, pre-operative sepsis due to acute inflammation of the bowel is a sign of decreased bowel integrity and portends poor ability of the bowel wall to hold suture. Strictureplasty in such a systemic inflammatory setting is highly likely to fail. Intraoperative findings of inflammatory pathology such as phlegmon, fistula or perforation is also a contraindication to strictureplasty. Additionally, performing a strictureplasty next to a site of planned resection can increase the likelihood of tension on closure of the strictureplasty and should be avoided [84, 85].

Techniques of Strictureplasty

Heinecke-Mikulicz

The Heineke-Mikulicz technique, described in 1888, was initially used for pyloroplasty. It popularized the concept of increasing the luminal diameter without resection, and remains a tenet of pyloroplasty in adults, primarily as a component of an acid-reducing operation [88, 89]. The procedure is most useful and safe for strictures under ten centimeters in length and begins with determination of the location of stricture. This is generally accomplished with palpation of the full length of small bowel, in combination with pre-operative radiologic imaging. Once the intestinal stricture is identified, a full-thickness longitudinal incision on the anti-mesenteric border of the bowel is made. The incision is then closed transversely in a two-layer fashion, generally with a running internal full thickness closure and outer interrupted lambert suture.

Finney and Jaboulay

The Finney strictureplasty is the approach of choice for small bowel strictures between 10-25cm in length. In this approach, the strictured segment is folded in a U-configuration with a stay suture placed at the base of the "U." An enterotomy is made, again on the antimesenteric aspect of bowel. The afferent and efferent limbs of the segment are then sewn together in a side-to-side fashion using a full-thickness running absorbable suture for reapproximation of the posterior aspect, and an interrupted closure of the anterior aspect [85]. Alternatively, the anastomosis can be stapled [90]. The Jaboulay strictureplasty technique is similar to the Finney strictureplasty. In the Jaboulay technique, the "U" shape is created, but two separate longitudinal incisions are made. The enteroenterostomy is then fashioned in a side-to-side fashion effectively bypassing the primary strictured region [84]. There have been multiple techniques reported that include variations of the Finney and Jaboulay strictureplasties as well.

Michelassi

In 1996, Michelassi reported a technique for longer-segment (>25cm) strictureplasty in patients with stricturing disease of the small bowel due to CD. The technique can be used for a long continuous stricture, or for multiple strictures in close proximity, as an alternative to the Heinecke-Mikulicz, Finney and Jaboulay approaches. In this technique, the portion of diseased bowel is isolated with atraumatic bowel clamps, first dividing the associated mesentery at its midpoint. The proximal and distal loops are apposed in a side-to-side fashion, and a formal enteroenterostomy is made. At this step, stenotic areas of one loop should be opposed to dilated areas of the other loop to avoid persistent narrowing. Two-layer closures of the enteroenterostomy and the blind ends are then made with non-absorbable sutures, in an interrupted fashion. This technique, or its variations, yields a side-to-side isoperistaltic strictureplasty [91].

Modifications have been made to these conventional approaches to strictureplasty. These techniques have recently been summarized by Campbell [92].

Surgical Approach

Minimally invasive techniques, including laparoscopy and robotic surgery, have been used successfully in the surgical management of CD. As discussed in other chapters in this text, minimally invasive resection offers at least equivalent intestinal outcomes to open surgery, while demonstrating improved perioperative outcomes, including reduced post operative pain, shorter hospital stays, and faster return to normal activities [93]. Minimally invasive techniques have been applied to the small bowel since the first laparoscopic ileocecal resections were described in the 1990s and are now considered the standard of care assuming the availability of appropriate surgical experience and expertise.

Laparoscopic Approach

Alabaz in 2000 identified several advantages to a laparoscopic ileocecal resection, including shorter length of hospital stay, improved abdominal wall cosmesis, and faster return to baseline activities, however, they demonstrated longer operative times in the laparoscopic group [94]. Numerous studies have since identified similar outcomes in laparoscopic cohorts of CD patients, including faster return to bowel function, lower hospital charges, and lower intra-operative blood loss with comparable rates of complications, operative morbidity, and 5-year recurrence rates compared to open surgery [95-100]. Additionally, as laparoscopic surgery has gained traction and surgeons have gained experience, operative times between laparoscopic and open approaches have equalized [101, 102]. Many patients will also require multiple operations over their lifetimes, and it is advantageous to minimize trauma to the abdominal wall during each incursion. Laparoscopic surgery has been shown in some studies to decrease in the extent of adhesion formation, which is of critical importance to these patients who often face multiple operations [103].

Laparoscopic approaches have also been demonstrated to be safe and effective in management of small bowel CD, as demonstrated by a Cochrane review (2011) on this subject [104]. Although only two randomized controlled trials were included, the reviewers found that there was a significant decrease in wound infection, intra-abdominal abscess, length of stay, and postoperative ileus with laparoscopic techniques. In addition, there was the suggestion that the risk of herniation was smaller in the laparoscopic group. A prospective observational study also demonstrated feasibility and safety of laparoscopic strictureplasty in management of CD [105].

Patients with penetrating CD or intra-abdominal abscess at time of operation are more likely to require conversion to open surgery, but a minimally invasive approach is still considered safe in patients with complex CD [106, 107]. Medically refractory disease, previous open resection, and longer operative times have also been associated with increased risk of conversion to open [108, 109].

Robotic Approach

A recent systematic review comparing outcomes in over 5000 patients (11 studies) undergoing robotic versus laparoscopic surgery for colorectal resections in patients with inflammatory bowel disease demonstrated similar outcomes with regards to conversion to open surgery, anastomotic leaks, post-operative ileus, abscess formation, and surgical site infection between the two groups. The main difference was the longer operative times appreciated in the robotic surgery group [110]. The safety of robotic surgery in terminal ileal CD was also demonstrated in a single institution review comparing laparoscopic to robotic ileocecal resection, finding similar rates of complications, leaks rates, and reoperation rates. Differences included a longer operative time (51 minutes), however, a faster return of bowel function (1 day) [111].

Intraoperative Considerations and Pitfalls

While minimally invasive approaches are safe and have been shown to improve perioperative outcomes in the management of CD, surgeons should be aware of the potential pitfalls inherent to this disease process. To begin with, the mesentery is deceptively thickened in many patients, and requires subtle changes in technique to ensure adequate hemostasis, as energy devices may prove inadequate. Secondly, identification of inflamed or stenotic segments of bowel becomes a visual exercise rather than a tactile one. Further, it is remarkably easy to traumatize the bowel while running the length laparoscopically, which may lead to iatrogenic enterotomies distant from the patient's disease. Lastly, estimation of the length of bowel may be inaccurate in the laparoscopic setting due to the well-known phenomenon of errors inherent in the magnification afforded by the laparoscope. For these reasons, many surgeons employ a laparoscopic-assisted approach for resection – mobilization of the diseased segment followed by exteriorization of the bowel allowing for extracorporeal management and division of the mesentery and creation of an anastomosis [97]. The advantages of minimally invasive surgery may be visualization and mobilization, not resection and anastomosis.

Postoperative Considerations

There are few clear guidelines regarding the medical management of patients with Crohn's in the immediate postoperative period with exception to the use of immunosuppressive medication. Regarding general care, we advocate for the prompt resumption of enteral/parenteral nutrition as soon as the patient can tolerate. Because some patients may have lost a significant portion of their terminal ileum, they may be at risk for vitamin B_{12} deficiency and bile malabsorption. B_{12} stores are readily treated with oral supplementation, whereas bile-acids may necessitate sequestrants to prevent diarrhea. Fluid balance should also be attended to appropriately.

Starting and stopping of immumodulatory drugs is nuanced, but a few key takeaways are noted. 5-Aminosalicylic acid (5-ASA) drugs may be restarted postoperative day two [112]. Resumption of thiopurine therapy can also commence on the second postoperative day, providing that renal function is within normal limits [112]. There is mixed data regarding the use of biologics in the perioperative setting, and when they should be resumed post-operatively.

Postoperative surveillance is essential to monitor for either endoscopic or clinical recurrence, both of which will be outlined in the following section. The current paradigm is that endoscopic recurrence is the first manifestation of recurrent CD, though not all endoscopic disease manifests clinically [113]. To monitor for endoscopic recurrence, the standard of care is to perform follow-up endoscopy six to twelve months postoperatively. De Cruz showed that "endoscopically targeted therapy," with appropriate escalation of treatment if there were identifiable areas of recurrence at 6-month endoscopy, resulted in superior outcomes to the standard of care [113-115].

Outcomes and Recurrent Disease

Recurrent CD can be stratified into endoscopic recurrence and clinical recurrence. Endoscopic recurrence is disappointingly common on routine follow-up endoscopy, most often occurs within one year postoperatively, and is a risk factor for clinical recurrence [116]. Endoscopic recurrence after ileocecal surgery has been reported to be 79% at 1-3 years post-ileocecectomy, and can be characterized by the Rutgeerts scoring system, a measure of severity of endoscopic lesions [117, 118]. A score of 0 reflects no lesions, 1 reflects <5 aphthous ulcers, and a spectrum of inflammatory lesions continues up to a score of 4, reflecting diffuse inflammation with large ulcers, nodules and narrowing. Generally, a score of 1 or greater indicates endoscopic recurrence [119, 120].

Clinical recurrence can be broadly defined as the recrudescence of severe symptoms after a primary operation, generally a resection. It can also be quantified by the CD activity index (CDAI), the most popular of the scores used to quantify clinical severity of disease. This index is calculated from eight patient-reported variables, including stool number and quality, abdominal pain severity, daily well-being scores, extraintestinal symptoms, antidiarrheal regimen, presence of an abnormal mass, hematocrit, and body weight [121]. A CDAI>150 is taken to indicate recurrent disease [120, 121]. Clinical recurrence rates in the absence of treatment are estimated at 10-30% during the first year postoperatively, and greater than 60% in the first decade postoperatively [116].

Reoperations for recurrence have been approximated to be about 20% at 5 years, 30% at 10 years and up to 60% at 20 years postoperatively [21, 122]. Patients undergoing a first or second reoperation tend to have similar long-term clinical courses as those without an additional procedure. However, postoperative complications are increased, and length of stay is longer in reoperative surgery [123]. Patients with multiple reoperations will continue to experience more frequent recurrences of active disease and have a shorter time until a permanent ileostomy is required [36, 124]. Cumulative reoperative rates after small bowel strictureplasty are between 22-45%, with a rate of re-stricture at the strictureplasty site estimated at 5-9%, higher at sites of ileocecal strictureplasties [36, 125-128].

There has been substantial research directed towards identifying risk factors that predispose one to recurrent disease to stratify patients. The most consistent risk factor in the literature is cigarette smoking, which has demonstrated a significant association with recurrence [113, 120, 129]. In addition, evidence suggests that a history of prior resection, perforating disease, and myenteric plexitis are independent risk factors for recurrence [113, 120, 129].

With the identification of risk factors and the advent of stratification, patients can receive more tailored therapy. In patients actively using tobacco, the first step for prevention of recurrent disease is smoking cessation. Medical therapies to prevent recurrence include drugs typically used in the treatment of CD. However, mesalamine and other similar 5-aminosalicylic (5-ASA) compounds provide only minor benefit in post-operative prevention across all risk categories [113, 120, 129]. Domenech suggested this benefit may be due to a delay in clinical symptoms, and not actually prevention of endoscopic recurrence[129]. It is generally accepted, however, that 5-ASA compounds are relatively well-tolerated and inexpensive, thus their use has been widespread. Thiopurines, including azathioprine and 6-mercaptopurine, are generally accepted to be first line therapy for low-risk patients. They exhibited a relative risk reduction for clinical recurrence vs. placebo of 0.59 (95% CI: 0.38-0.92) and endoscopic recurrence vs.

placebo of 0.64 (95% CI: 0.44-0.92) [113]. For high-risk patients, anti-TNF agents are recommended as they had a greater relative risk reduction compared to placebo, with the recommendation to start them two to three weeks after surgery [120, 129].

Not surprisingly, the most recent research suggests that anti-TNF agents are more efficacious than thiopruines in the prevention of recurrence [115]. Probiotics, interleukin-10, and steroids have all proven ineffective for postoperative prophylaxis [113, 115, 129]. There is some evidence that suggests nitroimidazole antibiotics, e.g., metronidazole, will decrease risk in the immediate postoperative setting when given for one month following the surgery, but side-effects and compliance often preclude the widespread use of these as an adjunctive therapy [113].

Conclusion

Crohn's disease is highly variable in its location and severity of presentation. Most patients, however, will require operative intervention during their clinical course. Small bowel involvement is quite common, particularly in the terminal ileum and cecum. While there are a variety of disease phenotypes and surgical indications, there remain guiding principles of surgical management of small bowel Crohn's disease. First, the goal of surgery is to make the operation as safe as possible. This involves directed preoperative imaging and optimization, as well as appropriate postoperative care including endoscopic followup [21]. Next, as serial operations are often necessary, conservation of bowel is paramount [21]. This can be accomplished by minimization of resection margins and consideration of strictureplasty for obstructing fibrostenotic disease, a technique that can be accomplished in a variety of ways based on stricture length. Finally, the surgeon must recognize that there is no surgical cure for Crohn's disease, and the decision to operate should be based on the presence of disease associated complications and severe symptoms. A multidisciplinary management strategy to identify appropriate timing of procedure, assure patient optimization, and to determine best operative approach and techniques can help improve both short term and long term post-operative outcomes [21].

References

[1] Wagner IJ, Rombeau JL. Nutritional support of surgical patients with inflammatory bowel disease. *Surg Clin North Am*. 2011;91(4):787-803, viii. doi: 10.1016/j.suc.2011.04.013.

[2] Peyrin-Biroulet L, Loftus EVJ, Colombel J, Sandborn WJ. The natural history of adult crohn's disease in population-based cohorts. *Am J Gastroenterol*. 2010;105(2):289-297. doi: 10.1038/ajg.2009.579.

[3] Delaney CP, Fazio VW. Crohn's disease of the small bowel. *Surg Clin North Am*. 2001;81(1):137-58, ix. doi: 10.1016/s0039-6109(05)70277-2.

[4] Kim YL, Park YS, Park EK, et al. Refractory duodenal crohn's disease successfully treated with infliximab. *Intest Res*. 2014;12(1):66-69. doi: 10.5217/ir.2014.12.1.66.

[5] Gonzalez AJ, Afraz S, Melendez-Rosado J, Schneider A. Isolated jejunal crohn's disease masquerading as gastroparesis. *Cureus*. 2022;14(6):e26333. doi: 10.7759/cureus.26333.

[6] Fichera A, Michelassi F. Surgical treatment of crohn's disease. *J Gastrointest Surg*. 2007;11(6):791-803. doi: 10.1007/s11605-006-0068-9.

[7] Freeman HJ. Natural history and long-term clinical course of crohn's disease. *World J Gastroenterol.* 2014;20(1):31-36. doi: 10.3748/wjg.v20.i1.31.

[8] Tonelli F, Alemanno G, Di Martino C, Focardi A, Gronchi G, Giudici F. Results of surgical treatment for jejunal crohn's disease: Choice between resection, strictureplasty, and combined treatment. *Langenbecks Arch Surg.* 2017;402(7):1071-1078. doi: 10.1007/s00423-016-1497-x.

[9] Task Force for Preoperative Cardiac Risk Assessment and Perioperative Cardiac Management in Non-cardiac Surgery, European Society of Cardiology (ESC) FAU -dermans, Don, Bax JJ, et al. Guidelines for pre-operative cardiac risk assessment and perioperative cardiac management in non-cardiac surgery. *Eur Heart J.* 2009;30(22):2769-2812. doi: 10.1093/eurheartj/ehp337.

[10] Sharma A, Chinn BT. Preoperative optimization of crohn disease. *Clin Colon Rectal Surg.* 2013;26(2):75-79. doi: 10.1055/s-0033-1348044.

[11] Makela JT, Kiviniemi H, Laitinen S. Risk factors for anastomotic leakage after left-sided colorectal resection with rectal anastomosis. *Dis Colon Rectum.* 2003;46(5):653-660. doi: 10.1007/s10350-004-6627-9.

[12] Zoli G, Care M, Parazza M, et al. A randomized controlled study comparing elemental diet and steroid treatment in crohn's disease. *Aliment Pharmacol Ther.* 1997;11(4):735-740. doi: 10.1046/j.1365-2036.1997.t01-1-00192.x.

[13] Takahashi H, Ando T, Watanabe O, et al. Usefulness of an elemental diet in crohn's disease. *Inflammopharmacology.* 2007;15(1):15-17. doi: 10.1007/s10787-006-1570-0.

[14] Macdonald A. Omega-3 fatty acids as adjunctive therapy in crohns disease. *Gastroenterol Nurs.* 2006;29(4):295-3. doi: 10.1097/00001610-200607000-00005.

[15] Tsujikawa T, Andoh A, Fujiyama Y. Enteral and parenteral nutrition therapy for crohn's disease. *Curr Pharm Des.* 2003;9(4):323-332. doi: 10.2174/1381612033391964.

[16] Jacobson S. Early postoperative complications in patients with crohn's disease given and not given preoperative total parenteral nutrition. *Scand J Gastroenterol.* 2012;47(2):170-177. doi: 10.3109/00365521.2011.648954.

[17] Cohen BL, Fleshner P, Kane SV, et al. Prospective cohort study to investigate the safety of preoperative tumor necrosis factor inhibitor exposure in patients with inflammatory bowel disease undergoing intra-abdominal surgery. *Gastroenterology.* 2022;163(1):204-221. doi: 10.1053/j.gastro.2022.03.057.

[18] Chilkoti GT, Singh A, Mohta M, Saxena AK. Perioperative "stress dose" of corticosteroid: Pharmacological and clinical perspective. *J Anaesthesiol Clin Pharmacol.* 2019;35(2):147-152. doi: 10.4103/joacp.JOACP_242_17.

[19] Sampietro GM, Casiraghi S, Foschi D. Perforating crohn's disease: Conservative and surgical treatment. *Dig Dis.* 2013;31(2):218-221. doi: 10.1159/000353373.

[20] Ripolles T, Martinez-Perez MJ, Paredes JM, Vizuete J, Garcia-Martinez E, Jimenez-Restrepo DH. Contrast-enhanced ultrasound in the differentiation between phlegmon and abscess in crohn's disease and other abdominal conditions. *Eur J Radiol.* 2013;82(10):525. doi: 10.1016/j.ejrad.2013.05.043.

[21] Yamamoto T, Watanabe T. Surgery for luminal crohn's disease. *World J Gastroenterol.* 2014;20(1):78-90. doi: 10.3748/wjg.v20.i1.78.

[22] Shapiro M, Greenstein AJ, Byrn J, et al. Surgical management and outcomes of patients with duodenal crohn's disease. *J Am Coll Surg.* 2008;207(1):36-42. doi: 10.1016/j.jamcollsurg.2007.12.049.

[23] Murray JJ, Schoetz DJJ, Nugent FW, Coller JA, Veidenheimer MC. Surgical management of crohn's disease involving the duodenum. *Am J Surg.* 1984;147(1):58-65. doi: 10.1016/0002-9610(84)90035-7.

[24] Fix OK, Soto JA, Andrews CW, Farraye FA. Gastroduodenal crohn's disease. *Gastrointest Endosc.* 2004;60(6):985-x. doi: 10.1016/s0016-5107(04)02200-x.

[25] Carbo AI, Sangster GP, Caraway J, Heldmann MG, Thomas J, Takalkar A. Acquired constricting and restricting lesions of the descending duodenum. *Radiographics.* 2014;34(5):1196-1217. doi: 10.1148/rg.345130055.

[26] Racz JM, Davies W. Severe stricturing crohn's disease of the duodenum: A case report and review of surgical options. *Int J Surg Case Rep.* 2012;3(7):242-245. doi: 10.1016/j.ijscr.2012.03.012.

[27] Butt WT, Ryan EJ, Boland MR, et al. Strictureplasty versus bowel resection for the surgical management of fibrostenotic crohn's disease: A systematic review and meta-analysis. *Int J Colorectal Dis*. 2020;35(4):705-717. doi: 10.1007/s00384-020-03507-z.

[28] Benoist S, Panis Y, Beaufour A, Bouhnik Y, Matuchansky C, Valleur P. Laparoscopic ileocecal resection in crohn's disease: A case-matched comparison with open resection. *Surg Endosc*. 2003;17(5):814-818. doi: 10.1007/s00464-002-9103-4.

[29] Tonelli F, Alemanno G, Bellucci F, Focardi A, Sturiale A, Giudici F. Symptomatic duodenal crohn's disease: Is strictureplasty the right choice? *J Crohns Colitis*. 2013;7(10):791-796. doi: 10.1016/j.crohns.2012.10.017.

[30] Fazio VW, Marchetti F, Church M, et al. Effect of resection margins on the recurrence of crohn's disease in the small bowel. A randomized controlled trial. *Ann Surg*. 1996;224(4):563-3. doi: 10.1097/00000658-199610000-00014.

[31] Michelassi F, Sultan S. Surgical treatment of complex small bowel crohn disease. *Ann Surg*. 2014;260(2):230-235. doi: 10.1097/SLA.0000000000000697.

[32] Hashemi M, Novell JR, Lewis AA. Side-to-side stapled anastomosis may delay recurrence in crohn's disease. *Dis Colon Rectum*. 1998;41(10):1293-1296. doi: 10.1007/BF02258231.

[33] Yamamoto T, Bain IM, Mylonakis E, Allan RN, Keighley MR. Stapled functional end-to-end anastomosis versus sutured end-to-end anastomosis after ileocolonic resection in crohn disease. *Scand J Gastroenterol*. 1999;34(7):708-713. doi: 10.1080/003655299750025921.

[34] Scarpa M, Angriman I, Barollo M, et al. Role of stapled and hand-sewn anastomoses in recurrence of crohn's disease. *Hepatogastroenterology*. 2004;51(58):1053-1057.

[35] McLeod RS, Wolff BG, Ross S, Parkes R, McKenzie M, Investigators of the CAST Trial. Recurrence of crohn's disease after ileocolic resection is not affected by anastomotic type: Results of a multicenter, randomized, controlled trial. *Dis Colon Rectum*. 2009;52(5):919-927. doi: 10.1007/DCR.0b013e3181a4fa58.

[36] Ramirez RL, Fleshner P. Reoperative inflammatory bowel disease surgery. *Clin Colon Rectal Surg*. 2006;19(4):195-206. doi: 10.1055/s-2006-956440.

[37] Scharl M, Rogler G. Pathophysiology of fistula formation in crohn's disease. *World J Gastrointest Pathophysiol*. 2014;5(3):205-212. doi: 10.4291/wjgp.v5.i3.205.

[38] Gecse K, Khanna R, Stoker J, et al. Fistulizing crohn's disease: Diagnosis and management. *United European Gastroenterol J*. 2013;1(3):206-213. doi: 10.1177/2050640613487194.

[39] Bouhnik Y, Panis Y. Therapeutic strategies of fistulous crohn's disease: Medical or surgical treatment? *Gastroenterol Clin Biol*. 2003;27(3 Suppl):98.

[40] Solem CA, Loftus EVJ, Tremaine WJ, Pemberton JH, Wolff BG, Sandborn WJ. Fistulas to the urinary system in crohn's disease: Clinical features and outcomes. *Am J Gastroenterol*. 2002;97(9):2300-2305. doi: 10.1111/j.1572-0241.2002.05983.x.

[41] Levy C, Tremaine WJ. Management of internal fistulas in crohn's disease. *Inflamm Bowel Dis*. 2002;8(2):106-111. doi: 10.1097/00054725-200203000-00007.

[42] Yoon YS, Yu CS, Yang S, Yoon SN, Lim S, Kim JC. Intra-abdominal fistulas in surgically treated crohn's disease patients. *World J Surg*. 2010;34(8):1924-1929. doi: 10.1007/s00268-010-0568-3.

[43] Lichtenstein GR. Treatment of fistulizing crohn's disease. *Gastroenterology*. 2000;119(4):1132-1147. doi: 10.1053/gast.2000.18165.

[44] Broe PJ, Bayless TM, Cameron JL. Crohn's disease: Are enteroenteral fistulas an indication for surgery? *Surgery*. 1982;91(3):249-253.

[45] Golabek T, Szymanska A, Szopinski T, et al. Enterovesical fistulae: Aetiology, imaging, and management. *Gastroenterol Res Pract*. 2013;2013:617967. doi: 10.1155/2013/617967.

[46] Su Y, Shih I, Tai H, et al. Surgical management in enterovesical fistula in crohn disease at a single medical center. *Int Surg*. 2014;99(2):120-125. doi: 10.9738/INTSURG-D-13-00038.1.

[47] Taxonera C, Barreiro-de-Acosta M, Bastida G, et al. Outcomes of medical and surgical therapy for entero-urinary fistulas in crohn's disease. *J Crohns Colitis*. 2016;10(6):657-662. doi: 10.1093/ecco-jcc/jjw016.

[48] O'Leary DP. Use of the greater omentum in colorectal surgery. *Dis Colon Rectum*. 1999;42(4):533-539. doi: 10.1007/BF02234183.

[49] Hanauer SB, Feagan BG, Lichtenstein GR, et al. Maintenance infliximab for crohn's disease: The ACCENT I randomised trial. *Lancet*. 2002;359(9317):1541-1549. doi: 10.1016/S0140-6736(02)08512-4.

[50] Sands BE, Anderson FH, Bernstein CN, et al. Infliximab maintenance therapy for fistulizing crohn's disease. *N Engl J Med*. 2004;350(9):876-885. doi: 10.1056/NEJMoa030815.

[51] Louis E, Reenaers CAC, Belaiche J. Does the phenotype at diagnosis (e.g., fibrostenosing, inflammatory, perforating) predict the course of crohn's disease? *Inflamm Bowel Dis*. 2008;14 Suppl 2:59. doi: 10.1002/ibd.20559.

[52] Bellolio F, Cohen Z, Macrae HM, et al. Outcomes following surgery for perforating crohn's disease. *Br J Surg*. 2013;100(10):1344-1348. doi: 10.1002/bjs.9212.

[53] Yamaguchi A, Matsui T, Sakurai T, et al. The clinical characteristics and outcome of intraabdominal abscess in crohn's disease. *J Gastroenterol*. 2004;39(5):441-448. doi: 10.1007/s00535-003-1317-2.

[54] Jawhari A, Kamm MA, Ong C, Forbes A, Bartram CI, Hawley PR. Intra-abdominal and pelvic abscess in crohn's disease: Results of noninvasive and surgical management. *Br J Surg*. 1998;85(3):367-371. doi: 10.1046/j.1365-2168.1998.00575.x.

[55] Gutierrez A, Lee H, Sands BE. Outcome of surgical versus percutaneous drainage of abdominal and pelvic abscesses in crohn's disease. *Am J Gastroenterol*. 2006;101(10):2283-2289. doi: 10.1111/j.1572-0241.2006.00757.x.

[56] Feagins LA, Holubar SD, Kane SV, Spechler SJ. Current strategies in the management of intra-abdominal abscesses in crohn's disease. *Clin Gastroenterol Hepatol*. 2011;9(10):842-850. doi: 10.1016/j.cgh.2011.04.023.

[57] Siddiki HA, Fidler JL, Fletcher JG, et al. Prospective comparison of state-of-the-art MR enterography and CT enterography in small-bowel crohn's disease. *AJR Am J Roentgenol*. 2009;193(1):113-121. doi: 10.2214/AJR.08.2027.

[58] Ananthakrishnan AN, McGinley EL. Treatment of intra-abdominal abscesses in crohn's disease: A nationwide analysis of patterns and outcomes of care. *Dig Dis Sci*. 2013;58(7):2013-2018. doi: 10.1007/s10620-013-2579-z.

[59] Gervais DA, Hahn PF, O'Neill MJ, Mueller PR. Percutaneous abscess drainage in crohn disease: Technical success and short- and long-term outcomes during 14 years. *Radiology*. 2002;222(3):645-651. doi: 10.1148/radiol.2223010554.

[60] Xie Y, Zhu W, Li N, Li J. The outcome of initial percutaneous drainage versus surgical drainage for intra-abdominal abscesses in crohn's disease. *Int J Colorectal Dis*. 2012;27(2):199-206. doi: 10.1007/s00384-011-1338-x.

[61] Rypens F, Dubois J, Garel L, Deslandres C, Saint-Vil D. Percutaneous drainage of abdominal abscesses in pediatric crohn's disease. *AJR Am J Roentgenol*. 2007;188(2):579-585. doi: 10.2214/AJR.06.0181.

[62] Freeman HJ. Spontaneous free perforation of the small intestine in adults. *World J Gastroenterol*. 2014;20(29):9990-9997. doi: 10.3748/wjg.v20.i29.9990.

[63] Ikeuchi H, Yamamura T. Free perforation in crohn's disease: Review of the japanese literature. *J Gastroenterol*. 2002;37(12):1020-1027. doi: 10.1007/s005350200172.

[64] Berg DF, Bahadursingh AM, Kaminski DL, Longo WE. Acute surgical emergencies in inflammatory bowel disease. *Am J Surg*. 2002;184(1):45-51. doi: 10.1016/s0002-9610(02)00879-6.

[65] Chirantan B, Niladri S, Madhumita M, Sabyasachi S, Sibaji D, Jay K. Crohn's perforation: Not so uncommon in the indian population. *Indian J Surg*. 2013;75(1):28-30. doi: 10.1007/s12262-012-0453-4.

[66] Gardiner KR, Dasari BVM. Operative management of small bowel crohn's disease. *Surg Clin North Am*. 2007;87(3):587-610. doi: 10.1016/j.suc.2007.03.011.

[67] Vanderhoof JA, Langnas AN. Short-bowel syndrome in children and adults. *Gastroenterology*. 1997;113(5):1767-1778. doi: 10.1053/gast.1997.v113.pm9352883.

[68] Buchman AL. Etiology and initial management of short bowel syndrome. *Gastroenterology*. 2006;130(2 Suppl 1):S5-S15. doi: 10.1053/j.gastro.2005.07.063.

[69] Williams NS, Evans P, King RF. Gastric acid secretion and gastrin production in the short bowel syndrome. *Gut*. 1985;26(9):914-919. doi: 10.1136/gut.26.9.914.

[70] Schalamon J, Mayr JM, Hollwarth ME. Mortality and economics in short bowel syndrome. *Best Pract Res Clin Gastroenterol*. 2003;17(6):931-942. doi: 10.1016/s1521-6918(03)00079-9.

[71] Brunicardi FC, Andersen DK, Cilliar TR, et al, eds. *Schwartz's principles of surgery.* 10th ed. New York, NY: McGraw-Hill Education; 2015.

[72] He X, Chen Z, Huang J, et al. Stapled side-to-side anastomosis might be better than handsewn end-to-end anastomosis in ileocolic resection for crohn's disease: A meta-analysis. *Dig Dis Sci*. 2014;59(7): 1544-1551. doi: 10.1007/s10620-014-3039-0.

[73] Fichera A, Mangrola AM, Olortegui KS, et al. Long-term outcomes of the kono-S anastomosis: A multicenter study. *Dis Colon Rectum*. 2024;67(3):406-413. doi: 10.1097/DCR.0000000000003132.

[74] Fichera A, Zoccali M, Kono T. Antimesenteric functional end-to-end handsewn (kono-S) anastomosis. *J Gastrointest Surg*. 2012;16(7):1412-1416. doi: 10.1007/s11605-012-1905-7.

[75] Kono T, Fichera A. Kono-S anastomosis for crohn's disease: Narrative - a video vignette. *Colorectal Dis*. 2014;16(10):833. doi: 10.1111/codi.12722.

[76] Kelm M, Reibetanz J, Kim M, et al. Kono-S anastomosis in crohn's disease: A retrospective study on postoperative morbidity and disease recurrence in comparison to the conventional side-to-side anastomosis. *J Clin Med*. 2022;11(23):6915. doi: 10.3390/jcm11236915. doi: 10.3390/jcm11236915.

[77] Alibert L, Betton L, Falcoz A, et al. Does kono-S anastomosis reduce recurrence in crohn's disease compared with conventional ileocolonic anastomosis? A nationwide propensity score-matched study from GETAID chirurgie group [KoCoRICCO study. *J Crohns Colitis*. 2024;18(4):525-532. doi: 10.1093/ecco-jcc/jjad176.

[78] Myrelid P, Soderholm JD, Olaison G, Sjodahl R, Andersson P. Split stoma in resectional surgery of high-risk patients with ileocolonic crohn's disease. *Colorectal Dis*. 2012;14(2):188-193. doi: 10.1111/j.1463-1318.2011.02578.x.

[79] D'Haens GR, Geboes K, Peeters M, Baert F, Penninckx F, Rutgeerts P. Early lesions of recurrent crohn's disease caused by infusion of intestinal contents in excluded ileum. *Gastroenterology*. 1998;114(2):262-267. doi: 10.1016/s0016-5085(98)70476-7.

[80] Winslet MC, Allan A, Poxon V, Youngs D, Keighley MR. Faecal diversion for crohn's colitis: A model to study the role of the faecal stream in the inflammatory process. *Gut*. 1994;35(2):236-242. doi: 10.1136/gut.35.2.236.

[81] Antoni L, Nuding S, Wehkamp J, Stange EF. Intestinal barrier in inflammatory bowel disease. *World J Gastroenterol*. 2014;20(5):1165-1179. doi: 10.3748/wjg.v20.i5.1165.

[82] Katariya RN, Sood S, Rao PG, Rao PL. Stricture-plasty for tubercular strictures of the gastro-intestinal tract. *Br J Surg*. 1977;64(7):496-498. doi: 10.1002/bjs.1800640713.

[83] Lee EC, Papaioannou N. Minimal surgery for chronic obstruction in patients with extensive or universal crohn's disease. *Ann R Coll Surg Engl*. 1982;64(4):229-233.

[84] Roy P, Kumar D. Strictureplasty. *Br J Surg*. 2004;91(11):1428-1437. doi: 10.1002/bjs.4804.

[85] Hesham W, Kann BR. Strictureplasty. *Clin Colon Rectal Surg*. 2013;26(2):80-83. doi: 10.1055/s-0033-1348045.

[86] Yamamoto T. The role of strictureplasty in the surgical management of duodenal crohn's disease. *J Crohns Colitis*. 2013;7(6):e237. doi: 10.1016/j.crohns.2012.12.001.

[87] Landerholm K, Reali C, Mortensen NJ, Travis SPL, Guy RJ, George BD. Short- and long-term outcomes of strictureplasty for obstructive crohn's disease. *Colorectal Dis*. 2020;22(9):1159-1168. doi: 10.1111/codi.15013.

[88] Fazio VW, Galandiuk S, Jagelman DG, Lavery IC. Strictureplasty in crohn's disease. *Ann Surg*. 1989;210(5):621-625. doi: 10.1097/00000658-198911000-00009.

[89] WILKINS FB. Pyloroplasty for gastric drainage with vagotomy. *Calif Med*. 1953;78(6):513-514.

[90] Keighley MR. Stapled strictureplasty for crohn's disease. *Dis Colon Rectum*. 1991;34(10):945-947. doi: 10.1007/BF02049714.

[91] Michelassi F, Hurst RD, Melis M, et al. Side-to-side isoperistaltic strictureplasty in extensive crohn's disease: A prospective longitudinal study. *Ann Surg*. 2000;232(3):401-408. doi: 10.1097/00000658-200009000-00012.

[92] Campbell L, Ambe R, Weaver J, Marcus SM, Cagir B. Comparison of conventional and nonconventional strictureplasties in crohn's disease: A systematic review and meta-analysis. *Dis Colon Rectum*. 2012;55(6):714-726. doi: 10.1097/DCR.0b013e31824f875a.

[93] Luglio, G., Cricrì, M., Tropeano, F., De Palma,G. Crohn's disease: Is minimally invasive surgery the gold standard? A narrative review. *Annals of Laparoscopic and Endoscopic Surgery*. 2023;8(0). https://ales.amegroups.org/article/view/9184.

[94] Alabaz O, Iroatulam AJ, Nessim A, Weiss EG, Nogueras JJ, Wexner SD. Comparison of laparoscopically assisted and conventional ileocolic resection for crohn's disease. *Eur J Surg*. 2000;166(3):213-217. doi: 10.1080/110241500750009302.

[95] Antoniou SA, Antoniou GA, Koch OO, Pointner R, Granderath FA. Is laparoscopic ileocecal resection a safe option for crohn's disease? best evidence topic. *Int J Surg*. 2014;12(5):22-25. doi: 10.1016/j.ijsu.2013.11.003.

[96] Tilney HS, Constantinides VA, Heriot AG, et al. Comparison of laparoscopic and open ileocecal resection for crohn's disease: A metaanalysis. *Surg Endosc*. 2006;20(7):1036-1044. doi: 10.1007/s00464-005-0500-3.

[97] Bemelman WA, Slors JF, Dunker MS, et al. Laparoscopic-assisted vs. open ileocolic resection for crohn's disease. A comparative study. *Surg Endosc*. 2000;14(8):721-725. doi: 10.1007/s00464 0000186.

[98] Duepree H, Senagore AJ, Delaney CP, Brady KM, Fazio VW. Advantages of laparoscopic resection for ileocecal crohn's disease. *Dis Colon Rectum*. 2002;45(5):605-610. doi: 10.1007/s10350-004-6253-6.

[99] Shore G, Gonzalez QH, Bondora A, Vickers SM. Laparoscopic vs conventional ileocolectomy for primary crohn disease. *Arch Surg*. 2003;138(1):76-79. doi: 10.1001/archsurg.138.1.76.

[100] Young-Fadok TM, HallLong K, McConnell EJ, Gomez Rey G, Cabanela RL. Advantages of laparoscopic resection for ileocolic crohn's disease. improved outcomes and reduced costs. *Surg Endosc*. 2001;15(5):450-454. doi: 10.1007/s004640080078.

[101] Tan JJY, Tjandra JJ. Laparoscopic surgery for crohn's disease: A meta-analysis. *Dis Colon Rectum*. 2007;50(5):576-585. doi: 10.1007/s10350-006-0855-0.

[102] Huilgol RL, Wright CM, Solomon MJ. Laparoscopic versus open ileocolic resection for crohn's disease. *J Laparoendosc Adv Surg Tech A*. 2004;14(2):61-65. doi: 10.1089/109264204322973808.

[103] Riss S, Schuster I, Papay P, Mittlbock M, Stift A. Repeat intestinal resections increase the risk of recurrence of crohn's disease. *Dis Colon Rectum*. 2013;56(7):881-887. doi: 10.1097/DCR.0b013e3 1828cb80c.

[104] Dasari BV, McKay D, Gardiner K. Laparoscopic versus open surgery for small bowel crohn's disease. *Cochrane Database Syst Rev*. 2011;(1):CD006956. doi(1):CD006956. doi: 10.1002/14651858.CD00 6956.pub2.

[105] Sampietro GM, Colombo F, Frontali A, et al. Strictureplasties performed by laparoscopic approach for complicated crohn's disease. A prospective, observational, cohort study. *Dig Liver Dis*. 2021;53(10):1286-1293. doi: 10.1016/j.dld.2021.01.023.

[106] Watanabe M, Hasegawa H, Yamamoto S, Hibi T, Kitajima M. Successful application of laparoscopic surgery to the treatment of crohn's disease with fistulas. *Dis Colon Rectum*. 2002;45(8):1057-1061. doi: 10.1007/s10350-004-6360-4.

[107] Alves A, Panis Y, Bouhnik Y, et al. Factors that predict conversion in 69 consecutive patients undergoing laparoscopic ileocecal resection for crohn's disease: A prospective study. *Dis Colon Rectum*. 2005;48(12):2302-2308. doi: 10.1007/s10350-005-0190-x.

[108] Emile SH, Freund MR, Horesh N, et al. Risk factors and predictors of 30-day complications and conversion to open surgery after repeat ileocolic resection of crohn's disease. *Surg Endosc*. 2023;37(2):941-949. doi: 10.1007/s00464-022-09557-4.

[109] Goyer P, Alves A, Bretagnol F, Bouhnik Y, Valleur P, Panis Y. Impact of complex crohn's disease on the outcome of laparoscopic ileocecal resection: A comparative clinical study in 124 patients. *Dis Colon Rectum*. 2009;52(2):205-210. doi: 10.1007/DCR.0b013e31819c9c08.

[110] Zaman S, Mohamedahmed AYY, Abdelrahman W, et al. Minimally invasive surgery for inflammatory bowel disease: A systematic review and meta-analysis of robotic versus laparoscopic surgical techniques. *J Crohns Colitis*. 2024. doi: 10.1093/ecco-jcc/jjae037.

[111] Aydinli HH, Anderson M, Hambrecht A, Bernstein MA, Grucela AL. Robotic ileocolic resection with intracorporeal anastomosis for crohn's disease. *J Robot Surg*. 2021;15(3):465-472. doi: 10.1007/s11701-020-01125-z.

[112] Kumar A, Auron M, Aneja A, Mohr F, Jain A, Shen B. Inflammatory bowel disease: Perioperative pharmacological considerations. *Mayo Clin Proc*. 2011;86(8):748-757. doi: 10.4065/mcp.2011.0074.

[113] Vaughn BP, Moss AC. Prevention of post-operative recurrence of crohn's disease. *World J Gastroenterol*. 2014;20(5):1147-1154. doi: 10.3748/wjg.v20.i5.1147.

[114] De Cruz P, Kamm MA, Prideaux L, Allen PB, Desmond PV. Postoperative recurrent luminal crohn's disease: A systematic review. *Inflamm Bowel Dis*. 2012;18(4):758-777. doi: 10.1002/ibd.21825.

[115] De Cruz P, Kamm MA, Hamilton AL, et al. Crohn's disease management after intestinal resection: A randomised trial. *Lancet*. 2015;385(9976):1406-1417. doi: 10.1016/S0140-6736(14)61908-5.

[116] Lee YW, Lee K, Chung WC, Paik CN, Sung HJ, Oh YS. Clinical and endoscopic recurrence after surgical resection in patients with crohn's disease. *Intest Res*. 2014;12(2):117-123. doi: 10.5217/ir.2014.12.2.117.

[117] Rutgeerts P, Geboes K, Vantrappen G, Beyls J, Kerremans R, Hiele M. Predictability of the postoperative course of crohn's disease. *Gastroenterology*. 1990;99(4):956-963. doi: 10.1016/0016-5085(90)90613-6.

[118] Rutgeerts P, Geboes K, Vantrappen G, Kerremans R, Coenegrachts JL, Coremans G. Natural history of recurrent crohn's disease at the ileocolonic anastomosis after curative surgery. *Gut*. 1984;25(6):665-672. doi: 10.1136/gut.25.6.665.

[119] Vantrappen G, Rutgeerts P. Recurrence of crohn's lesions in the neoterminal ileum after ileal resection and ileocolonic anastomosis. *Verh K Acad Geneeskd Belg*. 1990;52(5):373-5.

[120] Spinelli A, Sacchi M, Fiorino G, Danese S, Montorsi M. Risk of postoperative recurrence and postoperative management of crohn's disease. *World J Gastroenterol*. 2011;17(27):3213-3219. doi: 10.3748/wjg.v17.i27.3213.

[121] Best WR, Becktel JM, Singleton JW, Kern FJ. Development of a crohn's disease activity index. national cooperative crohn's disease study. *Gastroenterology*. 1976;70(3):439-444.

[122] Yamamoto T. Factors affecting recurrence after surgery for crohn's disease. *World J Gastroenterol*. 2005;11(26):3971-3979. doi: 10.3748/wjg.v11.i26.3971.

[123] Brouquet A, Blanc B, Bretagnol F, Valleur P, Bouhnik Y, Panis Y. Surgery for intestinal crohn's disease recurrence. *Surgery*. 2010;148(5):936-946. doi: 10.1016/j.surg.2010.02.001.

[124] Heimann TM, Greenstein AJ, Lewis B, Kaufman D, Heimann DM, Aufses AHJ. Comparison of primary and reoperative surgery in patients with crohns disease. *Ann Surg*. 1998;227(4):492-495. doi: 10.1097/00000658-199804000-00007.

[125] Dietz DW, Laureti S, Strong SA, et al. Safety and longterm efficacy of strictureplasty in 314 patients with obstructing small bowel crohn's disease. *J Am Coll Surg*. 2001;192(3):330-8. doi: 10.1016/s1072-7515(01)00775-x.

[126] Ozuner G, Fazio VW, Lavery IC, Milsom JW, Strong SA. Reoperative rates for crohn's disease following strictureplasty. long-term analysis. *Dis Colon Rectum*. 1996;39(11):1199-1203. doi: 10.1007/BF02055108.

[127] Hurst RD, Michelassi F. Strictureplasty for crohn's disease: Techniques and long-term results. *World J Surg*. 1998;22(4):359-363. doi: 10.1007/s002689900397.

[128] Futami K, Arima S. Role of strictureplasty in surgical treatment of crohn's disease. *J Gastroenterol*. 2005;40 Suppl 16:35-39. doi: 10.1007/BF02990577.

[129] Domenech E, Manosa M, Lobaton T, Cabre E. Optimizing post-operative crohn's disease treatment. *Ann Gastroenterol*. 2014;27(4):313-319.

Chapter 10

Colon Surgery*

Cassandra A. Cairns[1], MD, MS and Kerri Lopez[2,†], MD

[1]University of Maryland Medical Center, Baltimore, Maryland, USA
[2]University of Maryland School of Medicine, Baltimore, Maryland, USA

Abstract

Crohn's disease frequently involves the colon, and most individuals with colonic Crohn's disease will ultimately require surgical intervention. The management of Crohn's colitis includes a careful assessment of the patient's response to medical therapy and the anatomy of the involved segments. Treatment selection is based on preserving as much function and quality of life as possible. While surgery cannot cure Crohn's disease, it can remove life-threatening complications and provide excellent symptom relief. Surgical options for colonic Crohn's include ileocecectomy, segmental colectomy, total colectomy, proctocolectomy, and in very select patients, reconstruction with ileal pouch-anal anastomosis. The choice of surgical treatment requires a thorough knowledge of currently evolving literature. This section will discuss the current state of evidence-based clinical practice in the surgical management of Crohn's colitis.

Introduction

Crohn's disease (CD) is an ulcerogenic, transmural, inflammatory bowel disease that can affect any portion of the gastrointestinal tract. It is most frequently found in the terminal ileum or ileocolic region, but approximately 60% of Crohn's patients will have colon involvement [1]. The foundation of current treatment for CD, regardless of site, is medical therapy with aminosalicylates, immunomodulators, biologic agents, and steroids, with surgery reserved for complications of the disease and failure of medical management. Though the advent of newer immunomodulators and biologic therapies have lowered the rates of operative management, surgery remains an important treatment tool [2]. Eventually, approximately half of patients with colonic Crohn's will undergo surgery [3]. The failure of medical management remains the leading indication for surgery in Crohn's patients [4, 5]. Reasons for failure vary widely in patients from noncompliance to intolerable side effects, to lack of response to the medical

* Based off Chapter 8: Colon Surgery 1st Edition by Andrea C. Bafford.

† Corresponding Author's Email: klopez@som.umaryland.edu

In: Surgery for Crohn's Disease. Second Edition
Editors: Stephen M. Kavic, Rebecca Brown and Kerri Lopez
ISBN: 979-8-89530-676-5

regimen. Importantly, surgical intervention must not be considered a "failure," but rather, an opportunity to offer many patients a demonstrable improvement in their quality of life [6-8]. Therefore, surgeons and IBD specialists must work together to achieve the best possible patient outcomes.

Surgical care in this patient population is particularly challenging due to pre-operative morbidities, such as anemia, malnutrition, and immunosuppression, as well as intraoperative considerations including thick and friable mesentery, adhesions, abscesses, and fistulas. Given this, Crohn's patients are at risk of significant perioperative morbidity and poor healing [9]. In the following sections, we detail pathology, epidemiology, and surgical strategies to address colonic CD.

Crohn's Disease of the Colon

Between 19-51% of patients with Crohn's have isolated colonic disease [10]. While the breakdown of anatomic distributions varies across studies, a large Swedish series of colonic Crohn's found that approximately 40% of patients had segmental disease, 31% had pan-colonic disease, and 26% had isolated left-sided disease [3, 11]. Notably, up to 88% of patients who present with pancolitis have been demonstrated to have isolated colonic disease. There is evidence that patients with segmental colitis may suffer a more virulent clinical course when compared to patients presenting with pancolitis [12].

Isolated colonic CD is associated with pathologic and clinical characteristics that differ from patients with other disease distributions. Colonic Crohn's is more common in late onset disease (>55 years), and is more often associated with non-smoking, female sex, and contraceptive use when compared to ileal Crohn's [13, 14]. Patients with isolated colonic disease are more often carriers of the DRB1*0103 allelic polymorphism as compared to patients without colonic involvement [15]. Colonic Crohn's is also more closely associated with the presence of extra-intestinal manifestations [13].

Colonic disease can manifest in various ways including abdominal pain, bloating, hip or pelvic pain, extraintestinal manifestations, or malnutrition. More severe presentations requiring procedural intervention include abscess, bleeding, stricture, and fulminant colitis non-responsive to medical therapy [3, 11, 16].

Indications for Surgery

Acute

Obstruction

Most colonic obstructions in CD that require surgery are due to stricture. Other, less common, etiologies include anastomotic stricture and malignancy. Strictures can occur throughout the colon secondary to acute inflammation, characterized by edema and increased bowel wall thickness [17], or chronic fibrosis from repeated episodes of transmural inflammation [16, 18]. Magnetic resonance enterography (MRE) and computed tomography enterography (CTE) can often be helpful in distinguishing active inflammation from chronic, fibrotic scar.

Large bowel obstructions resulting from active CD can often be managed medically with medications, bowel rest, and decompression [18]. If these methods are unsuccessful, surgical management with resection or diversion is required. Chronic strictures are unlikely to respond to medical management and should be managed operatively [18]. For patients with single short segment strictures, endoscopic balloon dilation can be successful in the short term, although it rarely produces a durable response [19].

Hemorrhage

Acute severe lower gastrointestinal (GI) tract bleeding occurs in 0.6 – 5.5% of patients with CD, a relatively infrequent complication when compared to patients with Ulcerative Colitis [16, 20-22]. One small series demonstrated that lower GI tract bleeding sites in Crohn's are most commonly found in the left or sigmoid colon [23]. In contrast to Ulcerative Colitis, when bleeding typically indicates widespread and severe mucosal ulceration, bleeding in Crohn's frequently occurs in the setting of a focal ulcer [16]. Initial management includes resuscitation with intravenous fluids, blood transfusion, correction of any coagulopathy, and attempts to identify the source of hemorrhage within the GI tract. Endoscopic evaluation should be performed, if possible, but additional techniques including angiography or nuclear scintigraphy can also be useful.

If a Crohn's patient with a lower gastrointestinal bleed becomes hemodynamically unstable or has recurrent bleeding despite nonoperative measures, they should be managed surgically. The extent of resection is determined by successful identification of the bleeding source. In general, grossly affected colon should be resected, preserving as much future colorectal function as possible. In patients where the source of hemorrhage cannot be identified, total abdominal colectomy should be performed [24].

Abscess

Contained perforation leading to abscess or fistula complicates colonic CD much more frequently than free perforation. Between 10 – 30% of patients with CD will develop an abdominal or pelvic abscess [25]. Microperforation of transmural ulcerations with or without fistula formation is the accepted pathogenesis of perforating CD. Abscesses most frequently occur due to disease within the terminal ileum and cecum [25, 26].

Abscesses can remain intra-abdominal or can involve the abdominal wall or retroperitoneum. Septic arthritis of the hip from a psoas abscess is a rare but known complication of colonic Crohn's [16]. Following initial resuscitation and initiation of antibiotics, additional treatment for abscess depends on the patient's response and clinical stability. Hemodynamically unstable patients and those with generalized peritonitis should undergo immediate surgery.

For stable patients, percutaneous abscess drainage is typically the first line treatment [27]. The timing of and need for definitive surgery has been debated in the literature. Most authors recommend controlling infection with the methods discussed above followed by subsequent elective surgery to resect affected bowel. Gutierrez showed that one-third of patients who underwent successful percutaneous abscess drainage ultimately required surgery within one year's time [16]. However, 30% of patients may avoid surgery with percutaneous drainage and antibiotics alone, and those who ultimately do require surgery have decreased rates of stoma creation following initial percutaneous drainage [28, 29]. Interestingly, colonic disease phenotype is a risk factor for failure of percutaneous drainage as are steroid use and multiloculated abscess [16]. When managing Crohn's patients with intra-abdominal septic complications, a holistic review of the individual's disease course and a multidisciplinary approach to therapy is recommended [26, 30].

Though rare, free perforation can occur in patients with Crohn's colitis and is an emergent indication for surgical intervention [31]. In small bowel disease, perforation is most associated with obstruction or abscess. In patients with colonic disease, perforation is usually seen complicating toxic colitis [32, 33].

Toxic Colitis

Toxic megacolon, or toxic colitis, is a rare but life-threatening complication of CD with up to 20% mortality [16]. It presents with abdominal pain and diarrhea and can be the first presentation of inflammatory bowel disease. Factors that may precipitate toxic colitis include use of medications such as anti-diarrheal agents, belladonna, and opiates, hypokalemia, steroid withdrawal, bowel preparation, and barium enemas [16, 34]. Diagnostic criteria include colonic distension >6cm and at least three signs of systemic toxicity (including fever, tachycardia, leukocytosis, or anemia) and either dehydration, altered mental status, electrolyte disturbance, or hypotension [35].

Initial management includes aggressive resuscitation, bowel rest and decompression, immunosuppressants such as intravenous steroids, broad-spectrum antibiotics, and nutritional support. Perforation or impending perforation, lack of improvement within two or three days of conservative management, clinical deterioration, and development of sepsis or shock are indications for immediate operative intervention. Surgery for toxic colitis usually consists of total abdominal colectomy with end ileostomy [16].

Chronic

Failure of Medical Therapy

Some complications that lead to the failure of medical management occur due to adverse effects of the immunosuppressive medications themselves. When successful, steroid treatment typically elicits an effect within days of IV therapy and 3-7 weeks of PO therapy [36, 37]. Unfortunately, long-term corticosteroid use can result in suppression of adrenal function, hypertension, osteoporosis, infections – including increased rates of abdominopelvic abscesses, hypokalemia, and hyperglycemia [38]. Corticosteroids should therefore never be used for maintenance of disease remission. Of the patients who receive corticosteroids for acute symptoms, 50% will develop steroid "dependent" or "resistant" CD [39], with higher rates of resistance seen in smokers and patients with colonic involvement [40]. Half of these patients will progress to resistance and require surgery within one year [41].

The expected time to response is generally between 6 – 12 weeks for various biologic and monoclonal antibody therapies, and 4 weeks for aminosalicylates [37]. Continued or worsening symptoms despite escalation of medical therapy is often an indication for operative intervention.

Growth Retardation in Children

The metabolic consequences of CD can be especially severe in the pediatric population. Growth retardation occurs in 15 – 40% of children affected and may precede the clinical diagnosis of Crohn's by several years [42-44]. Failure of growth is due to malabsorption, decreased caloric intake, and increased nutrient loss as a result of the disease's effect on the GI tract. Surgical intervention, specifically resection of involved segments, has been shown in retrospective series to improve growth velocity and pubertal development in patients with growth retardation [45-48].

Stricture

Colonic strictures occur in 9-13% of patients with CD, mostly commonly at a single site. Stricturing disease is caused by chronic and severe inflammation of the bowel wall with up-regulation of extracellular matrix component deposition, including collagen and fibronectins, and mesenchymal cell expansion [49]. In contrast to inflammatory strictures, which are often responsive to medication, fibrotic strictures typically require procedural intervention. Short strictures less than 5 cm in length, without associated abscess or fistula, may be responsive to endoscopic dilation [18, 50]. However, up to 7% of colonic strictures in Crohn's patients may contain dysplasia or malignancy. Therefore, these lesions should always undergo brushing or biopsy [18, 51, 52]. In the absence of malignancy, many strictures can be treated conservatively. However, symptomatic strictures and strictures that preclude endoscopic surveillance should be managed with surgical intervention. The standard operation for a colonic stricture is segmental resection; strictureplasty is typically not performed due to the higher risk of underlying malignancy [16, 53].

Despite advancements in medical therapies over the past decade, stricturing disease remains a significant problem with up to 32% of biologic-naïve patients starting biologic treatment for Crohn's associated strictures requiring surgery within two years [54].

Malignant Transformation

As a pro-inflammatory disease, it is not surprising that patients with CD have a higher incidence of malignancy, especially colorectal cancer [55]. Screening colonoscopy with staging biopsies should begin eight years after Crohn's symptom onset [56]. When discovered, resectable malignancy remains an indication for surgical intervention. The extent of colonic resection required for Crohn's colitis patients with colorectal dysplasia or cancer is somewhat controversial and will be discussed later in this chapter.

Fistula

In patients with CD, the colon is sometimes affected by fistula formation (Figure 10.1) [57, 58]. Overall, fistulization is predictive of higher lifetime relative risk (1.7) of requiring surgical treatment [3], and is independently associated with decreased time to surgery (HR, 3.44, 95% CI 2.33 to 5.08 vs inflammatory disease) [58]. Given the transmural nature of CD, fistulous communication with other bowel [59], lung, vagina [60], bladder [61], and skin [62] have been reported in patients where the colon is the primary site of inflammation. Underlying fistula should be strongly suspected in individuals with abdominal wall abscesses [16]. The colon may also be involved secondarily with fistulous communications arising from the stomach, duodenum, or small bowel [62]. Fistulizing disease is associated with increased postoperative complications, a higher rate of conversion to open procedure, and a higher incidence of postoperative fistula formation, of which enteroenteric is the most common [63, 64]. Even with the development of anti-TNF agents, 75% of patients being treated for fistulizing CD still require surgical intervention [65].

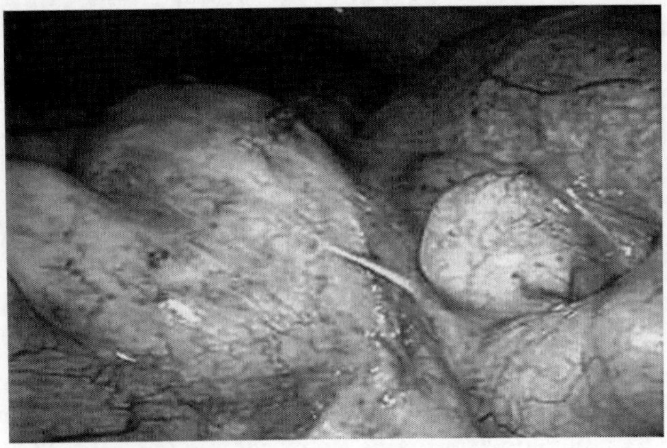

Figure 10.1. Ileal-sigmoid fistula secondary to Crohn's disease.

Extraintestinal Disease

Colonic CD has been associated with an increased risk of multiple extraintestinal manifestations including erythema nodosum, pyoderma gangrenosum, primary sclerosing cholangitis, peripheral arthritis, and ocular involvement [66]. In the Swiss IBD cohort, one-third of Crohn's patients with colonic Crohn's and extra-intestinal manifestations experienced cessation of symptoms after colectomy [67]. Surgery may therefore be indicated in patients with severe extra-intestinal disease [36, 68].

Preoperative Considerations

A thorough discussion of pre-operative management of patients with CD can be found in preceding chapters. Briefly, patients undergoing surgery for colonic Crohn's in non-urgent settings should receive pre-operative nutritional optimization, smoking cessation counseling, and "pre-habilitation" whenever possible [69]. Immunomodulators, monoclonal antibodies, and anti-TNF medications should be continued peri-operatively, and steroid doses >20mg daily should be weaned [28, 69].

Surgical Approaches to Colonic CD

When surgical treatment for colonic CD becomes necessary, the most important decision point is the extent of resection. Surgery for CD of the colon may include ileocolic resection, segmental colon resection, total colectomy, proctocolectomy, and proximal diversion (See Figure 10.2).

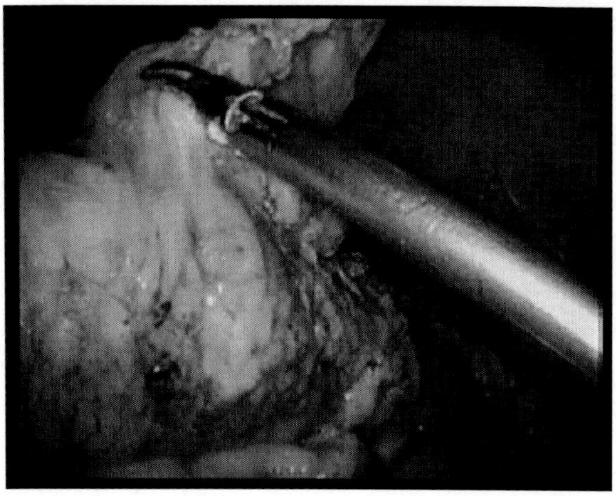

Figure 10.2. Severely inflamed transverse colon in a patient with Crohn's colitis.

Surgical Ileocolonic Disease

Indications for Surgery

Ileocolonic disease is both the most common presentation in CD and the leading cause of surgical intervention. The preferred method of surgical treatment is ileocecal resection to remove the diseased bowel. Operation for ileocolonic CD is indicated in any of the complications discussed above. Most patients with ileocolonic disease undergo surgery for either penetrating disease, which may be fistula or abscess, or stricturing disease, which may cause partial or complete obstruction.

As with penetrating disease, the most common locations for stricturing disease are the terminal ileum and ileocecal junction [70]. Penetrating and stricturing disease can be a continuum of disease pathogenesis, where perforation arises in areas of transmural inflammation due to increased pressure produced by downstream stricture, especially at the ileocecal junction [71]. Recently, studies have supported early surgical intervention followed by anti-TNF initiation for ileocolic CD with this approach resulting in fewer overall hospital admissions and a more benign disease course [72-74].

Minimally Invasive Ileocolic Resection

Laparoscopic surgery has increased significantly in popularity since the early 2000's and is generally accepted to reduce hospital stay and patient recovery without significant changes in surgical complications. Increased operative time is one drawback of laparoscopic surgery [10, 75, 76]. These results have been replicated in CD, where laparoscopic surgery has been shown to decrease postoperative complications, morbidity, length of stay, and time to return of bowel function [77-80]. Furthermore, Crohn's patients who underwent laparoscopic surgery experienced a similar or lower rate of disease recurrence, morbidity, and a lower rate of bowel obstruction at five years [78, 79, 81-83]. As such, laparoscopic ileocolic resection is considered to be the preferred surgical technique for these patients.

Robotic assisted surgery has been rapidly gaining popularity as a useful tool for the surgical treatment of CD [84]. It is purported to improve visualization and dexterity which is extremely important for CD patients, many of whom have had multiple operations and significant inflammation and thick, friable tissue [85]. For ileocolic resection, a robotic approach facilitates an intracorporeal anastomosis, minimizes the need for colon mobilization, and can decrease postoperative ileus rates and incisional hernias without significantly impacting rates of surgical site infection or overall 30-day postoperative complications [85]. While robotic assisted surgery appears to have benefits for ileocolic resection in Crohn's patients, it is not clear whether those benefits carry over to other colonic surgeries in CD [84].

Methods of Anastomosis

Outcomes in laparoscopic bowel resection appear to be influenced by several factors. Smoking, perianal disease, and presence of perforation all been associated with worse overall outcomes [86]. Pre-operative nutritional status, abdominal sepsis, medications, and specific surgical techniques have been all been identified as risk factors for anastomotic leak [87]. Stapled side-to-side anastomoses may reduce leak rate and overall postoperative complications when compared to hand-sewn end-to-end anastomosis, though these findings have been inconsistent across studies [8, 86, 88-92].

The Kono-S technique, a novel anti-mesenteric functional end-to-end anastomosis, was first published by Toru Kono in 2011 [93]. The development of this technique has challenged the perception of superiority of the side-to-side anastomosis. This technique is performed by creating a small window in the mesentery at the proximal and distal resection margins and dividing the mesentery close to the intestinal wall to preserve vascularization and innervation. The bowel is divided perpendicular to the intestinal lumen so the mesentery is in the center of the staple lines. The staple lines are then sewn together with interrupted silk suture to create a supporting column and an antimesenteric longitudinal enterotomy is created on each stump to create a 7-8cm transverse lumen which is then closed in two layers [87].

In the SuPREME-CD Study, the Kono-S anastomosis was compared to a stapled ileocolic side-to-side anastomosis. Among 79 patients with ileocolic CD, those who underwent Kono-S anastomosis had significant decrease in 6-month endoscopic recurrence (13.8% vs. 34.8%), and 24-month clinical (18% vs. 30.2%) and surgical (0% vs. 4.6%) recurrence at 24 months without any difference in postoperative outcomes [94]. Furthermore, Kono-S recipients reported significantly better bowel symptom scores and social functioning at 54 months after surgery when compared to the conventional side-to-side group [95]. These results are certainly promising, and continued positive studies may lead a more universal implementation of this approach.

Surgical Colonic Disease

Toxic Colitis

Toxic colitis or toxic megacolon is the most severe form of Crohn's colitis, and a frequent cause of urgent surgical intervention. Similar to in ulcerative colitis, toxic megacolon due to CD is initially treated with medical management, including aggressive resuscitation, antibiotics, and possibly immunosuppressive agents. Following adequate resuscitation, patients with perforation, uncontrolled bleeding, and clinical deterioration should undergo emergent surgical intervention [96].

Early operative management was with a loop ileostomy and "blowhole" transverse colostomy, as reported in 1970 by Turnbull [97]. However, this procedure was associated with high rates of mortality (71%) and complications, including ongoing severe bleeding [98]. The Turnbull procedure is therefore rarely performed.

Total proctocolectomy and subtotal colectomy with end ileostomy are the remaining options for surgical intervention. One study showed that in patients who received total proctocolectomy for toxic megacolon, complication and mortality rates were both 21%, whereas in those treated with subtotal colectomy with end ileostomy, the complication rate was 8% and the mortality rate was 6% [98]. The use of subtotal colectomy with end-ileostomy has greatly reduced the mortality of toxic colitis and remains the procedure of choice.

Segmental versus Subtotal Colectomy

Preservation of function with bowel-sparing is a primary goal in the surgical treatment of colonic CD. Despite the eventual choice of procedure, the literature is clear that segmental colectomy only requires resection to grossly normal bowel [99]. The choice of surgical procedure is governed largely by the anatomical presentation of the disease. Fichera published a prospective series of patients comparing the surgical outcomes of segmental colectomy, total abdominal colectomy, and total proctocolectomy [100]. Clinical characteristics were the same for all groups, except that the segmental colectomy patients were significantly younger. The authors found that patients with diffuse colonic involvement, distal colonic involvement, or multiple involved segments were significantly less likely to receive segmental colectomy. The literature has conflicting data regarding the rate of recurrence following the surgical options mentioned above.

In Fichera's study, segmental colectomy patients had a greater risk of recurrence than patients who underwent proctocolectomy, but not subtotal colectomy [100]. These results were confirmed in a large meta-analysis that compared segmental resection to subtotal colectomy with ileorectal anastomosis; no significant difference in the incidence of surgical recurrence was found between groups [101]. A more recent single institution series also demonstrated that segmental colectomy was not an independent predictor of disease recurrence [83]. There is some consensus that the speed of recurrence differs between surgical techniques. Fichera reported a significant difference in time to first recurrence between the three surgical groups, especially between segmental colectomy and total proctocolectomy [100]. Tekkis similarly found that the segmental resection group presented with recurrence approximately 4 years earlier [101]. Current guidelines recommend subtotal colectomy with ileorectal anastomosis over segmental colectomy for disease involving >2 segments of colon or for left sided disease [28].

One important consideration concerning patient quality of life is the need for a permanent stoma following colectomy. In Fischera's study, the need for permanent stoma was significantly higher in patients presenting with isolated distal colonic disease versus isolated proximal disease [100]. Kiran found no difference in stoma free survival between segmental colectomy (76.8%) and subtotal colectomy (84.2%) groups. A history of perianal sepsis and the presence of multiple comorbidities did reduce stoma-free survival [102]. These studies support the conclusion that both segmental and subtotal colectomies are reasonable options for treatment of Crohn's colitis when used in conjunction with careful patient selection and thorough review of patient disease course.

Colectomy for Dysplasia or Cancer

Crohn's patients are at 2-3x increased risk of colorectal malignancy given the chronic inflammation inherent to the disease [103]. Surveillance endoscopy should begin within 8 years of symptoms. When visible dysplasia is encountered on screening colonoscopy, it can be resected endoscopically and endoscopic surveillance is continued. Patients with invisible dysplasia on random biopsy should undergo high resolution colonoscopy and chromoendoscopy. Total colectomy or proctocolectomy is indicated for dysplasia that is endoscopically unresectable, multifocal, or found in surrounding flat mucosa as well as for adenocarcinoma due to the risk of synchronous disease [103].

Kiran evaluated 50 patients who underwent colectomy for Crohn's colitis-associated dysplasia. 44% of patients who underwent total proctocolectomy or subtotal colectomy had multifocal dysplasia. Of those patients who had a colorectal cancer, 40% had dysplasia remote from the cancer site. The authors therefore recommended total proctocolectomy as the treatment of choice in good-risk patients [104]. Maser found that 40% of patients who underwent segmental resection for colon cancer and 35% of patients who underwent subtotal colectomy for colon cancer developed metachronous cancer. 43% of patients who underwent segmental colectomy and 50% of patients who underwent subtotal colectomy for dysplasia developed a new dysplasia. They similarly concluded that total proctocolectomy should be considered in Crohn's patients with dysplasia or cancer due to high rates of metachronous disease [105]. Based upon limited data, proctocolectomy rather than segmental colectomy should be strongly considered in Crohn's colitis patients with colorectal dysplasia or cancer, though total colectomy can be considered in patients with rectal sparing disease [103].

Distal Colonic Disease

The management of CD affecting the distal colon is challenging. Patients with isolated distal disease are significantly more likely to require a permanent stoma than those with isolated proximal disease (54% vs 11%) [100]. Patients with distal involvement are also significantly more likely to undergo a more extensive resection than those with more proximal disease patterns.

Surgical indications for distal resection are dependent on the extent of inflammation and anatomy involved. Total proctocolectomy with end ileostomy is indicated when patients present with diffuse and extensive colorectal disease. In patients with rectal sparing, both total abdominal colectomy with ileorectal anastomosis and segmental resection can be considered. For patients with concomitant distal colonic and perianal CD, surgical options include proctectomy with end-colostomy, proctocolectomy, and proximal diversion with or without segmental or subtotal colectomy. The surgical management of perianal CD will be further discussed in a subsequent chapter.

Techniques in Crohn's Colitis with Rectal Sparing

Total Proctocolectomy with end Ileostomy

The management of Crohn's colitis with relative rectal sparing is an area of relative controversy in the literature. In patients with Crohn's colitis, involvement of the rectum and anal canal must be considered when choosing treatment. Total proctocolectomy is the most appropriate option for patients with extensive colitis and refractory perianal disease, despite the presence of rectal sparing. This procedure involves the removal of all colonic, rectal and perianal disease and therefore affords the lowest rates of recurrence, reoperation, and need for medical therapy postoperatively, though recurrence rates can be as high as 13-25% [16, 100, 106, 107].

On the other hand, many patients undergoing surgery for CD are relatively young, and the risk of pelvic nerve injury, including impact on sexual function and fertility, may not be acceptable [106, 108]. Further, total proctocolectomy results in a permanent end ileostomy, which can negatively impact patient satisfaction and quality of life given the inherent challenges of ostomy management and the potential for peristomal hernia [16, 109]. As a result, high levels of patient resistance to this procedure are frequently encountered. In recent years, intersphincteric proctectomy has been used to reduce the rates of sexual dysfunction related to dissection near the hypogastric nerve plexus and to minimize perineal wound complications [110].

Total Abdominal Colectomy with End Ileostomy

Proctocolectomy is preferred in patients with rectal involvement, but total abdominal colectomy with end ileostomy is an option for patients with an acute surgical indication if the degree of pelvic inflammation makes rectal dissection unsafe [16]. In these situations, the question of what to do with rectal stump is challenging. The stump may be closed and drained intra-abdominally or brought up as a mucus fistula. The incidence of pelvic sepsis is proportional to the length of remaining rectum, and therefore the surgeon must weigh the risk of stump blowout and septic complications. Secondary proctectomy will be required in most cases [16].

Total Abdominal Colectomy with Ileorectal Anastomosis

Total abdominal colectomy with ileorectal anastomosis is an option in patients with rectal sparing. It is preferred for patients with minimal to no perianal disease and good continence at baseline. A series of 833 patients with Crohn's colitis demonstrated relatively high rates of symptomatic recurrence when subtotal colectomy with ileorectal anastomosis and segmental colon resection were compared with subtotal colectomy and proctocolectomy with ileostomy (58% and 47% versus 24% and 37%, respectively). On multivariate analysis, perianal disease, ileorectal anastomosis, and segmental resection were all independent risk factors for recurrence [111]. Andersson also found similar rates of re-resection following segmental versus subtotal colectomy for Crohn's colitis. However, segmental colectomy patients had the advantages of fewer loose stools, better anorectal function, and fewer symptoms overall [112].

In contrast, a large meta-analysis examining 488 patients undergoing ileorectal anastomosis versus segmental colectomy showed that ileorectal anastomosis led to lower rates of postoperative complications and permanent stoma creation. Those patients with multiple affected colonic segments were less likely to need re-operation when they underwent ileorectal anastomosis [101]. Overall, total abdominal colectomy with ileorectal anastomosis carries an approximate 7.4% leak rate and 30% long-term risk of proctectomy [16].

Ileal Pouch-Anal Anastomosis (IPAA)

Ileal pouch-anal anastomosis (IPAA) may be an option for very select patients with both ileal and anal sparing CD. The more common setting is that patients who carry a preoperative diagnosis of ulcerative colitis undergo total proctocolectomy with IPAA and are then diagnosed with CD postoperatively. A study of 60 patients in this situation found that 35% developed disease recurrence, 40% reported issues with continence, and 12% ultimately required pouch excision [113]. Another study of 41 patients with ileal and rectal-sparing inflammation including 26 patients with a preoperative diagnosis of CD, demonstrated a 10% rate of pouch excision, and a 35% incidence of serious complications, including pouchitis, abscess, and fistula formation [114]. Many of these patients had improvement in symptoms with medical management, and therefore the authors concluded that IPAA may be considered in Crohn's patients meeting the criteria of ileal and anal sparing.

Several more contemporaneous studies found that the outcomes of IPAA in CD were not as favorable. One study published results showing that 56% of patients who underwent restorative proctocolectomy for Crohn's colitis required diversion or pouch excision compared to only 6% who had the procedure performed for ulcerative colitis [115]. Further, Braveman found that of 32 patients diagnosed with CD postoperatively after IPAA, 93% had significant complications, including fistula (63%), pouchitis (50%), and anal stricture (38%). Pouch excision or permanent diversion was required in 29% of patients [116].

Finally, meta-analyses of patients who underwent restorative proctocolectomy have demonstrated equivalent or higher rates of incontinence, anastomotic strictures, and pouch failure in Crohn's patients compared to Ulcerative Colitis [117, 118]. In summary, ileoanal pouch construction remains controversial due to significant variance in the rate of complications (35% to 93%) reported in the literature [113-116, 118] . Some studies have suggested better outcomes in those Crohn's colitis patients without perianal disease or small bowel involvement. Other investigators have not found any features predictive of outcome after an IPAA procedure [116].

Laparoscopic Techniques in Crohn's Colitis

Laparoscopic techniques have significantly improved the outcomes of patients undergoing colorectal surgery, both cosmetically and functionally [9]. There is an abundance of evidence showing advantages of laparoscopic colorectal surgery over open techniques, including reduced length of hospital stay, decreased postoperative narcotic use, reduced wound complications, and earlier return of postoperative bowel function [119]. Though its implementation was slow given the unique challenges in Crohn's patients, laparoscopic surgery is considered preferable given the young age of patients, the high likelihood of subsequent reoperation, the high rates of wound infections, and the debilitated state patients with CD often present in [85].

Studies comparing laparoscopic and open colectomy have demonstrated shorter length of stay, earlier return of bowel function, less intraoperative blood loss, and fewer complications in the laparoscopic group [120]. The literature-to-date supports the conclusion that laparoscopy is a safe and effective surgical option for patients with colonic CD.

Recurrent disease is a noteworthy challenge in the management of patients with Crohn's. As the indications for laparoscopic intervention in colonic CD grow, its use in difficult recrudescent cases is expected. There are several studies available which have investigated the use of laparoscopy in recurrent disease with favorable results [64, 121, 122]. In a study of 26 patients who underwent mixed small and large bowel procedures, laparoscopic and open techniques were compared. The authors found similar rates of blood loss, operative time, need for reoperation, time to return of bowel function, length of hospital stay, and readmission. They also found that laparoscopy was associated with a significantly lower rate of wound infection [123]. They concluded that while laparoscopy may have lower rates of wound infection, the similarity in surgical outcomes between laparoscopy and open procedures does not show a clear advantage to either approach.

The advancement of laparoscopic techniques for the management of CD has been augmented by several methods, including robotic assisted and hand-assisted laparoscopic surgery (HALS). Robotic assisted surgery in particular has gained significant attention in the treatment of colorectal disease. It has been shown to have a similar safety profile to laparoscopic surgery with lower conversion rates. Proponents of robotic assisted surgery describe improved visualization, useful computer technology, improved ergonomics, and added dexterity which is particularly advantageous in Crohn's patients who often have technically challenging anatomy [9, 85, 124].

A meta-analysis of 39 studies including 13 ileocecal resections, 220 right colectomies, 190 left and sigmoid resections, 440 anterior resections, 149 abdominoperineal resections, and 11 total or subtotal colectomies, demonstrated acceptable rates of conversion and morbidity [125]. Recently, a study of 17 robot assisted proctectomies and ileal pouch-anal anastomosis procedures in patients with Crohn's colitis demonstrated similar rates of operative blood loss, postoperative complications, and impact on bowel and sexual function, compared to their laparoscopic counterparts [126]. While the evidence for robotic and laparoscopic surgery in Crohn's patients continues to grow, the aforementioned challenges inherent to Crohn's patients demand that these technologies are used only by experienced colorectal and minimally invasive surgeons.

Post-Operative Considerations

Briefly, working as a multidisciplinary team in the peri-operative period is essential to ensuring the best outcomes in patients with CD. Enhanced Recovery After Surgery, (ERAS) protocols have been shown to offer significant benefit in postoperative recovery for patients with inflammatory bowel disease [9, 127-129]. Patients should receive appropriate nutritional counseling to ensure functional recovery and wound healing [69]. The patient's gastroenterologist should be consulted promptly in the post-operative period to ensure that medical therapy can be initiated or resumed to treat residual disease or maintain remission [73].

Conclusion

Crohn's disease is a complicated disease that affects the entire gastrointestinal tract and significantly impacts the health and quality of life of patients who suffer from it. Medical management has greatly improved over the past decades, and new medications are being actively developed. However, despite these improvements in medical therapy, the majority of CD patients will require surgical intervention at some point during their lifetime. Although surgery cannot cure CD, it continues to play a significant role in managing complications and improving disease symptomatology and patient quality of life. As discussed in this chapter, the management of Crohn's colitis is complex, and therefore treating surgeons must remain abreast of the relevant literature and facile in current surgical techniques. Minimization of morbidity, preservation of gastrointestinal function, and improvement in quality of life are all priorities when caring for patients with Crohn's disease.

References

[1] Mills S, Stamos M. Colonic Crohn's Disease. *Clin Colon Rectal Surg*. 2007;20(4):309-313. doi:10.1055/s-2007-991030.

[2] Lin CC, Lin HH, Chen HC, et al. Perioperative optimization of Crohn's disease. *Ann Gastroenterol Surg*. 2023;7(1):10-26. doi:10.1002/ags3.12621.

[3] Lapidus A, Bernell O, Hellers G, Löfberg R. Clinical course of colorectal Crohn's disease: a 35-year follow-up study of 507 patients. *Gastroenterology*. 1998;114(6):1151-1160. doi:10.1016/s0016-5085(98)70420-2.

[4] Penner RM, Madsen KL, Fedorak RN. Postoperative Crohn's disease. *Inflamm Bowel Dis*. 2005;11(8):765-777. doi:10.1097/01.mib.0000171273.09757.f2.

[5] Hancock L, Windsor AC, Mortensen NJ. Inflammatory bowel disease: the view of the surgeon. *Colorectal Dis*. 2006;8 Suppl 1:10-14. doi:10.1111/j.1463-1318.2006.00986.x.

[6] Thirlby RC, Land JC, Fenster LF, Lonborg R. Effect of Surgery on Health-Related Quality of Life in Patients With Inflammatory Bowel Disease. *Archives of Surgery*. 1998;133(8). doi:10.1001/archsurg.133.8.826.

[7] Silverstein MD, Loftus E V, Sandborn WJ, et al. Clinical course and costs of care for Crohn's disease: Markov model analysis of a population-based cohort. *Gastroenterology*. 1999;117(1):49-57. doi:10.1016/s0016-5085(99)70549-4.

[8] McLeod RS. Surgery for inflammatory bowel diseases. *Dig Dis*. 2003;21(2):168-179. doi:10.1159/000073248.

[9] Holder-Murray J, Marsicovetere P, Holubar SD. Minimally invasive surgery for inflammatory bowel disease. *Inflamm Bowel Dis*. 2015;21(6):1443-1458. doi:10.1097/MIB.0000000000000316.

[10] Dasari BV, McKay D, Gardiner K. Laparoscopic versus Open surgery for small bowel Crohn's disease. *Cochrane Database Syst Rev*. 2011;(1):CD006956. doi:10.1002/14651858.CD006956.pub2.

[11] Renison DM, Forouhar FA, Levine JB, Breiter JR. Filiform polyposis of the colon presenting as massive hemorrhage: an uncommon complication of Crohn's disease. *Am J Gastroenterol*. 1983;78(7): 413-416.

[12] Morpurgo E, Petras R, Kimberling J, Ziegler C, Galandiuk S. Characterization and Clinical Behavior of Crohn's Disease Initially Presenting Predominantly as Colitis. *Dis Colon Rectum*. 2003;46(7):918-924. doi:10.1007/s10350-004-6685-z.

[13] Dulai PS, Singh S, Vande Casteele N, et al. Should We Divide Crohn's Disease Into Ileum-Dominant and Isolated Colonic Diseases? *Clinical Gastroenterology and Hepatology*. 2019;17(13):2634-2643. doi:10.1016/j.cgh.2019.04.040.

[14] Soucy G, Wang HH, Farraye FA, et al. Clinical and pathological analysis of colonic Crohn's disease, including a subgroup with ulcerative colitis-like features. *Modern Pathology*. 2012;25(2):295-307. doi:10.1038/modpathol.2011.120.

[15] Hancock L, Beckly J, Geremia A, et al. Clinical and molecular characteristics of isolated colonic Crohn's disease. *Inflamm Bowel Dis*. 2008;14(12):1667-1677. doi:10.1002/ibd.20517.

[16] Harb WJ. Crohn's Disease of the Colon, Rectum, and Anus. *Surgical Clinics of North America*. 2015;95(6):1195-1210. doi:10.1016/j.suc.2015.07.005.

[17] Alfredsson J, Wick MJ. Mechanism of fibrosis and stricture formation in Crohn's disease. *Scand J Immunol*. 2020;92(6). doi:10.1111/sji.12990.

[18] Ford MM. Crohn's Disease Obstructions. *Clin Colon Rectal Surg*. 2021;34(04):227-232. doi:10.1055/s-0041-1729926.

[19] Bettenworth D, Gustavsson A, Atreja A, et al. A Pooled Analysis of Efficacy, Safety, and Long-term Outcome of Endoscopic Balloon Dilation Therapy for Patients with Stricturing Crohn's Disease. *Inflamm Bowel Dis*. 2017;23(1):133-142. doi:10.1097/MIB.0000000000000988.

[20] Daperno M, Sostegni R, Rocca R. Lower gastrointestinal bleeding in Crohn's disease: How (un-)common is it and how to tackle it? *Digestive and Liver Disease*. 2012;44(9):721-722. doi:10.1016/j.dld.2012.06.006.

[21] Kostka R, Lukás M. Massive, life-threatening bleeding in Crohn's disease. *Acta Chir Belg*. 2005;105(2):168-174.

[22] Tu T, Chen M, Zeng Z, et al. A comprehensive review and update on acute severe lower gastrointestinal bleeding in Crohn's disease: a management algorithm. *Gastroenterol Rep (Oxf)*. 2023;12. doi:10.1093/gastro/goae099.

[23] Belaiche J, Louis E, D'Haens G, et al. Acute Lower Gastrointestinal Bleeding in Crohn's Disease: Characteristics of A Unique Series of 34 Patients. *American Journal of Gastroenterology*. 1999;94(8):2177-2181. doi:10.1111/j.1572-0241.1999.01291.x.

[24] Raphaeli T, Menon R. Current treatment of lower gastrointestinal hemorrhage. *Clin Colon Rectal Surg*. 2012;25(4):219-227. doi:10.1055/s-0032-1329393.

[25] Yamaguchi A, Matsui T, Sakurai T, et al. The clinical characteristics and outcome of intraabdominal abscess in Crohn's disease. *J Gastroenterol*. 2004;39(5):441-448. doi:10.1007/s00535-003-1317-2.

[26] Alós R, Hinojosa J. Timing of surgery in Crohn's disease: a key issue in the management. *World J Gastroenterol*. 2008;14(36):5532-5539. doi:10.3748/wjg.14.5532.

[27] Gutierrez A, Lee H, Sands BE. Outcome of surgical versus percutaneous drainage of abdominal and pelvic abscesses in Crohn's disease. *Am J Gastroenterol*. 2006;101(10):2283-2289. doi:10.1111/j.1572-0241.2006.00757.x.

[28] Adamina M, Bonovas S, Raine T, et al. ECCO Guidelines on Therapeutics in Crohn's Disease: Surgical Treatment. *J Crohns Colitis*. 2020;14(2):155-168. doi:10.1093/ecco-jcc/jjz187.

[29] Moreira A da L, Stocchi L, Tan E, Tekkis PP, Fazio VW. Outcomes of Crohn's Disease Presenting with Abdominopelvic Abscess. *Dis Colon Rectum*. 2009;52(5):906-912. doi:10.1007/DCR.0b013e31819f27c3.

[30] Fleshman JW. Pyogenic complications of Crohn's disease, evaluation, and management. *J Gastrointest Surg*. 2008;12(12):2160-2163. doi:10.1007/s11605-008-0673-x.

[31] Gardiner KR, Dasari BVM. Operative management of small bowel Crohn's disease. *Surg Clin North Am*. 2007;87(3):587-610. doi:10.1016/j.suc.2007.03.011.

[32] Werbin N, Haddad R, Greenberg R, Karin E, Skornick Y. Free perforation in Crohn's disease. *Isr Med Assoc J*. 2003;5(3):175-177.

[33] Greenstein AJ, Sachar DB, Mann D, Lachman P, Heimann T, Aufses AH. Spontaneous free perforation and perforated abscess in 30 patients with Crohn's disease. *Ann Surg*. 1987;205(1):72-76. doi:10.1097/00000658-198701000-00013.

[34] Tariq S, Farooq A, Ali I, Wijesinghe H. Toxic colonoscopy--how investigating active inflammatory bowel disease can lead to the serious complication of toxic megacolon. *BMJ Case Rep*. 2015;2015. doi:10.1136/bcr-2015-209769.

[35] Jalan KN, Sircus W, Card WI, et al. An experience of ulcerative colitis. I. Toxic dilation in 55 cases. *Gastroenterology*. 1969;57(1):68-82.

[36] Heriot A, Smart P. Current Status of Segmental Colectomy in Select Crohn's Disease Patients. *Clin Colon Rectal Surg*. 2019;32(04):249-254. doi:10.1055/s-0039-1683906.

[37] Vasudevan A, Gibson PR, van Langenberg DR. Time to clinical response and remission for therapeutics in inflammatory bowel diseases: What should the clinician expect, what should patients be told? *World J Gastroenterol*. 2017;23(35):6385-6402. doi:10.3748/wjg.v23.i35.6385.

[38] Vavricka SR, Schoepfer AM, Scharl M, Rogler G. Steroid use in Crohn's disease. *Drugs*. 2014;74(3):313-324. doi:10.1007/s40265-014-0183-y.

[39] Munkholm P, Langholz E, Davidsen M, Binder V. Frequency of glucocorticoid resistance and dependency in Crohn's disease. *Gut*. 1994;35(3):360-362. doi:10.1136/gut.35.3.360.

[40] Franchimont DP, Louis E, Croes F, Belaiche J. Clinical pattern of corticosteroid dependent Crohn's disease. *Eur J Gastroenterol Hepatol*. 1998;10(10):821-825. doi:10.1097/00042737-199810000-00001.

[41] Faubion WA, Loftus E V, Harmsen WS, Zinsmeister AR, Sandborn WJ. The natural history of corticosteroid therapy for inflammatory bowel disease: a population-based study. *Gastroenterology*. 2001;121(2):255-260. doi:10.1053/gast.2001.26279.

[42] Shamir R, Phillip M, Levine A. Growth retardation in pediatric Crohn's disease: pathogenesis and interventions. *Inflamm Bowel Dis*. 2007;13(5):620-628. doi:10.1002/ibd.20115.

[43] Newby EA, Sawczenko A, Thomas AG, Wilson D. Interventions for growth failure in childhood Crohn's disease. *Cochrane Database Syst Rev*. 2005;2005(3):CD003873. doi:10.1002/14651858. CD003873.pub2.

[44] Cezard JP, Touati G, Alberti C, Hugot JP, Brinon C, Czernichow P. Growth in paediatric Crohn's disease. *Horm Res*. 2002;58 Suppl 1:11-15. doi:10.1159/000064759.

[45] Heuschkel R, Salvestrini C, Beattie RM, Hildebrand H, Walters T, Griffiths A. Guidelines for the management of growth failure in childhood inflammatory bowel disease. *Inflamm Bowel Dis*. 2008;14(6):839-849. doi:10.1002/ibd.20378.

[46] McLain BI, Davidson PM, Stokes KB, Beasley SW. Growth after gut resection for Crohn's disease. *Arch Dis Child*. 1990;65(7):760-762. doi:10.1136/adc.65.7.760.

[47] Griffiths AM, Wesson DE, Shandling B, Corey M, Sherman PM. Factors influencing postoperative recurrence of Crohn's disease in childhood. *Gut*. 1991;32(5):491-495. doi:10.1136/gut.32.5.491.

[48] Dokucu AI, Sarnacki S, Michel JL, et al. Indications and results of surgery in patients with Crohn's disease with onset under 10 years of age: a series of 18 patients. *Eur J Pediatr Surg*. 2002;12(3):180-185. doi:10.1055/s-2002-32725.

[49] Rieder F, Zimmermann EM, Remzi FH, Sandborn WJ. Crohn's disease complicated by strictures: a systematic review. *Gut*. 2013;62(7):1072-1084. doi:10.1136/gutjnl-2012-304353.

[50] Chutkan RK, Scherl E, Waye JD. Colonoscopy in inflammatory bowel disease. *Gastrointest Endosc Clin N Am*. 2002;12(3):463-483, viii. doi:10.1016/s1052-5157(02)00007-7.

[51] Yamazaki Y, Ribeiro MB, Sachar DB, Aufses AH, Greenstein AJ. Malignant colorectal strictures in Crohn's disease. *Am J Gastroenterol*. 1991;86(7):882-885.

[52] Itzkowitz SH, Present DH, Crohn's and Colitis Foundation of America Colon Cancer in IBD Study Group. Consensus conference: Colorectal cancer screening and surveillance in inflammatory bowel disease. *Inflamm Bowel Dis*. 2005;11(3):314-321. doi:10.1097/01.mib.0000160811.76729.d5.

[53] Strong SA. Strictureplasty in Complex Crohn's Disease: Beyond the Basics. *Clin Colon Rectal Surg*. 2019;32(04):243-248. doi:10.1055/s-0039-1683905.

[54] Sleiman J, El Ouali S, Qazi T, et al. Prevention and Treatment of Stricturing Crohn's Disease - Perspectives and Challenges. *Expert Rev Gastroenterol Hepatol*. 2021;15(4):401-411. doi:10.1080/17474124.2021.1854732.

[55] Grivennikov SI. Inflammation and colorectal cancer: colitis-associated neoplasia. *Semin Immunopathol*. 2013;35(2):229-244. doi:10.1007/s00281-012-0352-6.

[56] Clarke WT, Feuerstein JD. Colorectal cancer surveillance in inflammatory bowel disease: Practice guidelines and recent developments. *World J Gastroenterol*. 2019;25(30):4148-4157. doi:10.3748/wjg.v25.i30.4148.

[57] Steele SR. Operative management of Crohn's disease of the colon including anorectal disease. *Surg Clin North Am*. 2007;87(3):611-631. doi:10.1016/j.suc.2007.03.006.

[58] Lakatos PL, Golovics PA, David G, et al. Has there been a change in the natural history of Crohn's disease? Surgical rates and medical management in a population-based inception cohort from Western Hungary between 1977-2009. *Am J Gastroenterol*. 2012;107(4):579-588. doi:10.1038/ajg.2011.448.

[59] El-Hajj II, Abdul-Baki H, El-Zahabi LM, Barada KA. Primary coloduodenal fistula in Crohn's disease. *Dig Dis Sci*. 2007;52(1):59-63. doi:10.1007/s10620-006-9227-9.

[60] Barisiae G, Krivokapiae Z, Adziae T, Pavloviae A, Popoviae M, Gojniae M. Fecopneumothorax and colopleural fistula - uncommon complications of Crohn's disease. *BMC Gastroenterol*. 2006;6:17. doi:10.1186/1471-230X-6-17.

[61] Garcea G, Majid I, Sutton CD, Pattenden CJ, Thomas WM. Diagnosis and management of colovesical fistulae; six-year experience of 90 consecutive cases. *Colorectal Dis*. 2006;8(4):347-352. doi:10.1111/j.1463-1318.2005.00928.x.

[62] Poritz LS, Gagliano GA, McLeod RS, MacRae H, Cohen Z. Surgical management of entero and colocutaneous fistulae in Crohn's disease: 17 year's experience. *Int J Colorectal Dis*. 2004;19(5):481-485; discussion 486. doi:10.1007/s00384-004-0580-x.

[63] Pinto RA, Shawki S, Narita K, Weiss EG, Wexner SD. Laparoscopy for recurrent Crohn's disease: how do the results compare with the results for primary Crohn's disease? *Colorectal Dis*. 2011;13(3):302-307. doi:10.1111/j.1463-1318.2009.02133.x.

[64] Brouquet A, Bretagnol F, Soprani A, Valleur P, Bouhnik Y, Panis Y. A laparoscopic approach to iterative ileocolonic resection for the recurrence of Crohn's disease. *Surg Endosc*. 2010;24(4):879-887. doi:10.1007/s00464-009-0682-1.

[65] Poritz LS, Rowe WA, Koltun WA. Remicade does not abolish the need for surgery in fistulizing Crohn's disease. *Dis Colon Rectum*. 2002;45(6):771-775. doi:10.1007/s10350-004-6296-8.

[66] Khrom M, Long M, Dube S, et al. Comprehensive Association Analyses of Extraintestinal Manifestations in Inflammatory Bowel Disease. *Gastroenterology*. 2024;167(2):315-332. doi:10.1053/j.gastro.2024.02.026.

[67] Roth R, Vavricka S, Scharl M, et al. The impact of colectomy on the course of extraintestinal manifestations in Swiss inflammatory bowel disease cohort study patients. *United European Gastroenterol J*. 2021;9(7):773-780. doi:10.1002/ueg2.12125.

[68] Guy TS, Williams NN, Rosato EF. Crohn's Disease of the Colon. *Surgical Clinics of North America*. 2001;81(1):159-168. doi:10.1016/S0039-6109(05)70278-4.

[69] Sebastian S, Segal JP, Hedin C, et al. ECCO Topical Review: Roadmap to Optimal Peri-Operative Care in IBD. *J Crohns Colitis*. 2023;17(2):153-169. doi:10.1093/ecco-jcc/jjac129.

[70] Gasche C, Scholmerich J, Brynskov J, et al. A simple classification of Crohn's disease: report of the Working Party for the World Congresses of Gastroenterology, Vienna 1998. *Inflamm Bowel Dis*. 2000;6(1):8-15. doi:10.1097/00054725-200002000-00002.

[71] Oberhuber G, Stangl PC, Vogelsang H, Schober E, Herbst F, Gasche C. Significant association of strictures and internal fistula formation in Crohn's disease. *Virchows Arch*. 2000;437(3):293-297. doi:10.1007/s004280000226.

[72] An V, Cohen L, Lawrence M, Thomas M, Andrews J, Moore J. Early surgery in Crohn's disease a benefit in selected cases. *World J Gastrointest Surg*. 2016;8(7):492. doi:10.4240/wjgs.v8.i7.492.

[73] Axelrad JE, Li T, Bachour SP, et al. Early Initiation of Antitumor Necrosis Factor Therapy Reduces Postoperative Recurrence of Crohn's Disease Following Ileocecal Resection. *Inflamm Bowel Dis*. 2023;29(6):888-897. doi:10.1093/ibd/izac158.

[74] Stevens TW, Haasnoot ML, D'Haens GR, et al. Laparoscopic ileocaecal resection versus infliximab for terminal ileitis in Crohn's disease: retrospective long-term follow-up of the LIR!C trial. *Lancet Gastroenterol Hepatol*. 2020;5(10):900-907. doi:10.1016/S2468-1253(20)30117-5.

[75] Milsom JW, Lavery IC, Böhm B, Fazio VW. Laparoscopically assisted ileocolectomy in Crohn's disease. *Surg Laparosc Endosc*. 1993;3(2):77-80.

[76] Maartense S, Dunker MS, Slors JFM, et al. Laparoscopic-assisted versus open ileocolic resection for Crohn's disease: a randomized trial. *Ann Surg*. 2006;243(2):143-149; discussion 150-3. doi:10.1097/01.sla.0000197318.37459.ec.

[77] Lee Y, Fleming FJ, Deeb A -P., Gunzler D, Messing S, Monson JRT. A laparoscopic approach reduces short-term complications and length of stay following ileocolic resection in Crohn's disease: an analysis of outcomes from the NSQIP database. *Colorectal Disease*. 2012;14(5):572-577. doi:10.1111/j.1463-1318.2011.02756.x.

[78] Tan JJY, Tjandra JJ. Laparoscopic surgery for Crohn's disease: a meta-analysis. *Dis Colon Rectum*. 2007;50(5):576-585. doi:10.1007/s10350-006-0855-0.

[79] Rosman AS, Melis M, Fichera A. Metaanalysis of trials comparing laparoscopic and open surgery for Crohn's disease. *Surg Endosc*. 2005;19(12):1549-1555. doi:10.1007/s00464-005-0114-9.

[80] Tilney HS, Constantinides VA, Heriot AG, et al. Comparison of laparoscopic and open ileocecal resection for Crohn's disease: a metaanalysis. *Surg Endosc*. 2006;20(7):1036-1044. doi:10.1007/s00464-005-0500-3.

[81] Lowney JK, Dietz DW, Birnbaum EH, Kodner IJ, Mutch MG, Fleshman JW. Is there any difference in recurrence rates in laparoscopic ileocolic resection for Crohn's disease compared with conventional surgery? A long-term, follow-up study. *Dis Colon Rectum*. 2006;49(1):58-63. doi:10.1007/s10350-005-0214-6.

[82] Stocchi L, Milsom JW, Fazio VW. Long-term outcomes of laparoscopic versus open ileocolic resection for Crohn's disease: follow-up of a prospective randomized trial. *Surgery*. 2008;144(4):622-627; discussion 627-8. doi:10.1016/j.surg.2008.06.016.

[83] Bergamaschi R, Pessaux P, Arnaud JP. Comparison of conventional and laparoscopic ileocolic resection for Crohn's disease. *Dis Colon Rectum*. 2003;46(8):1129-1133. doi:10.1007/s10350-004-7292-8.

[84] Radomski SN, Stem M, Consul M, et al. National trends and feasibility of a robotic surgical approach in the management of patients with inflammatory bowel disease. *Surg Endosc*. 2023;37(10):7849-7858. doi:10.1007/s00464-023-10333-1.

[85] Gunnells D, Cannon J. Robotic Surgery in Crohn's Disease. *Clin Colon Rectal Surg*. 2021;34(5):286-291. doi:10.1055/s-0041-1729862.

[86] Ikeuchi H, Kusunoki M, Yamamura T. Long-Term Results of Stapled and Hand-Sewn Anastomoses in Patients with Crohn's Disease. *Dig Surg*. 2000;17(5):493-496. doi:10.1159/000051946.

[87] Kann BR. Anastomotic Considerations in Crohn's Disease. *Clin Colon Rectal Surg*. 2023;36(1):63-73. doi:10.1055/s-0042-1758770.

[88] Guo Z, Li Y, Zhu W, Gong J, Li N, Li J. Comparing Outcomes Between Side-to-Side Anastomosis and Other Anastomotic Configurations After Intestinal Resection for Patients with Crohn's Disease: A Meta-Analysis. *World J Surg*. 2013;37(4):893-901. doi:10.1007/s00268-013-1928-6.

[89] He X, Chen Z, Huang J, et al. Stapled Side-to-Side Anastomosis Might Be Better Than Handsewn End-to-End Anastomosis in Ileocolic Resection for Crohn's Disease: A Meta-Analysis. *Dig Dis Sci*. 2014;59(7):1544-1551. doi:10.1007/s10620-014-3039-0.

[90] Simillis C, Purkayastha S, Yamamoto T, Strong SA, Darzi AW, Tekkis PP. A meta-analysis comparing conventional end-to-end anastomosis vs. other anastomotic configurations after resection in Crohn's disease. *Dis Colon Rectum*. 2007;50(10):1674-1687. doi:10.1007/s10350-007-9011-8.

[91] Muñoz-Juárez M, Yamamoto T, Wolff BG, Keighley MR. Wide-lumen stapled anastomosis vs. conventional end-to-end anastomosis in the treatment of Crohn's disease. *Dis Colon Rectum.* 2001;44(1):20-25; discussion 25-6. doi:10.1007/BF02234814.

[92] Resegotti A, Astegiano M, Farina EC, et al. Side-to-side stapled anastomosis strongly reduces anastomotic leak rates in Crohn's disease surgery. *Dis Colon Rectum.* 2005;48(3):464-468. doi:10.1007/s10350-004-0786-6.

[93] Kono T, Ashida T, Ebisawa Y, et al. A New Antimesenteric Functional End-to-End Handsewn Anastomosis: Surgical Prevention of Anastomotic Recurrence in Crohn's Disease. *Dis Colon Rectum.* 2011;54(5):586-592. doi:10.1007/DCR.0b013e318208b90f.

[94] Luglio G, Rispo A, Imperatore N, et al. Surgical Prevention of Anastomotic Recurrence by Excluding Mesentery in Crohn's Disease: The SuPREMe-CD Study - A Randomized Clinical Trial. *Ann Surg.* 2020;272(2):210-217. doi:10.1097/SLA.0000000000003821.

[95] Cricrì M, Tropeano FP, Rispo A, et al. Impact of Kono-S anastomosis on quality of life after ileocolic resection in Crohn's disease: an analysis from the SuPREMe-CD trial. *Colorectal Dis.* Published online June 16, 2024. doi:10.1111/codi.17073.

[96] Autenrieth DM, Baumgart DC. Toxic megacolon. *Inflamm Bowel Dis.* 2012;18(3):584-591. doi:10.1002/ibd.21847.

[97] Turnbull RB, Weakley FL, Hawk WA, Schofield P. Choice of Operation for the Toxic Megacolon Phase of Nonspecific Ulcerative Colitis. *Surgical Clinics of North America.* 1970;50(5):1151-1169. doi:10.1016/S0039-6109(16)39254-4.

[98] Ausch C, Madoff RD, Gnant M, et al. Aetiology and surgical management of toxic megacolon. *Colorectal Disease.* 2006;8(3):195-201. doi:10.1111/j.1463-1318.2005.00887.x.

[99] PENNINGTON L, HAMILTON SR, BAYLESS TM, CAMERON JL. Surgical Management of Crohn's Disease. *Ann Surg.* 1980;192(3):311-318. doi:10.1097/00000658-198009000-00006.

[100] Fichera A, McCormack R, Rubin MA, Hurst RD, Michelassi F. Long-Term Outcome of Surgically Treated Crohn's Colitis: A Prospective Study. *Dis Colon Rectum.* 2005;48(5):963-969. doi:10.1007/s10350-004-0906-3.

[101] Tekkis PP, Heriot AG, Smith O, Smith JJ, Windsor ACJ, Nicholls RJ. Long-term outcomes of restorative proctocolectomy for Crohn's disease and indeterminate colitis. *Colorectal Disease.* 2005;7(3):218-223. doi:10.1111/j.1463-1318.2005.00800.x.

[102] Kiran RP, Nisar PJ, Church JM, Fazio VW. The Role of Primary Surgical Procedure in Maintaining Intestinal Continuity for Patients With Crohn's Colitis. *Ann Surg.* 2011;253(6):1130-1135. doi:10.1097/SLA.0b013e318212b1a4.

[103] Lightner AL, Vogel JD, Carmichael JC, et al. The American Society of Colon and Rectal Surgeons Clinical Practice Guidelines for the Surgical Management of Crohn's Disease. *Dis Colon Rectum.* 2020;63(8):1028-1052. doi:10.1097/DCR.0000000000001716.

[104] Kiran RP, Nisar PJ, Goldblum JR, et al. Dysplasia Associated with Crohn's Colitis. *Ann Surg.* 2012;256(2):221-226. doi:10.1097/SLA.0b013e31825f0709.

[105] Maser EA, Sachar DB, Kruse D, Harpaz N, Ullman T, Bauer JJ. High Rates of Metachronous Colon Cancer or Dysplasia After Segmental Resection or Subtotal Colectomy in Crohn's Colitis. *Inflamm Bowel Dis.* Published online May 2013:1. doi:10.1097/MIB.0b013e318289c166.

[106] Yamamoto T. Proctocolectomy Is Associated with a Higher Complication Rate but Carries a Lower Recurrence Rate Than Total Colectomy and Ileorectal Anastomosis in Crohn Colitis. *Scand J Gastroenterol.* 1999;34(12):1212-1215. doi:10.1080/003655299750024724.

[107] Ritchie JK. The results of surgery for large bowel Crohn's disease. *Ann R Coll Surg Engl.* 1990;72(3):155-157.

[108] Yamamoto T, Bain IM, Allan RN, Keighley MRB. Persistent perineal sinus after proctocolectomy for Crohn's disease. *Dis Colon Rectum.* 1999;42(1):96-101. doi:10.1007/BF02235190.

[109] Aboulian A. Ostomy Complications in Crohn's Disease. *Clin Colon Rectal Surg.* 2019;32(04):314-322. doi:10.1055/s-0039-1683924.

[110] Leicester RJ, Ritchie JK, Wadsworth J, Thomson JPS, Hawley PR. Sexual function and perineal wound healing after intersphincteric excision of the rectum for inflammatory bowel disease. *Dis Colon Rectum.* 1984;27(4):244-248. doi:10.1007/BF02553795.

[111] Bernell O, Lapidus A, Hellers G. Recurrence after colectomy in Crohn's colitis. *Dis Colon Rectum*. 2001;44(5):647-654. doi:10.1007/BF02234559.

[112] Andersson P, Olaison G, Hallböök O, Sjödahl R. Segmental Resection or Subtotal Colectomy in Crohn's Colitis? *Dis Colon Rectum*. 2002;45(1):47-53. doi:10.1007/s10350-004-6113-4.

[113] Hartley JE, Fazio VW, Remzi FH, et al. Analysis of the Outcome of Ileal Pouch-Anal Anastomosis in Patients With Crohn's Disease. *Dis Colon Rectum*. 2004;47(11):1808-1815. doi:10.1007/s10350-004-0644-6.

[114] Regimbeau JM, Panis Y, Pocard M, et al. Long-term results of ileal pouch-anal anastomosis for colorectal Crohn's disease. *Dis Colon Rectum*. 2001;44(6):769-776. doi:10.1007/BF02234693.

[115] Brown CJ, MacLean AR, Cohen Z, MacRae HM, O'Connor BI, McLeod RS. Crohn's Disease and Indeterminate Colitis and the Ileal Pouch-Anal Anastomosis: Outcomes and Patterns of Failure. *Dis Colon Rectum*. 2005;48(8):1542-1549. doi:10.1007/s10350-005-0059-z.

[116] Braveman JM, Schoetz DJ, Marcello PW, et al. The Fate of the Ileal Pouch in Patients Developing Crohn's Disease. *Dis Colon Rectum*. 2004;47(10):1613-1619. doi:10.1007/s10350-004-0645-5.

[117] Lightner AL, Jia X, Zaghiyan K, Fleshner PR. IPAA in Known Preoperative Crohn's Disease: A Systematic Review. *Dis Colon Rectum*. 2021;64(3):355-364. doi:10.1097/DCR.0000000000001918.

[118] Reese GE, Lovegrove RE, Tilney HS, et al. The Effect of Crohn's Disease on Outcomes After Restorative Proctocolectomy. *Dis Colon Rectum*. 2007;50(2):239-250. doi:10.1007/s10350-006-0777-x.

[119] A Comparison of Laparoscopically Assisted and Open Colectomy for Colon Cancer. *New England Journal of Medicine*. 2004;350(20):2050-2059. doi:10.1056/NEJMoa032651.

[120] Umanskiy K, Malhotra G, Chase A, Rubin MA, Hurst RD, Fichera A. Laparoscopic Colectomy for Crohn's Colitis. A Large Prospective Comparative Study. *Journal of Gastrointestinal Surgery*. 2010;14(4):658-663. doi:10.1007/s11605-010-1157-3.

[121] Chaudhary B, Glancy D, Dixon AR. Laparoscopic surgery for recurrent ileocolic Crohn's disease is as safe and effective as primary resection. *Colorectal Disease*. 2011;13(12):1413-1416. doi:10.1111/j.1463-1318.2010.02511.x.

[122] Carmichael H, Peyser D, Baratta VM, et al. The role of laparoscopic surgery in repeat ileocolic resection for Crohn's disease. *Colorectal Dis*. 2021;23(8):2075-2084. doi:10.1111/codi.15675.

[123] Aytac E, Stocchi L, Remzi FH, Kiran RP. Is laparoscopic surgery for recurrent Crohn's disease beneficial in patients with previous primary resection through midline laparotomy? A case-matched study. *Surg Endosc*. 2012;26(12):3552-3556. doi:10.1007/s00464-012-2361-x.

[124] Dalsgaard T, Jensen MD, Hartwell D, Mosgaard BJ, Jørgensen A, Jensen BR. Robotic Surgery Is Less Physically Demanding Than Laparoscopic Surgery. *Ann Surg*. 2020;271(1):106-113. doi:10.1097/SLA.0000000000002845.

[125] Antoniou SA, Antoniou GA, Koch OO, Pointner R, Granderath FA. Robot-assisted laparoscopic surgery of the colon and rectum. *Surg Endosc*. 2012;26(1):1-11. doi:10.1007/s00464-011-1867-y.

[126] Miller AT, Berian JR, Rubin M, Hurst RD, Fichera A, Umanskiy K. Robotic-Assisted Proctectomy for Inflammatory Bowel Disease: A Case-Matched Comparison of Laparoscopic and Robotic Technique. *Journal of Gastrointestinal Surgery*. 2012;16(3):587-594. doi:10.1007/s11605-011-1692-6.

[127] Peng D, Cheng YX, Tao W, Tang H, Ji GY. Effect of enhanced recovery after surgery on inflammatory bowel disease surgery: A meta-analysis. *World J Clin Cases*. 2022;10(11):3426-3435. doi:10.12998/wjcc.v10.i11.3426.

[128] Vigorita V, Cano-Valderrama O, Celentano V, et al. Inflammatory Bowel Diseases Benefit from Enhanced Recovery After Surgery [ERAS] Protocol: A Systematic Review with Practical Implications. *J Crohns Colitis*. 2022;16(5):845-851. doi:10.1093/ecco-jcc/jjab209.

[129] Spinelli A, Sacchi M, Bazzi P, Leone N, Danese S, Montorsi M. Laparoscopic Surgery for Recurrent Crohn's Disease. *Gastroenterol Res Pract*. 2012;2012:1-6. doi:10.1155/2012/381017.

Chapter 11

Perianal Disease

John J. Newland[1,*], MD, MD
Leah Sukri[1], MD
and Kerri E. Lopez[2], MD
[1]University of Maryland Medical Center, Baltimore, Maryland, USA
[2]University of Maryland School of Medicine, Baltimore, Maryland, USA

Abstract

Perianal manifestations of Crohn's disease are common; up to 30% of patients develop a perianal complication at some point in the disease process. These can severely affect a patient's quality of life. While medical management of CD is paramount in the primary prevention of perianal disease and its complications, most patients eventually require a surgical intervention. The goal of surgical therapy is to minimize symptoms, control sepsis, and to preserve continence. Interventions may range from simple incision and drainage of an abscess to diverting ostomy or proctectomy for severe, unrelenting disease. It is critical to approach these patients from a multi-disciplinary perspective, as the combination of appropriate medical therapy and judicious surgical intervention results in the most optimal outcomes.

Introduction

Perianal manifestations of Crohn's Disease (CD) are relatively common, with up to 30% of patients developing at least one perianal fistula during their lifetime [1–3]. Other manifestations include skin tags, atypical anal fissures, ulcers, abscesses, and strictures. Patients can suffer from chronic pain, drainage and incontinence, which can be debilitating and have a significant effect on quality of life [4, 5]. Appropriate management of perianal CD depends on a thorough understanding of the involved anatomy, recognition of the manifestations of the disease process, and accurate localization using physical examination and imaging techniques. Diagnostic techniques include exam under anesthesia (EUA), magnetic resonance imaging (MRI), and endorectal ultrasound (ERUS).

It is important to remember that CD is not curable by medical or surgical therapy. The goal of surgical therapy for perianal CD is to minimize patient symptoms and disability by controlling sepsis and preserving continence. It is critical to avoid overly aggressive surgical

[*] Corresponding Author's Email: jnewland@som.umaryland.edu

In: Surgery for Crohn's Disease. Second Edition
Editors: Stephen M. Kavic, Rebecca Brown and Kerri Lopez
ISBN: 979-8-89530-676-5

interventions which may result in an outcome worse than the original problem. Management of these patients requires a multi-disciplinary effort, with close collaboration between the gastroenterologist, radiologist and surgeon.

Fistulizing Complications

Perianal abscess and fistula are common in CD; approximately 20% of patients with Crohn's will develop at least one anorectal fistula in their lifetime [1]. While idiopathic anal fistulas likely arise from intersphincteric mucus gland infection, fistulas in Crohn's are thought to occur as a sequela of mucosal inflammation and ulceration. Their incidence increases with greater severity and duration of disease, and recurrence rates are high [6, 7].

Fistulizing perianal disease can be difficult to manage and can significantly impair quality of life for Crohn's patients. As with other manifestations of CD, management should be approached in a multidisciplinary manner.

Anatomy and Classification of Disease

Perianal CD can present in a wide variety of locations and patterns, making classification systems a necessity to communicate vital information such as disease location and severity. Historically, the Parks classification system, developed in 1976, was used to characterize disease based on its relation to the sphincteric complex [8] listed in Figure 11.1 [9]. Fistulas are further classified as "low" if the internal opening is found below the dentate line, or "high" if the internal opening is at or above the dentate line.

The American Gastroenterological Association (AGA) proposed a simpler classification system, characterizing fistulas as either complex or simple [10]. Superficial, low intersphincteric or transsphincteric fistulas with one external opening and no associated abscess were classified as simple. Fistulas with an internal opening above the dentate line, multiple external openings or branches, and rectovaginal fistulas were all considered complex fistulas [10].

Imaging and Diagnosis

The location and extent of Crohn's-related abscesses and fistulas can be difficult to delineate with physical exam alone. ERUS and MRI of the pelvis can be very useful adjuncts in defining the anatomy and guiding treatment. A 2001 study compared EUA, ERUS, and MRI and found that all were able to accurately describe the anatomy of the disease in over 85% of patients, improving to 100% accuracy if two of the imaging modalities were used [11]. Although none of the three modalities demonstrated statistically significant superiority, EUA demonstrated the highest overall accuracy of 90%.

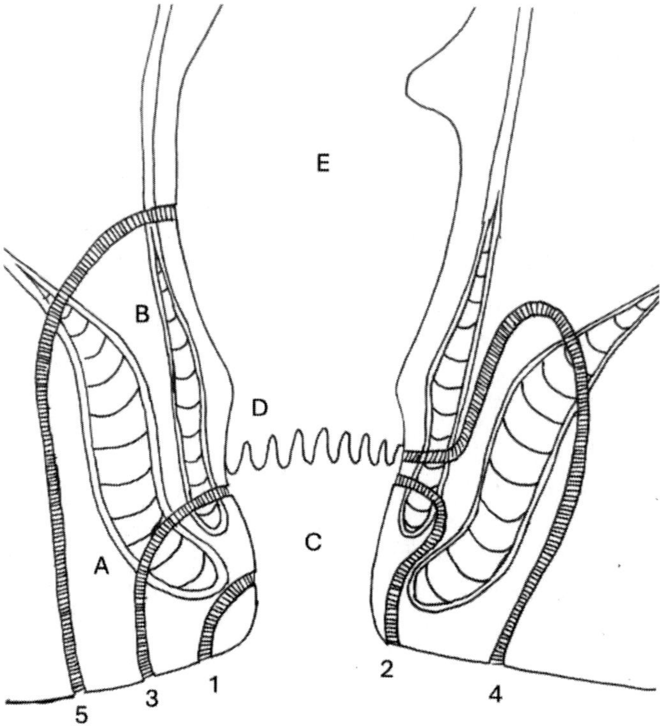

Figure 11.1. Parks Classification of Anal Fistula. 1. Superficial fistula, 2. Intersphincteric fistula, 3. Transsphincteric fistula, 4. Suprasphincteric fistula, 5. Extrasphinteric fistula, A. External anal sphincter, B. Internal anal sphincter, C. Anal canal, D. Dentate line, E. Rectum.

Choosing between imaging modalities depends on several factors. ERUS historically was more readily available and less expensive than MRI. However, it is operator-dependent, can be uncomfortable for patients, and tends to give less information about the surrounding anatomy compared to MRI. In comparison, MRI can give a great deal of information about the surrounding soft tissue and offers excellent visualization of the fistula tracts and their relationship to the rectum or anus. Patients with a high BMI, claustrophobia, or metallic implants may have relative or absolute contraindications to MRI.

In the absence of definitive data supporting one modality over the other, the use of ERUS versus MRI should be dictated by individual institution and patient factors. Specifically, metallic implants or claustrophobia argue in favor of endoanal ultrasound. On the other hand, discomfort with endoscopy or a lack of ultrasound expertise may suggest MRI as the preferred modality.

Medical Therapy

As with other manifestations of CD, the mainstay of perianal Crohn's treatment is medical therapy. Treatment is focused on symptom relief and clinical remission, as findings on imaging may persist for up to a year after clinical resolution. Although previous chapters discuss the medical management of CD thoroughly, we will review some of the specific agents used for patients with perianal disease.

Antibiotics

Antibiotics, particularly metronidazole and ciprofloxacin, have historically been the first line medical options for Crohn's perianal fistulas. However, data supporting their use as a monotherapy remains sparse and may be limited only to simple fistulas [12]. Studies have shown a decrease in pain and drainage after treatment with antibiotics alone, but have also reported immediate recurrence of symptoms after discontinuation [13]. Therefore, antibiotics may have a role as an adjunct for symptomatic improvement but are unlikely to lead to healing on their own.

Biologics

Tumor necrosis factor (TNF) inhibitors, such as infliximab and adalimumab, have become well-established in the management of perianal disease. They target the inflammatory pathways known to be active in fistula development and have substantial evidence as an effective treatment for fistulizing perianal CD. They have been demonstrated to improve rates of fistula closure and disease remission. In the seminal New England Journal of Medicine study, the use of infliximab resulted in a significant reduction in the number of draining fistulas when compared to placebo, as well as in the number of patients achieving complete response (55% vs. 13%, $p = 0.001$). The average time to response was two weeks from initiation of treatment [14]. The ACCENT-II trial examined the efficacy of maintenance infliximab and showed that patients who had experienced initial remission with induction were more likely to have sustained remission with maintenance dosing (36% vs. 19%, $p = 0.009$) [15]. Precise timing, doing, and duration of treatment remain variable in practice [16].

There may be a synergistic effect of administering TNF-inhibitors along with ciprofloxacin, as higher rates of fistula closure have been shown with combination therapy compared to adalimumab monotherapy (71% vs 47%, $p = 0.047$) [17]. Notably, this effect seems to disappear after discontinuation of ciprofloxacin.

Vedolizumab, an $\alpha 4\beta 7$ integrin monoclonal antibody, and Ustekinumab, an anti-IL23/23 IgG1 kappa monoclonal antibody, have both been shown to have some efficacy in fistula closure and may be options for patients with disease refractory to anti-TNF agents [18–20].

Other Medications

Thiopurines such as azathioprine and 6-mercaptopurine have demonstrated some efficacy in closing fistulas and decreasing symptoms when compared to placebo [21, 22]. However, the lack of evidence supporting their use and their long response times (over three months) have limited their independent application in perianal disease. Thiopurines are sometimes still used in conjunction with other medications. Similarly, calcineurin inhibitors such as tacrolimus and cyclosporine may also have a limited role in select patients. Tacrolimus has been shown to improve drainage but is not effective in fistula closure [23]. Cyclosporine has demonstrated significant rates of fistula closure in some studies, but recurrence occurs quickly with discontinuation and significant medication side effects make long term use unappealing [24]. Steroids, commonly used to induce remission in active luminal CD, have minimal use in perianal CD and may in fact predispose patients to abscess formation [25, 26].

Surgical Management

Abscess

Patients with perianal abscesses usually present with anorectal pain, erythema, swelling, and drainage, or a combination thereof. Crohn's-related abscesses tend to be more complex, occurring more frequently in the supralevator or ischiorectal spaces. These may present with minimal external signs, and imaging studies may be required for diagnosis. ERUS, computed tomography (CT), and MRI are all useful adjuncts for diagnosis, although results should be interpreted carefully, as CT can miss up to 23% of perianal abscesses [27–32].

The initial management of Crohn's related abscesses is generally the same as for cryptoglandular disease. The goal of surgery is threefold. First and foremost, the primary goal is to control sepsis. The second priority is to preserve continence. Third, surgeons must attempt to minimize the complexity of any subsequent fistulas that may develop. To achieve this last goal, incisions should be radially oriented and placed as close to the anus as possible. Intersphincteric abscesses should be drained internally.

There is some debate over the management of an internal opening at the time of initial abscess drainage. It is widely accepted that an aggressive search for an internal opening should not be performed in the acute setting due to the friable nature of inflamed tissue and the risk of creating false passages. Several small series suggest that drainage alone can result in healing in 25 – 50% of Crohn's patients with perirectal abscesses [33]. There is certainly a role for drainage without seton placement in some patients. However, in the case of a recurrent abscess, care should be taken to identify the fistula tract and address it either by seton placement or fistulotomy, as discussed later in this chapter. A mushroom-tip, or Malecot catheter can be a useful tool for draining deeper infections, particularly high ischiorectal abscesses. These drains are generally well-tolerated by the patient, with similar quality of life scores compared to packing, and they are likely more effective in preventing recurrence than incision and drainage alone [30, 34].

The role for antibiotics is abscess management is limited, as the mainstay of treatment is surgical drainage. Antibiotics may be warranted if significant cellulitis is present, though the optimal duration of treatment has not been established. Similarly, cultures will generally be polymicrobial and are of little utility unless significant cellulitis is present.

Anorectal Fistulas

Fistulas are the most common perianal disease manifestation in patients with CD [35]. These are defined as a chronic track of inflammatory tissue that connects the anus or rectum with the skin, vagina, or urinary tract. Patients with active proctitis are at high risk for developing perianal fistulas as a direct sequala of mucosal inflammation and erosion [36]. When compared to cryptoglandular fistulas, perianal fistulas in patients with CD are more likely to be painless, occur laterally or deep, or have multiple complex branching fistulas tracts.

Up to 90% of patients with fistulas will eventually require surgical treatment [37]. If an operation is indicated, the goals of surgery include achieving symptomatic relief and/or definitive therapy while avoiding overly aggressive operations that could result in incontinence.

Fistulotomy

Primary fistulotomy is performed by laying open a fistula tract. This procedure is typically done in the operating room under anesthesia – a probe is passed into the fistula tract and the soft tissue overlying the probe is divided with electrocautery. Due to potential wound complications and impact on continence, it is only considered in very low and simple fistulas with minimal overlying tissue and no concurrent active proctitis [38–42].

Setons

Draining setons are a mainstay of treatment for complex fistulas in CD. The seton, typically a silastic vessel loop, is threaded into a fistula tract and secured to itself loosely. This allows for patency of the tract and prevention of recurrent abscesses while allowing for medical therapy, typically a TNF inhibitor, to treat the active inflammation [43–48]. After anti-TNF therapy has been started and proctitis has resolved, seton removal can be trialed in select patients and is often successful, even without concurrent definitive fistula surgery.

The ideal timing of seton removal is not established – reports range from 3 weeks to 3 months of treatment prior to attempted removal. A recent study of Crohn's patients with anorectal fistulas showed that 57% of patients experienced sustained fistula closure with infliximab treatment and seton removal, and that these outcomes did not differ between patients who underwent seton removal alone and those that underwent seton removal combined with additional surgery (such as fistulotomy, advancement flap, and fistula plug) [49]. A recent systematic review published a range of fistula closure rates between 13.6% and 100% in patients who were managed with draining setons and anti-TNF therapy, with recurrence rates ranging between 0 – 83% [43, 46, 50–53]. This suggests that seton removal alone may be a reasonable approach for patients on infliximab maintenance therapy who have experienced resolution of their proctitis [48, 54–57].

For patients with recurrent fistulas on anti-TNF treatment, a seton should be replaced and consideration of alternative approaches should be undertaken. For some patients with complex and recurrent fistulas, there may be no surgical options with a reasonable chance of cure. Cutting setons, setons that are sequentially tightened in an attempt to superficialize a tract, result in high rates of incontinence and recurrent disease and do not have a role in the treatment of Crohn's related fistulas [58, 59].

Ligation of Intersphincteric Fistula Tract (LIFT)

The LIFT procedure for transsphincteric fistulas was first described by Rojanasakul in 2007 [60]. The technique consists of making an incision in the intersphincteric groove, isolating the fistula tract, ligating it on both sides, curetting out the external tract and widening the external opening to allow for drainage, and closing the incision. The healing rates after LIFT in CD range between 45 – 67%. One study found healing rates of 60% at 2 months and 67% at 12 months [61, 62]. Factors associated with success were lateral location and longer fistula length.

This procedure is appealing in its relative simplicity and complete sparing of the sphincter muscles. Additionally, failure of LIFT often results in an intersphincteric fistula; a successful reduction in complexity that can allow for fistula closure in the future. LIFT has also been demonstrated to have lower rates of incontinence as compared to endorectal flap advancement [63]. However, it is typically only indicated in relatively simple transsphincteric fistulas, so many of the complex, branching fistulas found in Crohn's patients may be unsuitable for the LIFT approach. Like other interventions, it should only be performed after resolution of proctitis.

Endorectal Advancement Flap

The endorectal advancement flap involves excising a fistula's internal opening and mobilizing a partial-thickness or full-thickness pedicle of rectal mucosa to cover the tract. This approach can be applied to a broader portion of Crohn's related fistulas including non-transsphincteric fistulas, LIFT failures, and fistulas with higher openings. Efficacy of advancement flaps in CD patients ranges from 50 – 85%, with a recent review article suggesting a 64% success rate and 9.4% risk of incontinence [64, 65]. Complications reported with advancement flaps include hematoma, recurrence, continence issues, and flap retraction [65]. A recent systematic review published a 61% overall success rate for Crohn's related fistula patients undergoing advancement flap, with a recurrence rate of 18% [66]. The same review cited higher rates of incontinence with advancement flap when compared to LIFT. However, the association with incontinence is likely dependent on depth of flap used; it is certainly more sphincter sparing when only the mucosal layers are included.

Fistula Plug

Fistula plugs provide a scaffold to be populated by connective tissue to heal a fistula tract. They are typically installed into the internal opening of a fistula after the tract is debrided. They have reported use in transsphincteric, anovaginal, intersphincteric, and extrasphincteric fistulas [67]. Although they are an appealing alternative in the management of complex fistulas, as the procedure is technically straightforward to perform and there is no muscle division involved, there have been limited studies demonstrating convincing efficacy. In 2009, Garg performed a systematic review of the literature in which they concluded that the data was heterogenous and inconclusive [68]. A later randomized control trial demonstrated no benefit in healing over placebo at one year, dampening the enthusiasm for this approach [69].

More recently, the STOMP trial evaluated the efficacy of bioabsorbable fistula plugs to deliver mesenchymal stem cells in patients with CD who failed conventional therapies. A clinical response was observed in 77% of patients at 6 months and 76% at 12 months. Larger studies will be needed to determine ideal patient populations and treatment protocols, but this may represent a potential path forward for fistula plug use [70].

Fibrin Glue

The use of fibrin glue to heal complex fistulas is also appealing in its simplicity. This method consists of injecting a slurry of biodegradable products into the external opening of a fistula to precipitate fibrin clot formation. Data on the efficacy of this technique has varied widely with remission rates ranging from 0 – 85% [71–77]. While most evidence is limited to small case series,' the use of fibrin glue is of minimal risk and may offer an appealing first step in attempting definitive management of Crohn's related fistulas.

Rectovaginal Fistula

Rectovaginal fistulas (RVF) are unfortunately highly common in women with CD – they occur in approximately 10% of women with Crohn's. While some patients stay relatively asymptomatic, many have significant symptoms such as seepage, vaginal and perianal irritation, urinary tract infections, sexual dysfunction, and social distress. As with other acute fistulas, primary initial treatment includes EUA with possible seton placement and optimization of medical therapy [78]. Many repair options exist for RVF – including advancement flaps from either the anal or vaginal side, episioproctotomy, and interposition flaps. Diversion is also a frequent consideration and can be temporary to allow for resolution of inflammation prior to and after repair. However, up to half of patients eventually require a permanent stoma for recurrent or refractory disease [79].

Fecal Diversion and Proctectomy

Fecal diversion via a defunctioning ostomy may be necessary to control unrelenting perineal disease, particularly when maximal medical therapy is unsuccessful, and quality of life suffers. Colostomies are typically preferred over ileostomies from a functional standpoint, but the choice of ostomy is typically dictated by the status of the patient's luminal disease. Up to half of these stomas will become permanent, especially in patients with colonic disease or anal stenosis [79, 80]. When feasible, laparoscopic stoma formation is straightforward and well-tolerated.

Proctectomies are typically reserved for patients with severe debilitating disease not amenable to medical or local therapy whose perianal symptoms severely affect their quality of life. Approximately 7 – 20% of patients with perianal CD ultimately require proctectomy [10, 81]. Proctectomies are not without their own complications including wound healing difficulties and chronic sinus formation [82]. During proctectomy, consideration should given to intersphincteric dissection and a vascularized muscle flap to minimize the size and morbidity of the perineal wound [83, 84].

Non-Fistulizating Manifestations

Anal Fissures

Anal fissures are common in CD. These may be either a sequalae of Crohn's related inflammation or may be related to anal canal trauma, similar to those in patients without IBD. Unlike idiopathic fissures, the atypical fissures associated with the inflammation and mucosal ulceration inherent to Crohn's are not considered to be a sequalae of increased internal sphincter tone. This shifts the treatment algorithm significantly when compared to treatment of idiopathic fissures. Atypical fissures in Crohn's are more likely to be deep, multiple in number, and located in positions other than the posterior midline [36]. These fissures are asymptomatic at times, but are most often associated with bleeding and discomfort [85].

Available evidence suggests that up to 80% of fissures associated with Crohn's will heal spontaneously [6]. For symptomatic patients, medical management remains the first line of treatment. In the setting of frequent, loose bowel movements, the focus should be on improving frequency and stool bulk. This may be accomplished by the addition of soluble fiber, anti-diarrheal medications, and medications directed toward addressing the underlying IBD. Topical agents such as nitrates and calcium channel blockers can be trialed in symptomatic patients and may be associated with improved healing [86–92]. For patients not already on anti-TNF treatment, consideration should be given to a trial of these medications, as they are associated with resolution in up to 70% of cases [93].

Surgical management of anal fissures is generally avoided in Crohn's due to a higher risk of complications such as non-healing wounds, recurrence, fistula formation and incontinence [94]. In the absence of high internal sphincter tone, surgical interventions aimed at decreasing tone should not be pursued – they are unlikely to provide benefit and can have lasting effects on continence in a patient population already prone to frequent, loose stools and control issues. Persistent or recurrent fissuring disease is often representative of poorly controlled CD, and escalation of medical treatment may be the best path toward resolution.

Ulcers

Cavitating ulcers are also frequently associated with proctitis – they can be found within the rectum, anal canal, and perianal skin. Like atypical fissures, the primary treatment is medical. There is some evidence that topical agents such as metronidazole and Tacrolimus may provide some symptomatic relief [95, 96]. However, systemic treatment results in much higher rates of healing, with up to 83% of patients demonstrating complete healing with anti-TNF agents [93]. Unfortunately, cavitating ulcers refractory to medical management may ultimately require proctectomy [97].

Hemorrhoids

Hemorrhoidal disease is relatively uncommon in the setting of IBD [98]. Much like the other anal pathologies seen in CD patients, conservative management is generally preferred. Soluble fiber supplementation, sitz baths, and minimizing time spent on the toilet should be the primary first-line interventions. Historically, studies have demonstrated a high rate of complications following surgical intervention for hemorrhoids in Crohn's patients. A recent meta-analysis of retrospective case series studies performed between 1977 and 2020 showed a complication rate of 11% after the surgical treatment of hemorrhoidal disease in patients with Crohn's. The most common complications were anal abscess or fistula (4.8%), followed by anal stenosis (3.6%), bleeding (2.4%), and non-healing wounds (2.4%) [99]. These complications rates are markedly lower than those reported by previous authors, perhaps due to more stringent inclusion criteria. For Crohn's patients with quiescent rectal disease and severely symptomatic hemorrhoidal disease refractory to conservative therapy, surgical intervention may have a reasonable risk-benefit profile. In the appropriate patients, there is some evidence to suggest that rubber band ligation and doppler-guided hemorrhoid artery ligation may be safer techniques with a lower rate of complications [126, 127].

Skin Tags

Anal skin tags in Crohn's can be classified based on their appearance in accordance with the AGA classification. Type 1 skin tags are large, edematous, tender, and cyanotic and typically arise in the setting of healed fissures or ulcers. Type 2, "elephant ear," skin tags are painless, and often are flat and soft with a broad base [6]. The 10-year cumulative probability of developing perianal skin tags of any kind in Crohn's is 19% - higher than for ulcers, fissures, or strictures [100]. These are often symptomatic, and patients may present for consideration of surgical excision. Type 2 skin tags can typically be safely excised, especially in patients with controlled disease without active proctitis. Excision of Type 1 skin tags is more likely to result in poor wound healing. For patients with active proctitis and symptomatic Type 1 tags, the focus should be on systemic treatments to improve control of inflammation.

Strictures

Anorectal strictures are common in perianal CD, occurring in approximately 17% of patients with perianal Crohn's [97]. They may be inflammatory or fibrotic in nature and are highly associated with proctitis [101]. Crohn's patients with strictures may remain asymptomatic due to their tendency toward loose stools, they may have obstructive signs, or they may experience symptoms that are difficult to distinguish from the underlying proctitis itself. Like other perianal manifestations of Crohn's, inflammatory strictures typically respond well to systemic anti-TNF treatment [93]. Fibrotic strictures without underlying proctitis should undergo dilation under anesthesia. This may be done manually or with balloon or Hegar dilators. Patients may require repeat procedures, which can be performed if symptomatic relief continues to be obtained. However, even in the era of anti-TNF treatment, up to 32% of patients with anorectal structuring will ultimately require diversion or proctectomy [102].

Conclusion

The ultimate role of the surgeon in perianal disease is one of restraint; in patients with active disease, medical management should be the primary focus, and the extent of surgical intervention should be limited. Optimal timing for surgery hinges on obtaining disease quiescence, with the understanding that operative intervention may be performed urgently in certain scenarios. The treating surgeon must have a clear understanding about the goals of therapy and use these goals to guide treatment. Infection and symptomatic disease must be addressed in a way that preserves continence and function. In patients with active perianal disease, the use of anti-TNF agents should be strongly considered and steroids should be avoided. Definitive surgery for Crohn's-related fistulas should be deferred in the face of active proctitis, and the surgeon should approach surgical management of fissures, hemorrhoids, and skin tags with caution in this population. Optimized patients can be considered for definitive procedures such as LIFT or advancement flaps, but long-term seton use may be the best treatment option in many situations. Diversion can be an appropriate component of management, but can become permanent in many patients. Proctectomy may ultimately be required in some patients with severe or refractory disease, especially those with severe anal stricturing. Close collaboration between surgeons and gastroenterologists is absolutely essential for optimal outcomes.

References

[1] Schwartz DA, Loftus EV, Tremaine WJ, Panaccione R, Harmsen WS, Zinsmeister AR, et al. The natural history of fistulizing Crohn's disease in Olmsted County, Minnesota. *Gastroenterology*. 2002 Apr;122(4):875–80.

[2] Hellers G, Bergstrand O, Ewerth S, Holmström B. Occurrence and outcome after primary treatment of anal fistulae in Crohn's disease. *Gut*. 1980 Jun;21(6):525–7.

[3] Vasudevan A, van Langenberg DR. Editorial: delving into the natural history of Crohn's disease and the impact of medical therapy. *Aliment Pharmacol Ther*. 2022 Jan;55(1):108–9.

[4] Kasparek MS, Glatzle J, Temeltcheva T, Mueller MH, Koenigsrainer A, Kreis ME. Long-term quality of life in patients with Crohn's disease and perianal fistulas: influence of fecal diversion. *Dis Colon Rectum*. 2007 Dec;50(12):2067–74.

[5] Ng SC, Plamondon S, Gupta A, Burling D, Kamm MA. Prospective assessment of the effect on quality of life of anti-tumour necrosis factor therapy for perineal Crohn's fistulas. *Aliment Pharmacol Ther*. 2009 Oct;30(7):757–66.

[6] Sandborn WJ, Fazio VW, Feagan BG, Hanauer SB. AGA technical review on perianal Crohn's disease. *Gastroenterology*. 2003 Nov;125(5):1508–30.

[7] Makowiec F, Jehle EC, Starlinger M. Clinical course of perianal fistulas in Crohn's disease. *Gut*. 1995 Nov;37(5):696–701.

[8] Parks AG, Gordon PH, Hardcastle JD. A classification of fistula-in-ano. *Br J Surg*. 1976 Jan;63(1):1–12.

[9] Lunniss PJ, Armstrong P, Barker PG, Reznek RH, Phillips RK. Magnetic resonance imaging of anal fistulae. *Lancet Lond Engl*. 1992 Aug;340(8816):394–6.

[10] American Gastroenterological Association. American gastroenterological association medical position statement: perianal Crohn's disease1. *Gastroenterology*. 2003 Nov;125(5):1503–7.

[11] Schwartz DA, Wiersema MJ, Dudiak KM, Fletcher JG, Clain JE, Tremaine WJ, et al. A comparison of endoscopic ultrasound, magnetic resonance imaging, and exam under anesthesia for evaluation of Crohn's perianal fistulas. *Gastroenterology*. 2001 Nov;121(5):1064–72.

[12] Parian AM, Obi M, Fleshner P, Schwartz DA. Management of Perianal Crohn's Disease. *Am J Gastroenterol.* 2023 Aug;118(8):1323–31.

[13] Wise PE, Schwartz DA. Management of Perianal Crohn's Disease. *Clin Gastroenterol Hepatol.* 2006 Apr;4(4):426–30.

[14] Present DH, Rutgeerts P, Targan S, Hanauer SB, Mayer L, van Hogezand RA, et al. Infliximab for the treatment of fistulas in patients with Crohn's disease. *N Engl J Med.* 1999 May;340(18):1398–405.

[15] Sands BE, Anderson FH, Bernstein CN, Chey WY, Feagan BG, Fedorak RN, et al. Infliximab Maintenance Therapy for Fistulizing Crohn's Disease. *N Engl J Med.* 2004 Feb;350(9):876–85.

[16] Vasudevan A, Bruining DH, Edward V Loftus J, Faubion W, Ehman EC, Raffals L. Approach to medical therapy in perianal Crohn's disease. *World J Gastroenterol.* 2021 Jul;27(25):3693.

[17] Dewint P, Hansen BE, Verhey E, Oldenburg B, Hommes DW, Pierik M, et al. Adalimumab combined with ciprofloxacin is superior to adalimumab monotherapy in perianal fistula closure in Crohn's disease: a randomised, double-blind, placebo controlled trial (ADAFI). *Gut.* 2014 Feb;63(2):292–9.

[18] Feagan BG, Schwartz D, Danese S, Rubin DT, Lissoos TW, Xu J, et al. Efficacy of Vedolizumab in Fistulising Crohn's Disease: Exploratory Analyses of Data from GEMINI 2. *J Crohns Colitis.* 2018 Feb;12(5):621.

[19] Ma C, Fedorak RN, Kaplan GG, Dieleman LA, Devlin SM, Stern N, et al. Clinical, endoscopic and radiographic outcomes with ustekinumab in medically-refractory Crohn's disease: real world experience from a multicentre cohort. *Aliment Pharmacol Ther.* 2017 May;45(9):1232–43.

[20] Khorrami S, Ginard D, Marín-Jiménez I, Chaparro M, Sierra M, Aguas M, et al. Ustekinumab for the Treatment of Refractory Crohn's Disease: The Spanish Experience in a Large Multicentre Open-label Cohort. *Inflamm Bowel Dis*. 2016 Jul;22(7):1662–9.

[21] Present DH, Korelitz BI, Wisch N, Glass JL, Sachar DB, Pasternack BS. Treatment of Crohn's Disease with 6-Mercaptopurine [Internet]. *N Engl J Med.* 1980 May doi: 10.1056/NEJM198005013021801

[22] Pearson DC, May GR, Fick GH, Sutherland LR. Azathioprine and 6-mercaptopurine in Crohn disease. A meta-analysis. *Ann Intern Med. 1*995 Jul;123(2):132–42.

[23] Sandborn WJ, Present DH, Isaacs KL, Wolf DC, Greenberg E, Hanauer SB, et al. Tacrolimus for the treatment of fistulas in patients with Crohn's disease: a randomized, placebo-controlled trial. *Gastroenterology*. 2003 Aug;125(2):380–8.

[24] Present DH, Lichtiger S. Efficacy of cyclosporine in treatment of fistula of Crohn's disease. *Dig Dis Sci*. 1994 Feb;39(2):374–80.

[25] Wetwittayakhlang P, Khoury AA, Hahn GD, Lakatos PL. The Optimal Management of Fistulizing Crohn's Disease: Evidence beyond Randomized Clinical Trials. *J Clin Med*. 2022 May;11(11):3045.

[26] Shergill AK, Terdiman JP. Controversies in the treatment of Crohn's disease: The case for an accelerated step-up treatment approach. *World J Gastroenterol WJG*. 2008 May;14(17):2670.

[27] Yamamoto T, Nakase H, Watanabe K, Shinzaki S, Takatsu N, Fujii T, et al. Diagnosis and Clinical Features of Perianal Lesions in Newly Diagnosed Crohn's Disease: Subgroup Analysis from Inception Cohort Registry Study of Patients with Crohn's Disease (iCREST-CD). *J Crohns Colitis.* 2023 Aug;17(8):1193–206.

[28] el Mouaaouy A, Tolksdorf A, Starlinger M, Becker HD. Endoscopic sonography of the anorectum in inflammatory rectal diseases. *Z Gastroenterol.* 1992 Jul;30(7):486–94.

[29] Giovannini M, Bories E, Moutardier V, Pesenti C, Guillemin A, Lelong B, et al. Drainage of deep pelvic abscesses using therapeutic echo endoscopy. *Endoscopy*. 2003 Jun;35(6):511–4.

[30] Viganò C, Losco A, Caprioli F, Basilisco G. Incidence and clinical outcomes of intersphincteric abscesses diagnosed by anal ultrasonography in patients with crohn's disease. *Inflamm Bowel Dis.* 2011 Oct;17(10):2102–8.

[31] Bennett AL, Schwartz DA. Endoscopic Evaluation and Management of Perianal Disease. *Gastrointest Endosc Clin N Am*. 2022 Oct;32(4):747–59.

[32] Caliste X, Nazir S, Goode T, Street JH, Hockstein M, McArthur K, et al. Sensitivity of computed tomography in detection of perirectal abscess. *Am Surg. 2*011 Feb;77(2):166–8.

[33] Michelassi F, Melis M, Rubin M, Hurst RD. Surgical treatment of anorectal complications in Crohn's disease. *Surgery*. 2000 Oct;128(4):597–603.

[34] Zhu DA, Houlihan LM, Mohan HM, McCourt M, Andrews E. Packing versus mushroom catheters following incision and drainage in anorectal abscess. *Ir J Med Sci.* 2019 Nov;188(4):1343–8.

[35] Eglinton TW, Barclay ML, Gearry RB, Frizelle FA. The spectrum of perianal Crohn's disease in a population-based cohort. *Dis Colon Rectum.* 2012 Jul;55(7):773–7.

[36] Ingle SB, Loftus EV. The natural history of perianal Crohn's disease. *Dig Liver Dis Off J Ital Soc Gastroenterol Ital Assoc Study Liver.* 2007 Oct;39(10):963–9.

[37] Williams JL, Shaffer VO. Modern Management of Perianal Crohn's Disease: A Review. *Am Surg.* 2021 Sep;87(9):1361–7.

[38] Hämäläinen KP, Sainio AP. Cutting seton for anal fistulas: high risk of minor control defects. *Dis Colon Rectum.* 1997 Dec;40(12):1443–6; discussion 1447.

[39] Ritchie RD, Sackier JM, Hodde JP. Incontinence rates after cutting seton treatment for anal fistula. *Colorectal Dis Off J Assoc Coloproctology G B Irel.* 2009 Jul;11(6):564–71.

[40] Nordgren S, Fasth S, Hultén L. Anal fistulas in Crohn's disease: incidence and outcome of surgical treatment. *Int J Colorectal Dis.* 1992 Dec;7(4):214–8.

[41] Matos D, Lunniss PJ, Phillips RK. Total sphincter conservation in high fistula in ano: results of a new approach. *Br J Surg.* 1993 Jun;80(6):802–4.

[42] Park MY, Yoon YS, Kim HE, Lee JL, Park IJ, Lim S-B, et al. Surgical options for perianal fistula in patients with Crohn's disease: A comparison of seton placement, fistulotomy, and stem cell therapy. *Asian J Surg.* 2021 Nov;44(11):1383–8.

[43] Williams JG, Rothenberger DA, Nemer FD, Goldberg SM. Fistula-in-ano in Crohn's disease. Results of aggressive surgical treatment. *Dis Colon Rectum.* 1991 May;34(5):378–84.

[44] Halme L, Sainio AP. Factors related to frequency, type, and outcome of anal fistulas in Crohn's disease. *Dis Colon Rectum.* 1995 Jan;38(1):55–9.

[45] Sangwan YP, Schoetz DJ, Murray JJ, Roberts PL, Coller JA. Perianal Crohn's disease. Results of local surgical treatment. *Dis Colon Rectum.* 1996 May;39(5):529–35.

[46] Faucheron JL, Saint-Marc O, Guibert L, Parc R. Long-term seton drainage for high anal fistulas in Crohn's disease--a sphincter-saving operation? *Dis Colon Rectum.* 1996 Feb;39(2):208–11.

[47] Pearl RK, Andrews JR, Orsay CP, Weisman RI, Prasad ML, Nelson RL, et al. Role of the seton in the management of anorectal fistulas. *Dis Colon Rectum.* 1993 Jun;36(6):573–7; discussion 577-579.

[48] Thornton M, Solomon MJ. Long-term indwelling seton for complex anal fistulas in Crohn's disease. *Dis Colon Rectum.* 2005 Mar;48(3):459–63.

[49] Bouguen G, Siproudhis L, Gizard E, Wallenhorst T, Billioud V, Bretagne J-F, et al. Long-term outcome of perianal fistulizing Crohn's disease treated with infliximab. *Clin Gastroenterol Hepatol Off Clin Pract J Am Gastroenterol Assoc.* 2013 Aug;11(8):975-981.e1-4.

[50] de Groof EJ, Sahami S, Lucas C, Ponsioen CY, Bemelman WA, Buskens CJ. Treatment of perianal fistula in Crohn's disease: a systematic review and meta-analysis comparing seton drainage and anti-tumour necrosis factor treatment. *Colorectal Dis Off J Assoc Coloproctology G B Irel.* 2016 Jul;18(7):667–75.

[51] Bolshinsky V, Church J. Management of Complex Anorectal and Perianal Crohn's Disease. *Clin Colon Rectal Surg.* 2019 Jul;32(4):255.

[52] Eitan A, Koliada M, Bickel A. The use of the loose seton technique as a definitive treatment for recurrent and persistent high trans-sphincteric anal fistulas: a long-term outcome. *J Gastrointest Surg Off J Soc Surg Aliment Tract.* 2009 Jun;13(6):1116–9.

[53] Motamedi MAK, Serahati S, Rajendran L, Brown CJ, Raval MJ, Karimuddin A, et al. Long-term outcomes after seton placement for perianal fistulas with and without Crohn's disease. *Colorectal Dis Off J Assoc Coloproctology G B Irel.* 2021 Sep;23(9):2407–15.

[54] Steele SR, Kumar R, Feingold DL, Rafferty JL, Buie WD, Standards Practice Task Force of the American Society of Colon and Rectal Surgeons. Practice parameters for the management of perianal abscess and fistula-in-ano. *Dis Colon Rectum.* 2011 Dec;54(12):1465–74.

[55] Whiteford MH, Kilkenny J, Hyman N, Buie WD, Cohen J, Orsay C, et al. Practice parameters for the treatment of perianal abscess and fistula-in-ano (revised). *Dis Colon Rectum.* 2005 Jul;48(7):1337–42.

[56] Galis-Rozen E, Tulchinsky H, Rosen A, Eldar S, Rabau M, Stepanski A, et al. Long-term outcome of loose seton for complex anal fistula: a two-centre study of patients with and without Crohn's disease. *Colorectal Dis Off J Assoc Coloproctology G B Irel.* 2010 Apr;12(4):358–62.

[57] Takesue Y, Ohge H, Yokoyama T, Murakami Y, Imamura Y, Sueda T. Long-term results of seton drainage on complex anal fistulae in patients with Crohn's disease. *J Gastroenterol.* 2002;37(11):912–5.

[58] Singh B, George BD, Mortensen NJM. Surgical therapy of perianal Crohn's disease. *Dig Liver Dis Off J Ital Soc Gastroenterol Ital Assoc Study Liver.* 2007 Oct;39(10):988–92.

[59] Wasmann KA, de Groof EJ, Stellingwerf ME, D'Haens GR, Ponsioen CY, Gecse KB, et al. Treatment of Perianal Fistulas in Crohn's Disease, Seton Versus Anti-TNF Versus Surgical Closure Following Anti-TNF [PISA]: A Randomised Controlled Trial. *J Crohns Colitis.* 2020 Sep;14(8):1049–56.

[60] Rojanasakul A. LIFT procedure: a simplified technique for fistula-in-ano. *Tech Coloproctology.* 2009 Sep;13(3):237–40.

[61] Wood T, Truong A, Mujukian A, Zaghiyan K, Fleshner P. Increasing experience with the LIFT procedure in Crohn's disease patients with complex anal fistula. *Tech Coloproctology.* 2022 Mar;26(3):205–12.

[62] Gingold DS, Murrell ZA, Fleshner PR. A prospective evaluation of the ligation of the intersphincteric tract procedure for complex anal fistula in patients with Crohn's disease. *Ann Surg.* 2014 Dec;260(6):1057–61.

[63] Kamiński JP, Zaghiyan K, Fleshner P. Increasing experience of ligation of the intersphincteric fistula tract for patients with Crohn's disease: what have we learned? *Colorectal Dis Off J Assoc Coloproctology G B Irel.* 2017 Aug;19(8):750–5.

[64] Soltani A, Kaiser AM. Endorectal advancement flap for cryptoglandular or Crohn's fistula-in-ano. *Dis Colon Rectum.* 2010 Apr;53(4):486–95.

[65] Lee MJ, Heywood N, Adegbola S, Tozer P, Sahnan K, Fearnhead NS, et al. Systematic review of surgical interventions for Crohn's anal fistula. *BJS Open.* 2017 Jun;1(3):55–66.

[66] Stellingwerf ME, van Praag EM, Tozer PJ, Bemelman WA, Buskens CJ. Systematic review and meta-analysis of endorectal advancement flap and ligation of the intersphincteric fistula tract for cryptoglandular and Crohn's high perianal fistulas. *BJS Open.* 2019 Jun;3(3):231–41.

[67] Corman M. The surgisis® AFP™ anal fistula plug: report of a consensus conference. *Colorectal Dis.* 2008;10(1):17–20.

[68] Garg P, Song J, Bhatia A, Kalia H, Menon GR. The efficacy of anal fistula plug in fistula-in-ano: a systematic review. *Colorectal Dis Off J Assoc Coloproctology G B Irel.* 2010 Oct;12(10):965–70.

[69] Senéjoux A, Siproudhis L, Abramowitz L, Munoz-Bongrand N, Desseaux K, Bouguen G, et al. Fistula Plug in Fistulising Ano-Perineal Crohn's Disease: a Randomised Controlled Trial. *J Crohns Colitis.* 2016 Feb;10(2):141–8.

[70] Dozois EJ, Lightner AL, Dietz AB, Fletcher JG, Lee YS, Friton JJ, et al. Durable Response in Patients With Refractory Fistulizing Perianal Crohn's Disease Using Autologous Mesenchymal Stem Cells on a Dissolvable Matrix: Results from the Phase I Stem Cell on Matrix Plug Trial. *Dis Colon Rectum.* 2023 Feb;66(2):243.

[71] Buchanan GN, Bartram CI, Phillips RKS, Gould SWT, Halligan S, Rockall TA, et al. Efficacy of fibrin sealant in the management of complex anal fistula: a prospective trial. *Dis Colon Rectum.* 2003 Sep;46(9):1167–74.

[72] Tinay OEY, El-Bakry AA. Treatment of chronic fistula-in-ano using commercial fibrin glue. *Saudi Med J.* 2003 Oct;24(10):1116–7.

[73] Zmora O, Neufeld D, Ziv Y, Tulchinsky H, Scott D, Khaikin M, et al. Prospective, multicenter evaluation of highly concentrated fibrin glue in the treatment of complex cryptogenic perianal fistulas. *Dis Colon Rectum.* 2005 Dec;48(12):2167–72.

[74] Grimaud J-C, Munoz–Bongrand N, Siproudhis L, Abramowitz L, Sénéjoux A, Vitton V, et al. Fibrin Glue Is Effective Healing Perianal Fistulas in Patients with Crohn's Disease. *Gastroenterology.* 2010 Jun;138(7):2275-2281.e1.

[75] Vitton V, Gasmi M, Barthet M, Desjeux A, Orsoni P, Grimaud JC. Long-term healing of Crohn's anal fistulas with fibrin glue injection. *Aliment Pharmacol Ther.* 2005 Jun;21(12):1453–7.

[76] Cirocchi R, Farinella E, Mura FL, Cattorini L, Rossetti B, Milani D, et al. Fibrin glue in the treatment of anal fistula: a systematic review. *Ann Surg Innov Res.* 2009 Nov;3:12.

[77] Vidon M, Munoz-Bongrand N, Lambert J, Maggiori L, Zeitoun J-D, Corte H, et al. Long-term efficacy of fibrin glue injection for perianal fistulas in patients with Crohn's disease. *Colorectal Dis Off J Assoc Coloproctology G B Irel.* 2021 Apr;23(4):894–900.

[78] Hannaway CD, Hull TL. Current considerations in the management of rectovaginal fistula from Crohn's disease. *Colorectal Dis.* 2008;10(8):747–55.

[79] Mueller MH, Geis M, Glatzle J, Kasparek M, Meile T, Jehle EC, et al. Risk of fecal diversion in complicated perianal Crohn's disease. *J Gastrointest Surg Off J Soc Surg Aliment Tract.* 2007 Apr;11(4):529–37.

[80] Galandiuk S, Kimberling J, Al-Mishlab TG, Stromberg AJ. Perianal Crohn disease: predictors of need for permanent diversion. *Ann Surg.* 2005 May;241(5):796–801; discussion 801-802.

[81] Munster LJ, Pronk AJM, Mundt MW, Hompes R, Bemelman WA, van der Bilt JDW, et al. Prolonged Time to Diagnosis of Crohn's Disease in Patients With Perianal Fistulas Negatively Affects Long-Term Outcomes. *J Crohns Colitis.* 2024 Sep;jjae146.

[82] Yamamoto T, Bain IM, Allan RN, Keighley MR. Persistent perineal sinus after proctocolectomy for Crohn's disease. *Dis Colon Rectum.* 1999 Jan;42(1):96–101.

[83] Rius J, Nessim A, Nogueras JJ, Wexner SD. Gracilis transposition in complicated perianal fistula and unhealed perineal wounds in Crohn's disease. *Eur J Surg Acta Chir.* 2000 Mar;166(3):218–22.

[84] Oomen JWPM, Spauwen PHM, Bleichrodt RP, van Goor H. Guideline proposal to reconstructive surgery for complex perineal sinus or rectal fistula. *Int J Colorectal Dis.* 2007 Feb;22(2):225–30.

[85] Fleshner PR, Schoetz DJ, Roberts PL, Murray JJ, Coller JA, Veidenheimer MC. Anal fissure in Crohn's disease: a plea for aggressive management. *Dis Colon Rectum.* 1995 Nov;38(11):1137–43.

[86] Evans J, Luck A, Hewett P. Glyceryl trinitratevs. lateral sphincterotomy for chronic anal fissure. *Dis Colon Rectum.* 2001 Jan;44(1):93–7.

[87] Kennedy ML, Sowter S, Nguyen H, Lubowski DZ. Glyceryl trinitrate ointment for the treatment of chronic anal fissure: results of a placebo-controlled trial and long-term follow-up. *Dis Colon Rectum.* 1999 Aug;42(8):1000–6.

[88] Libertiny G, Knight JS, Farouk R. Randomised trial of topical 0.2% glyceryl trinitrate and lateral internal sphincterotomy for the treatment of patients with chronic anal fissure: long-term follow-up. *Eur J Surg Acta Chir.* 2002;168(7):418–21.

[89] Lund JN, Scholefield JH. Glyceryl trinitrate is an effective treatment for anal fissure. *Dis Colon Rectum.* 1997 Apr;40(4):468–70.

[90] Oettlé GJ. Glyceryl trinitrate vs. sphincterotomy for treatment of chronic fissure-in-ano: a randomized, controlled trial. *Dis Colon Rectum.* 1997 Nov;40(11):1318–20.

[91] Werre AJ, Palamba HW, Bilgen EJ, Eggink WF. Isosorbide dinitrate in the treatment of anal fissure: a randomised, prospective, double blind, placebo-controlled trial. *Eur J Surg Acta Chir.* 2001 May;167(5):382–5.

[92] Scholefield JH, Bock JU, Marla B, Richter HJ, Athanasiadis S, Pröls M, et al. A dose finding study with 0.1%, 0.2%, and 0.4% glyceryl trinitrate ointment in patients with chronic anal fissures. *Gut.* 2003 Feb;52(2):264–9.

[93] Bouguen G, Trouilloud I, Siproudhis L, Oussalah A, Bigard M-A, Bretagne J-F, et al. Long-term outcome of non-fistulizing (ulcers, stricture) perianal Crohn's disease in patients treated with infliximab. *Aliment Pharmacol Ther.* 2009;30(7):749–56.

[94] D'Ugo S, Franceschilli L, Cadeddu F, Leccesi L, Blanco GDV, Calabrese E, et al. Medical and surgical treatment of haemorrhoids and anal fissure in Crohn's disease: a critical appraisal. *BMC Gastroenterol.* 2013 Mar;13:47.

[95] Stringer EE, Nicholson TJ, Armstrong D. Efficacy of topical metronidazole (10 percent) in the treatment of anorectal Crohn's disease. *Dis Colon Rectum.* 2005 May;48(5):970–4.

[96] Hart AL, Plamondon S, Kamm MA. Topical tacrolimus in the treatment of perianal Crohn's disease: exploratory randomized controlled trial. *Inflamm Bowel Dis.* 2007 Mar;13(3):245–53.

[97] Keighley MR, Allan RN. Current status and influence of operation on perianal Crohn's disease. *Int J Colorectal Dis.* 1986 Apr;1(2):104–7.

[98] Jeffery PJ, Parks AG, Ritchie JK. Treatment of haemorrhoids in patients with inflammatory bowel disease. *Lancet Lond Engl*. 1977 May;1(8021):1084–5.

[99] Grossi U, Gallo G, Tanna GLD, Bracale U, Ballo M, Galasso E, et al. Surgical Management of Hemorrhoidal Disease in Inflammatory Bowel Disease: A Systematic Review with Proportional Meta-Analysis. *J Clin Med.* 2022 Jan;11(3):709.

[100] Peyrin-Biroulet L, Loftus EV, Tremaine WJ, Harmsen WS, Zinsmeister AR, Sandborn WJ. Perianal Crohn's disease findings other than fistulas in a population-based cohort. *Inflamm Bowel Dis*. 2012 Jan;18(1):43–8.

[101] Bouguen G, Siproudhis L, Bretagne J-F, Bigard M-A, Peyrin-Biroulet L. Nonfistulizing perianal Crohn's disease: clinical features, epidemiology, and treatment. *Inflamm Bowel Dis.* 2010 Aug;16(8):1431–42.

[102] Brochard C, Siproudhis L, Wallenhorst T, Cuen D, d'Halluin PN, Garros A, et al. Anorectal stricture in 102 patients with Crohn's disease: natural history in the era of biologics. *Aliment Pharmacol Ther.* 2014 Oct;40(7):796–803.

Chapter 12

Special Situations: Pediatric Disease and Pregnancy

Rebecca Kowalski[1], MD
John J. Kessler II[1], MD
and Laura E. Cooper[2,*], MD
[1]University of Maryland Medical Center, Baltimore, Maryland, USA
[2]Penn State Milton Hershey S. Medical Center, Hershey, Pennsylvania, USA

Abstract

Crohn's Disease (CD) often presents during childhood, sometimes with serious complications and and/or extraintestinal manifestations. There are several unique considerations to acknowledge when caring for the pediatric patient. Emerging data continues to shape our guidelines for the optimal medical and surgical management of pediatric CD. The fertility of female patients with CD is similar to that of the general population, though fecundity is affected by disease activity. Remission prior to conception should be sought to optimize pregnancy outcomes. Patients with CD are also at risk for developing a variety of symptoms unrelated to the gastrointestinal system. Extraintestinal manifestations may precede the diagnosis of CD, creating diagnostic confusion. Each patient should be asked about arthralgias, aphthous ulceration, uveitis, pyoderma gangrenosum, and erythema nodosum. Treatment of CD should improve aphthous stomatitis, EN, and Type I arthropathy. In cases where EIMs are suspected, expert consultation may be warranted.

Pediatric Crohn's Disease

Epidemiology

The US prevalence of Crohn's Disease (CD) is 398 per 100,000 people, or about 1.011 million individuals nationwide [1]. At the pediatric level, the prevalence of CD internationally can be up to 47.5 per 100,000 children, with the highest prevalence noted in North America [2]. From 2011 to 2020, prevalence of Inflammatory Bowel Disease (IBD) has increased gradually, a trend that is reflected in the pediatric population [1, 2]. The U.S. incidence of IBD in the 21st century has been estimated at 10.9 per 100,000 person-years [1]. The overall incidence of ulcerative colitis (UC) is higher than that of CD, estimated at 6.3 and 4.1, respectively, but in

* Corresponding Author's Email: lcooper2@pennstatehealth.psu.edu

In: Surgery for Crohn's Disease. Second Edition
Editors: Stephen M. Kavic, Rebecca Brown and Kerri Lopez
ISBN: 979-8-89530-676-5

children, this finding is reversed [1, 2]. Internationally, incidence of pediatric CD is increasing and varies from 0.2-15.3 per 100,000 person years, with highest rates reported in North America and Northern Europe [2].

Most commonly, patients are diagnosed with CD in the second or third decade of life, but patients have been diagnosed as early as infancy and as late as the ninth decade [1,3]. Data from a multicenter pediatric IBD registry including six centers across the US showed that between January 2000 and November 2002, among 1,370 children with IBD, the mean age at diagnosis of IBD was 10 years old [3]. The incidence of very early onset IBD (VEO-IBD, age <6 years at diagnosis) varies from 0.2-3.3 per 100,000 person years internationally, representing 3-20% of pediatric IBD across studies in Canada, Singapore, and France [2, 4]. In Canada, the incidence of VEO-IBD is the fastest growing among pediatric IBD [5].

The most frequent (53-63%) disease location at diagnosis is the terminal ileum/colon [6, 7]. In a large European cohort, the proportion of other isolated locations of disease at diagnosis included terminal ileum (16%), colon (27%), and upper tract (4%) [7]. Isolated colonic disease was a more common presentation in younger (<10 years) patients. Of those with lower tract disease at diagnosis, 30% had concomitant upper gastrointestinal (GI) disease, including esophagoduodenal and jejunal/proximal ileal disease. Perianal disease was present in 9% of children at diagnosis [7]. Compared with adults, children with IBD appear more likely to present with extensive intestinal involvement and have rapid clinical progression with disease extension to include at least one additional segment in up to 31% of children at follow-up [6].

The prevalence of complicated disease (e.g., fistulae, strictures) at diagnosis of pediatric CD is approximately 30 percent [6, 8]. Younger patients (<10 years old) are more likely to present with uncomplicated disease [7]. Patients with any terminal ileal involvement (with or without colon involvement) were more likely to present with stricturing disease, with prevalence of approximately 1 in 5 children [7]. The development of pediatric CD complications has also been demonstrated to increase over time, with cumulative incidence rates of CD complications after diagnosis of 13.0% at one year and 37.9% at 10 years [7]. It should be kept in mind, however, that medical therapy since the time of this study has evolved significantly, likely altering the progression of disease observed here.

Approximately 30% of children with IBD have a family history of IBD. There is clearly an important genetic component in the pathogenesis of IBD [3]. This is particularly true in VEO-IBD and even moreso in infantile (<2 years of age) onset IBD [4]; even so, only about a third of the VEO-IBD have an identified genetic cause [9]. Furthermore, lack of concordance of disease among monozygotic twins and differences in rates of IBD among migrant populations support a role for environmental factors in the development of IBD [10]. Definitive genetic testing for CD in children as well as adults remains elusive. Notably, there is also evidence that non-genetic factors play a role in the pathogenesis of CD; epidemiologically, incidence of pediatric CD globally is modified by population-level characteristics such as the human development growth index, gross domestic product, and presence of universal health coverage [11].

Symptoms and Signs

As in the adult population, children with CD may present with intestinal and/or extraintestinal manifestations. Intestinal manifestations are more common, most often abdominal pain (44%), diarrhea (39%), weight loss (23%), and rectal bleeding (21%) [12]. Notably, only a quarter of pediatric patients present with the classic triad of abdominal triad, diarrhea, and weight loss [13]. Less than 10% present with perianal disease, including fistula, abscess, or ulcer, and only 40% of pediatric CD patients present with rectal bleeding [13]. Other symptoms include fever, fatigue, nausea, vomiting, and joint pains. Symptoms typically begin insidiously with fatigue and diarrhea with or without blood or mucus [14]. Infrequently, children may have a more fulminant presentation with severe abdominal pain, hematochezia, tenesmus, or fevers. Initial symptoms may be difficult to distinguish from conditions such as functional abdominal pain or infectious gastroenteritis. Delay in diagnosis is common, with 27% experiencing a greater than one year difference between onset of symptoms and diagnosis [13].

Growth failure is a common feature of pediatric CD. The earliest form of growth failure is a decrease in height velocity, which is defined as (1) a fall in the height percentile of more than 0.3 standard deviations per year, (2) growth velocity of less than 5 cm per year, or (3) a decrease in the growth velocity of $\geq$ 2 cm compared with the previous year during early to mid-puberty. Growth failure leads to short stature for age, delayed bone age, and pubertal delay. In general, growth failure is more common in pediatric patients with CD than UC [15]. Previously, up to 30-50% of pediatric CD patients had growth failure [16, 17], but more recent studies from the 2010s suggest the prevalence of growth failure in pediatric onset CD has decreased to 6-10% [15]. Growth outcomes improve with treatment, particularly steroid-sparing approaches like elemental enteral nutrition and immunotherapeutic agents [15].

Presence of complicated behavior may affect symptomatic presentation [6, 8]. Fistulae can develop between diseased bowel and adjacent tissue or organs, such as enteroenteric, enterovesicular, and enterocutaneous fistulae. Enteroenteric fistulae may be asymptomatic or present with diarrhea and malabsorption or small intestinal bacterial overgrowth. Enterovesicular fistulae present with pneumaturia and recurrent urinary tract infections. Enterocutaneous fistulae are most common in the perianal region and present with drainage or abscesses, which commonly occur adjacent to inflamed bowel loops. Patients with intra-abdominal abscesses often present with fever, abdominal pain, and leukocytosis. Depending on their location and degree, strictures may cause partial or complete bowel obstruction, commonly presenting with nausea, vomiting, and abdominal pain.

Diagnosis

Differentiating CD from UC can be challenging. Features that are uniquely suggestive of CD include: non-contiguous "skip" lesions, gastrointestinal noncaseating granulomas not proximal to ruptured cysts, presence of gross lesions of proximal GI tract, bowel stricture, cobblestoning, linear ileal ulcerations, and ileal inflammation with normal cecum [18]. Diagnostic schema such as the Porto criteria incorporate clinical features, laboratory values, imaging, endoscopic findings, and histopathologic findings to categorize disease phenotypes; these criteria may be useful in the setting of diagnostic ambiguity [18–20].

Laboratory Evaluation

In children suspected of IBD, several lab tests are warranted for both the diagnostic work-up and evaluation of known associated abnormalities. European Society for Paediatric Gastroenterology Hepatology and Nutrition (ESPGHAN) 2014 guidelines recommend labs to (a) rule out enteral infectious causes, (b) identify intestinal inflammation, and (c) screen for extraintestinal manifestations (18). Enteral infectious work-up should include Salmonella, Shigella, Yersinia, Campylobacter, and Clostridium difficile toxins; assessment for ova, cysts, and parasites may be warranted for those with relevant travel histories [18, 21]. Intestinal inflammatory evaluation should include complete blood count, inflammatory markers (e.g., erythrocyte sedimentation rate (ESR) and C-reactive protein (CRP)), albumin, and fecal calprotectin or lactoferrin. Of these, fecal calprotectin is the most sensitive for detection of intestinal inflammation, though it is non-specific among other causes of bowel inflammation [21]. Recommended tests to screen for extra-intestinal manifestations include transaminases and gamma-glutamyl transferase (GGT) [18].

While a standard component of the diagnostic work-up, serologic evaluation including serum anti-saccharomyces cerevisiae antibodies (ASCA) and perinuclear antineutrophil cytoplasmic antibodies (pANCA) may be useful for IBD diagnosis and discrimination between UC and CD (22). ASCA is found in 40 - 80 % of patients with CD and tends to identify those with terminal ileum and cecal involvement [14], whereas pANCA is more specific for UC [22]. In adults, the presence of either antibody is helpful to distinguish between IBD and non-IBD with sensitivity and specificity of 62.6% and 92.6%, respectively. The combination of ASCA positivity and pANCA negativity was associated with 55% sensitivity and 93% specificity for CD diagnosis in adults, but this combination has not been assessed in the pediatric population [22]. ASCA positivity alone has a sensitivity of 43% and specificity 96% for CD diagnosis in pediatric patients, and thus ASCA negativity can essentially rule out CD as a possible diagnosis [22]. As with any screening test, the positive predictive value depends on the likelihood of disease based on symptoms and population incidence. False-positive results are more likely in asymptomatic patients or in populations with a low incidence of CD, such as the pediatric population. Practice guidelines do not currently advocate for antibody testing to aid in establishing a diagnosis [14, 23].

Blood-based biomarkers to predict disease progression are emerging, but not yet clinically available. One study found that two sets of serum proteins including several interleukins, matrix metalloproteinase-10, and other signaling molecules and cell-receptors were more predictive of the development of complicated pediatric CD (stricturing and fistulizing, respectively) than serologic or clinical evaluations [24]. These biomarkers may ultimately be helpful in identifying cohorts of patients who may benefit from early biologic therapy.

Imaging Evaluation

All initial diagnostic work-up for pediatric CD, as with adults, should include imaging to assess the small bowel for active disease and its complications such as strictures, fistulae, and abscesses. This can be performed as standard computed tomography (CT), CT enterography (CTE), magnetic resonance enterography (MRE), upper gastrointestinal series with small bowel follow-through, intestinal ultrasound, or video capsule endoscopy depending on the presenting symptoms. ESPGHAN recommends MRE for all pediatric patients undergoing IBD work-up unless it is not practical, in which case capsule endoscopy is the next best option. Ultrasound can be utilized as a screening tool, but these guidelines recommend complementing it with additional small bowel imaging [18].

Upper GI series with small bowel follow-through (UGI/SBFT) can be used to evaluate the small bowel for strictures and fistulas, although in recent years has been used less often given the increasing availability of CTE and MRE. In addition to detecting strictures, MRE can also identify fistulae and abscesses. MRE is often preferred over UGI/SBFT and CT, particularly in the pediatric population, because it does not subject patients to radiation. Patients with CD are at high risk for an unacceptable cumulative radiation exposure over the course of their lifetime [25]. CT with contrast provides good visualization of the lumen and luminal wall as well as any extraintestinal complications such as abscesses and fistulas. The radiation dose is higher than that of UGI/SBFT and is not generally recommended unless MRE is not available. Like CTE, a large volume of oral contrast is administered to patients undergoing MRE to optimally distend the small bowel. In addition, MRE requires breath holding to obtain optimal imaging. Consequently, MRE can be challenging to perform in very young children who may not be able to comply with these instructions.

Intestinal ultrasound (IUS) is an emerging tool for disease monitoring, which overcomes practical limitations of other imaging modalities like the radiation of CT scans and the need to hold breath for MRE [26]. Gastroenterologists trained in IUS can utilize it at the bedside during clinic visits, obviating the need for a separate visit for additional diagnostic testing. IUS parameters of interest are bowel wall thickness (and associated ratio of submucosa to total wall thickness, which can be helpful to identify mild disease where thickness is normal) and hyperemia. Additionally, while less well-studied, proximal luminal dilation and hyperperistalsis may indicate the presence of a distal stricture. The mesentery can also be evaluated for creeping fat and, while nonspecific, the presence of mesenteric lymphadenopathy. Complications such as fistulae and abscesses can also be detected [27]. The localization, length, and continuity of affected segments can be characterized. The utilization of this modality is limited by availability of trained practitioners to complete the examination.

Video capsule endoscopy (VCE) is increasingly used in adult IBD patients for CD diagnosis and severity assessment, particularly if lower endoscopy is normal but CD is still suspected. Validated indices – Capsule Endoscopy Crohn's Disease Activity Index (CECDAI) and the Lewis Score – can be utilized to characterize small bowel disease location and activity [21]. The use of VCE is limited if there are concerns for luminal strictures due to the risk of capsule retention [28, 29]. VCE retention rates in CD patients have been reported between 2-13%, and in cases where stenosis is a concern, dissolvable patency capsules can be utilized to screen for likelihood of pill impaction prior to VCE administration [21]. VCE has been approved by the US FDA for use in children older than 10 years.

Regarding diagnostic accuracy of the available modalities, IUS and MRE have similarly excellent sensitivity, specificity, positive predictive value, and negative predictive value (all over 90%) when compared against ileocolonoscopy and/or surgical findings. However, MRE outperforms IUS for CD extension (especially for enteroenteric fistula detection) and in some studies, is slightly more accurate than IUS [30, 31]. IUS diagnostic accuracy is improved with utilization of enteral contrast [27]. In children with IBD, the Simple Pediatric Activity Ultrasound Score (SPAUSS), which utilizes the parameters bowel wall thickness, inflammatory mesenteric fat, and hyperemia, has been shown to have excellent accuracy (91.6-100% for identifying active disease in colon or ileum) when compared to standard ileocolonoscopy [26]. VCE has comparable diagnostic accuracy to MRE and IUS, and may be superior for proximal small bowel assessment [21]. VCE, IUS, MRE, and CTE are diagnostically superior to UGI/SBFT [32].

Endoscopy

ESPGHAN 2021 guidelines recommended both esophagogastroduodenal (EGD) and ileocolonic endoscopic evaluation for diagnosis in children with suspected IBD [18]. Endoscopy is generally well tolerated by the pediatric population. Most endoscopists prefer anesthesiologist-driven sedation such as propofol or general anesthesia to improve patient comfort. In a registry of children undergoing colonoscopy, the rate of short-term complications such as hypoxia, arrhythmia, gastrointestinal bleeding, and perforation, among others, was approximately 1% [33].

Ileocolonoscopy should include at least two biopsies from each the ileum, ascending, transverse, descending, sigmoid colon, and rectum [18]. Macroscopic findings suggestive of CD include ulceration, stenosis/stricture, cobblestoning, skip lesions, and stricture/fistula formation; notably, architecture can be preserved in early IBD [21]. EGD should be completed even in the absence of upper gastrointestinal symptoms (unlike the recommendation in adults to only screen those who are symptomatic) and should include at least two biopsies from each the esophagus, stomach, and duodenum [18, 21]. EGD findings can help differentiate IBD phenotypes when lower endoscopy is non-specific and may identify CD-specific abnormalities (e.g., aphthae, ulcerations, cobblestoning, stenosis) in up to a quarter of patients under investigation for pediatric IBD [7].

Histopathology

Noncaseating granulomas in a patient with IBD are diagnostic of CD unless they are adjacent to ruptured crypts. However, mucosal biopsies reveal granulomas in only 25 - 50% of patients with CD [14]. Transmural lymphoid aggregates are also diagnostic, but these can only be identified on surgical specimens from small bowel resections or colectomy. Detailed pathologic criteria have been developed for CD diagnosis but are beyond the scope of this chapter.

Differential Diagnosis

Infectious causes should be ruled out with routine stool culture as well as Clostridium difficile toxin testing. Gastroenteritis is far more common than CD in children. Infectious colitis can mimic IBD. Consequently, the presence of an enteric pathogen does not necessarily exclude underlying IBD, as the enteric pathogen can often trigger disease flares [18]. Patients who fail to respond to treatment should undergo further investigation. In cases of refractory disease, cytomegalovirus (CMV) colitis should also be considered. Infants (<2 years) diagnosed with IBD should undergo investigation for a primary immune deficiency [18].

Medical Therapy

Approach to Treatment

The goal of medical therapy for pediatric CD has shifted significantly from symptom control to mucosal healing, which can be achieved with either a "step-up" or "top down" approach, as these patients are believed to have better long-term outcomes [34, 35]. Top-down therapy utilizes high potency immunosuppressive medications early in an attempt to induce remission rapidly [36]. Step-up therapy uses low potency medications initially with escalation of medical therapy until remission is achieved. Recent evidence shows the top-down approach is associated with higher steroid and surgery-free remission, high rates of mucosal healing, and lower risk of complications (stricture or penetrating disease), though head-to-head comparisons of the two approaches are still underway [37]. In either case, treatment of active CD involves an induction regimen with transition to a maintenance regimen once remission is achieved.

The ECCO-ESPGHAN 2021 Guidelines have outlined an algorithm for medical therapy of pediatric CD that will be summarized here [37]. The first step is to determine the patient's risk of need for early surgical intervention or rapid progression of injury to the bowel. Those with penetrating or stricturing disease, pan-enteric involvement, deep ulcerations of the colon, or perianal fistulas were considered high risk. Those with growth delay or who did not achieve remission 12 weeks after induction therapy were considered medium risk. The remainder were deemed low risk. Following the algorithm, those determined to be medium or high risk should begin with anti-tumor necrosis factor (anti-TNF) therapy such as infliximab or adalimumab. Those that start with infliximab should also be given an immunomodulator such as a thiopurine or methotrexate to reduce the risk of developing anti-drug antibodies.

Patients deemed to be low risk should start with exclusive enteral nutrition (EEN), corticosteroids if response to EEN is inadequate or the diet is not tolerated, or 8 weeks of combination antibiotic therapy with azithromycin and metronidazole (though the evidence for this last approach is limited). For all patients, anti-TNF therapy should be monitored, adjusted, and optimized. If remission is not possible after optimal therapy, alternative biologics should be considered such as ustekinumab or vedolizumab. Failure to achieve remission after induction therapy is a predictor for poor outcome. Once remission is achieved, maintenance therapy should be continued in the form of biologics or immunomodulators. Probiotics and fecal microbiota transplants have no role in the treatment of pediatric CD.

Approach to Disease Monitoring

Mucosal healing is optimally assessed with endoscopic evaluation. Scoring systems like the Endoscopic Score for Crohn's Disease (SES-CD) and the Crohn's Disease Endoscopic Index of Severity (CDEIS) can aid in this evaluation. In adults, endoscopic or cross-sectional evaluation are recommended within 6 months of therapy initiation, but no such recommendations exist in the pediatric guidelines [21].

While endoscopy should be utilized to evaluate mucosal healing, more frequent assessments with less invasive measures are more practical. European adult IBD guidelines recommend chemical and biochemical re-evaluation within 12 weeks of therapy initiation [21]. The ECCO-ESPGHAN pediatric CD guidelines suggest fecal calprotectin coupled with an improvement in clinical symptoms can be a useful marker of treatment response. Fecal calprotectin correlates with endoscopically identified disease activity, and has been shown to predict disease relapse in adults with IBD; fecal calprotectin's diagnostic utility is well established for colonic CD, and newer evidence suggests that it has reasonable accuracy for small bowel inflammation, too [38, 39]. Regarding clinical symptoms, patients should be queried regarding diarrhea, abdominal pain, nausea, vomiting, weight loss (or lack of weight gain), and extraintestinal symptoms. Height velocity should be calculated to determine if growth failure is present. Disease activity may also be quantified using the pediatric CD activity index (PCDAI), a numerical scoring system ranging that measures well-being, abdominal pain, number of bowel movements, weight gain, linear growth, physical exam findings, and laboratory parameters including hematocrit, ESR, and serum albumin. A score of 0 to 10 correlates with inactive disease, 11 to 30 with mild disease, and > 30 with moderate to severe disease. A decrease in PCDAI of greater than 12.5 indicates clinical response, but notably this score does not adequately reflect mucosal healing [40]. In patients with clinical remission, a rising fecal calprotectin may be an early indicator of a disease flare; this finding should prompt further investigation and may warrant treatment escalation [37]. Of note, CRP does not reliably correlate with mucosal healing [21].

Transmural disease activity should be monitored with imaging, though monitoring intervals are again undefined. VCE, IUS, and MRE have utility in assessment of transmural healing as a response to treatment, and this has been demonstrated for the latter two modalities specifically in the pediatric CD population; CTE should not be utilized for serial evaluation due to the cumulative radiation risk [21, 41]. Perianal CD monitoring should couple clinical assessment with imaging, as external closure may mask residual internal fistulae patency [21].

Specific post-surgical disease monitoring recommendations exist for some CD-related procedures. Following ileocecal resection, endoscopic re-evaluation should be completed between 6-12 months post-operatively [37]. Special attention should be paid to the mucosa proximal to the anastomosis, as this is most commonly where mucosal lesions are visualized. If the anastomosis is unable to be reached endoscopically, alternative evaluation should be sought with video capsule endoscopy, MRE, or intestinal ultrasound. This re-evaluation has important treatment implications - if the endoscopy reveals features that are high risk for disease recurrence (as can be quantified with the Rutgeerts score), initiation of anti-TNF therapy should be considered.

Induction Therapy

The three commonly utilized approaches to induction therapy for pediatric CD are exclusive enteral nutrition, steroids, and anti-TNF agents. The selection of induction therapy is driven by disease severity.

Exclusive enteral nutrition (EEN) is recommended by international clinical guidelines as the first line therapy for the induction of remission in children with active luminal CD because of its superior mucosal healing rates and side effect profile compared to alternatives [37, 42, 43]. Patients on EEN receive all nutrition via elemental and/or polymeric formula by mouth, nasogastric tube, or gastrostomy tube. While adherence is a concern, newer formulas that include solid food may be better tolerated by patients [44, 45]. The typical duration of EEN for induction therapy is 6 to 8 weeks, though an alternative strategy should be sought if some improvement is not observed in the first 2 to 4 weeks [37].

Glucocorticoids may be used to induce remission in moderate to severe disease. Steroids should be used infrequently and for short periods of time in children, as long-term exposure is associated with a variety of side effects including growth failure, osteopenia, diabetes, adrenal suppression, psychosis, hirsutism, and cataracts among others. Induction with steroid therapy should serve as a bridge to long-term non-steroid therapies using medications such as immunosuppressants (azathioprine, 6-mercaptopurine, methotrexate) or biologic therapy (anti-TNF agents).

For patients with mild to moderate disease, oral prednisone or budesonide can be used. The starting dose of prednisone is 1 to 2 mg/kg per day to 40 mg daily, and a dose increase to 1.5 mg/kg to 60 mg daily can be considered if response is unsatisfactory [42]. Budesonide is a steroid with fever systemic side effects than other steroids given its extensive first-pass metabolism. Budesonide is most active in the distal ileum and right colon, making it a great option for patients with ileocolonic CD. As the initial response rate to budesonide may be lower than prednisone, prednisone can be utilized as a rescue therapy for non-responders [46]. The initial dose of budesonide is 9 mg daily, although doses up to 12 mg daily for four weeks have been used in children for induction of remission [42].

For those who do not respond to oral steroids or with severe disease, intravenous (IV) methylprednisolone can be considered. Once remission is achieved, patients can be converted to oral therapy and a slow steroid taper should be initiated after a non-steroid maintenance agent has been selected. Up to one quarter of patients may become steroid-dependent and over one third may require surgery despite intensive medical therapy [47]. For those patients on long-term, supraphysiologic doses of steroids, adrenal insufficiency should be assumed to be present and managed appropriately perioperatively [37].

For pediatric patients with higher risk disease (e.g., growth failure, fistulizing perianal disease, ulcerating colonic disease, extensive small bowel disease, or steroid-unresponsive disease), anti-TNF agents have been shown to be superior to steroids, EEN, or immunosuppressants in inducing remission, facilitating mucosal healing, and mitigating penetrating or stricturing complications [14, 37, 48, 49]. Thus, anti-TNF agents are recommended as a first-line induction therapy for higher risk patients [37]. These medications can be paired with corticosteroids in severe cases. For induction, infliximab is typically administered as 3 intravenous doses over 6 weeks, and adalimumab as two subcutaneous injections over two weeks, followed by maintenance therapy in both cases [37].

Maintenance Therapy

Several maintenance options exist for pediatric patients who have achieved remission, including thiopurines, methotrexate, biologic therapies, and combinations of these. Other strategies have proven less effective. Aminosalicylates are no longer recommended for use in pediatric CD due to their high relapse rates [50]. Maintenance enteral nutrition, wherein more than half of the daily calorie needs are derived from an elemental formula, has poor long-term adherence and evidence of its effectiveness in the pediatric CD population is limited [37].

Methotrexate (MTX), a folic acid antagonist, is moderately effective as a maintenance therapy, demonstrating one-year remission rates for pediatric CD between 25-53% [37]. MTX can be administered intramuscularly, subcutaneously, or orally once weekly. MTX can be used in conjunction with TNF antagonists without increasing risk of lymphoma, unlike combination therapy with thiopurines and TNF antagonists [42, 51]. Side effects include myelosuppression, infection, hepatitis, and oral ulcers. MTX is strictly contraindicated in pregnancy and should be discontinued for 6 months for females and 3 months for males prior to conception. Laboratory monitoring including complete blood counts (CBC) and liver function tests (LFTs) should be performed monthly for the first 4 months of therapy and then every 3 months. Folic acid supplementation reduces side effects including, nausea, vomiting, and oral ulcers and should be given in conjunction with MTX.

Thiopurines include azathioprine (AZA) and mercaptopurine (6-MP). Remission rates for thiopurines vary in the literature from 30-90%, and most studies in pediatric CD are small and/or observational [37, 52, 53]. Thiopurines are associated with a side effect profile including nausea and vomiting, transaminitis, hematologic toxicity, pancreatitis, hypersensitivity reactions, and a small but evident increased risk of lymphoma and non-melanoma skin cancer development [37, 54–57]. Before treatment with thiopurines, routine laboratory monitoring should include CBC and LFTs, and these should be repeated at 2, 4, 8, and 12 weeks after initiating therapy. Once stable, these laboratory values can be rechecked every three months or two to three weeks after changes in dosage. Dose reduction or treatment cessation is recommended for significant leukopenia (WBC <3,000). Due to the increased susceptibility to bacterial and viral infections associated with thiopurines, pediatric patients must have the appropriate vaccinations prior to starting therapy.

Anti-TNF agents (infliximab and adalimumab) have both been shown to be effective and durable maintenance therapies compared to thiopurines or methotrexate alone, with up to two-thirds of patients remaining in remission 5 years following drug initiation [48, 58, 59]. Prior to initiating therapy, testing for tuberculosis, hepatitis B & C, varicella zoster (VZV), and human immunodeficiency virus (HIV) should be completed; VZV vaccination should be offered to seronegative patients without a history of chickenpox if treatment can be postponed several weeks [60]. After induction, infliximab is administered as an infusion every 8 weeks and adalimumab as a subcutaneous injection every other week. For both infliximab and adalimumab, drug levels should be monitored and regimen adjustments (e.g., more frequent administration) should be made to achieve therapeutic levels prior to switching drug classes for treatment failure; dose escalation may be required over time [37, 60]. Notably, higher trough levels of infliximab may be required for effective treatment of fistulizing perianal disease [60].

Antibody development to infliximab is an important concern. Combination therapy of infliximab with either a thiopurine or MTX is recommended as it mitigates antibody formation against infliximab, likely due to alterations in the pharmacokinetics and higher anti-TNF drug concentrations with combination therapy [37, 61]. Importantly, the increased lymphoma risk associated with thiopurines is heightened when paired as combination therapy with infliximab (but is not observed with infliximab alone), so the risks of long-term combination therapy should be weighed against its benefits [51, 56]. Immunomodulator combination therapy with adalimumab does not appear to confer the same benefit regarding antibody development as it does with infliximab, and thus combination therapy is not recommended with this drug unless patients are otherwise high risk for antibody development [37, 62, 63]. The side effect profile of these anti-TNF agents is similar and includes infusion reactions, serious infections, and rarely, hemophagocytic lymphohistiocytosis [60]. A third anti-TNF agent, golimumab, has very preliminary data in children and thus far does not appear to have sustained therapeutic effect [64].

Additional biologic agents have shown promise for disease refractory to anti-TNF therapy, though data in pediatric CD is still limited. In small trials, ustekinumab has shown durable remission rates in nearly half of patients up to one year, though has higher remission rates for patients with no prior biologic exposure [65, 66]. Ustekinumab may be a particularly helpful therapy for CD patients with extraintestinal skin manifestations [60]. Vedolizumab may be useful for refractory pediatric CD, and like ustekinumab, the drug has greater efficacy for biologic-naive patients [60, 67]. Vedolizumab may take up to four months to take effect, in which case bridging with steroids may be helpful [37]. In a case series of pediatric CD patients receiving vedolizumab who underwent surgical management, a high postoperative wound healing complication rate was reported, which warrants further study [68]. Neither ustekinumab or vedolizumab have high rates of antibody development and thus combination therapy with an immunomodulator does not increase efficacy [37]. Finally, natalizumab is an anti-integrin monoclonal antibody that is more commonly used to treat multiple sclerosis and has very limited data in pediatric CD. A small case series demonstrated early CD symptom improvement, but longitudinal follow-up was limited [69]. Because natalizumab is associated with an increased risk for developing progressive multifocal leukoencephalopathy, vedolizumab has gained more momentum as a lower-risk alternative for pediatric CD [70].

Antibiotic administration should be limited to perianal or colonic involvement in mild pediatric CD, and is not a typical maintenance regimen. Ciprofloxacin and metronidazole have been shown to have similar efficacy to steroids in adults [71]. Peripheral neuropathy, metallic taste, and disulfiram reactions can all occur with administration of metronidazole. Although studies do not show any increase in birth defects [72, 73], prolonged use in pregnancy is controversial as some studies have found metronidazole to be carcinogenic in rodents [74]. Side effects of ciprofloxacin include allergic reaction, abdominal pain, *Clostridium difficile* colitis, tendonitis, or tendon rupture. Overall, antibiotics are tolerated well.

Surgery

Overview

Surgical treatment of pediatric CD is typically reserved for disease refractory to medical therapy, complications of disease, or growth failure, especially when the growth failure occurs in early to mid-puberty to mitigate poor catch-up growth [75–77]. The most common indications for surgery are stricturing disease (60%), which causes obstruction in over half of patients, and unresponsive luminal disease (22%) [78, 79]. Although CD has no surgical cure, the goal of surgery is to reset to a new baseline of no active disease in order to obtain deep remission.

Over the past decade, as biologic therapies have become more numerous, more accessible, and better studied, the treatment paradigm has been altered with many advocating for a more aggressive, "top-down" approach to medical management prior to pursuing surgery [36, 61, 80, 81]. Because of this, the majority of pediatric CD patients are exposed to immunomodulators, steroids, and at least one biologic therapy prior to surgical intervention [82, 83]. Despite this, the need for surgical intervention has remained the same [84]. This holds true whether considering ileocolic resection, small bowel resection, colon resection, or perianal drainage procedures, though the rate of ileostomy creation has increased overtime [84].

Among pediatric patients with CD, 20 - 30% undergo surgery within 10 years of initial diagnosis [83, 85–87]. The risk of surgery increases with time from diagnosis, with cumulative probabilities of surgery of <10% at 1 year, one in five at 3 years, and a third at 5 years from diagnosis [6, 83]. Stricturing and penetrating phenotypes at diagnosis, perianal disease, and complications during follow-up were associated with increased likelihood of undergoing surgery [83]. Treatment with steroids may be associated with increased risk for needing surgery, and treatment whereas treatment with AZA, 5-aminosalicylic acid, and infliximab have been associated with decreased risk, though these medication associations should be interpreted with caution due to confounding by timing of medication initiation and disease severity [6, 88]. Surgery earlier in the course of disease (<3 years) has been associated with lower rates of medication requirement in the years to follow, as well as improved catch-up growth [89].

Surgical Approaches

Of the patients requiring surgery for CD, most (85%) operations are intra-abdominal surgery (hemicolectomy, subtotal colectomy, small bowel resection, stoma creation and others) with a small proportion requiring surgery for perianal disease (14%) [78]. Since the early 2000s, the laparoscopic approach has been associated with no increase in complications, lower narcotic use, faster dietary recovery, and shorter hospital stays in pediatric CD and the proportion of laparoscopic operations has increased [77, 84]. The safety of single-incision laparoscopic ileocecectomies and robotic-assisted laparoscopic colon resections has been demonstrated in children, but data have not yet demonstrated clear advantages over traditional laparoscopic surgery [77].

Strictures, which arise from prolonged inflammation and subsequent fibrosis, are typically managed with resection of the strictured segment or strictureplasty. For extensive or long strictures, resection with primary anastomosis is often required. There is limited pediatric evidence on the comparative effectiveness of different anastomotic techniques, including stapled vs handsewn, Kono-S vs side-to-side anastomosis vs mesenteric excision [77]. Strictureplasty may be attempted for shorter strictures and has the benefit of bowel conservation. Of note, strictureplasty should not be formed in the setting of concurrent bowel perforation, malnutrition, multifocal strictures within a short segment, or proximity to bowel that is planned to be resected [77]. Balloon dilation of ileocolic strictures has also been performed, but effects tend to be transient and patients usually require multiple dilations [79]. Still, this approach deserves consideration in pediatric CD, where disease has a high likelihood of recurrence and multiple resections [77]. While data is limited to case series, the endoscopic placement of lumen-apposing stents for pediatric CD patients is a promising alternative to stricture resection [90].

For colonic disease, limited retrospective data suggests that proximal strictures may be effectively managed with limited resection and primary anastomosis, but that subtotal colectomy is warranted for strictures distal to the transverse as a high rate of reintervention was observed; further study of this strategy is needed [91]. If subtotal colectomy with ileorectal anastomosis is pursued for pancolitis with rectal sparing, a temporary diverting ileostomy should be created due to otherwise high anastomotic leak rates [77]. For patients with pancolitis and severe rectal disease, the standard treatment remains total proctocolectomy with end ileostomy; ileal pouch anal anastomosis (IPAA) can be cautiously considered for patients without distal small bowel or perianal disease, but the outcomes of this procedure are less successful in CD than UC due to higher rates of pouchitis and pouch failure in CD patients [77].

Penetrating complications, including perforation, intra-abdominal or pelvic abscesses, and fistulas, typically require surgical management. Greater than 10% of patients with CD develop an intra-abdominal or pelvic abscess during their lifetime [92]. Abscesses must be drained surgically or percutaneously. Due to the transmural nature of CD, fistula formation occurs frequently. Enteroenteric, enterocutaneous, enterovesicular, and rectovaginal fistulas often require surgical therapy to correct [93].

Perianal CD remains a challenging condition to treat across all ages. These patients should undergo an exam under anesthesia and lower endoscopy, and pre-operative MRI should be considered for evaluation of fistulae and abscesses [77]. Fissures, fistulas, and abscesses may be multiple and recurrent. Repeat operations predispose patients to anal sphincter damage and subsequent incontinence [94]. If symptomatic fistulous tracts are identified, non-cutting setons should be placed to allow complete epithelialization of the tract and to prevent premature skin closure and formation of recurrent abscesses, and the patient should be initiated on infliximab [77, 95]. In patients with severe perianal disease and destruction of the sphincter, diverting ileostomy is the most appropriate strategy, though approximately of these patients go on to require further colorectal resection or perineal reconstruction, and many of them are unable to have reversal of their ostomies [77, 96, 97]. Management of low rectal and anal strictures is evolving and available evidence is limited to case studies; reported approaches include serial dilation with Hegar dilators, endoscopic balloon dilation, local injections of steroids or anti-TNF agents, transanal strictureplasty, proctectomy with diversion, and either transanal or transabdominal rectosigmoid resection with pull-through and coloanal anastomosis [77].

Pre-Operative Considerations and Post-Operative Course

Preoperative considerations include determining the extent of intestinal disease with recent imaging and endoscopic evaluation. Steroid therapy should be tapered as much as possible preoperatively. Historically, anti-TNF therapy was thought to be associated with increased postoperative complications, resulting in the recommendation that biologic therapies should be held 4-6 weeks preoperatively for elective procedures [77]. Newer data, however, suggests that preoperative anti-TNF therapy is not associated with an increase in postoperative infectious complications, so the decision to delay elective procedures for an anti-TNF drug holiday should be individualized [98, 99]. Nutritional status should be optimized prior to surgery and may require administration of total parenteral nutrition. Pediatric patients in whom a stoma is being considered often benefit from preoperative counseling and meeting a stoma nurse to manage postoperative expectations [100].

After initial surgical management, recurrence rates remain high: up to 30% of patients develop clinical and endoscopic disease recurrence within one year, which increases to 60% by five years [101]. Factors associated with increased risk of recurrence include age < 14 years, severe or upper gastrointestinal disease at the time of surgery, high PCDAI scores, and pre-operative thiopurine use, and this recurrence may occur sooner in patients with colonic CD (rather than ileocecal or diffuse disease) [78, 89, 101]. Recurrence often requires additional intestinal resection, with rates estimated to be <10% at 2 years and up to 29% at 10 years, which increases the risk of developing short bowel syndrome [78, 89, 102].

Postoperative maintenance therapy can include thiopurines for patients not previously receiving anti-TNF therapy or resumption of preoperative anti-TNF therapy within 4 weeks of the procedure [37, 103, 104]. Prophylactic medical therapy with anti-TNF agents should be considered for patients at higher risk of recurrence, which can be initiated 2 to 4 weeks after surgery [37].

Despite high rates of surgical disease, post-operative disease recurrence, and need for additional resection, quality of life appears to be comparable with peers who do not have IBD. In a retrospective study of 36 children who had undergone bowel resection, despite surgical complications occurring for 3 in 4 patients and half of patients requiring an additional resection, 96% of pediatric patients were satisfied with the outcome of the surgery [102].

Pregnancy and IBD

Inflammatory bowel disease predominantly affects younger patients. At the time of diagnosis, many women are of child-bearing age [105]. If pregnancy is pursued, women and their physicians should consider the status of their CD, the potential impact of medical therapy on their pregnancy, mode of delivery, and implications for breast-feeding. Many women with IBD deliver early [106]. Caesarean section (c-section) is generally recommended in patients with active perianal disease or prior ileo-anal pouch surgery [106]. The following section will discuss issues pertinent to the management of pregnant patients with CD.

Fertility

In females with CD, the fertility rate is largely preserved and approximates that of the general population [107]. However, the ability to conceive may be lower in the period following a disease flare [106, 107]. Additionally, meta-analyses indicate that ileo-pouch anal anastomosis (IPAA) increases risk of infertility 2-5 fold, most likely due to the development of adhesions within the pelvis [108–110]. Infertility rates may be lower in patients who undergo laparoscopic IPAA, possibly due to reduced formation of adnexal adhesions [111, 112]. *In vitro* fertilization (IVF) has similar success in patients with CD compared to the general population [106]. History of prior surgical procedures for IBD may reduce the likelihood of success with IVF, but these studies have only included patients with UC [113, 114]. Patients with IBD have fewer children than the general population, which may be attributable to higher rates of voluntary childlessness, occurring in 17-38% of patients with IBD [106].

Males with CD may have difficulty conceiving due to the effects of active disease and medications on sperm. Compared to males in remission, those with active disease are more likely to report difficulty conceiving which may be related to decreased sperm motility [115, 116]. Sulfasalazine is associated with lower sperm counts and motility compared to mesalazine, though patients should be made aware that some mesalazine products contain phthalate and should be avoided due to its association with lower sperm motility [117, 118]. The effect of sulfasalazine on sperm is reversible within approximately 2 months after stopping the medication [119]. Paternal methotrexate exposure is associated with reversible oligospermia but is not associated with congenital malformations or still birth [120–122]. Anti-TNF medications, steroids, and thiopurines do not appear to be associated with sperm abnormalities [106, 116, 117, 123]. Finally, erectile dysfunction is prevalent among men with IBD, and the incidence of erectile dysfunction and retrograde ejaculation may be increased after IPAA [119, 124, 125].

Impact of IBD on Pregnancy

While many pregnancies in CD are uncomplicated, CD does increase the risk of many pregnancy complications. Rates of preterm delivery, stillbirth, small for gestational age (SGA) infants, and low birth weight (LBW) infants are elevated compared to the general population, while rates of early pregnancy loss are similar [106]. Ectopic pregnancies appear to be more common (1.1%) in patients with CD, and this risk may be higher still for those with a surgical history [106, 126]. The risk of developing gestational diabetes is also slightly higher for patients with CD, though the incidence remains low [127]. The prevalences of placental diseases are similar to those of the general population, with the exception of an increased risk of specifically severe preeclampsia [127, 128]. The incidence of preterm premature rupture of membranes (PPROM) has been shown to be higher for patients with CD (14%) compared to the general population, especially for patients who experience a disease flare during pregnancy [106, 127]. C-section rates are similar in CD to the general population, though prior intestinal or perianal surgery and active perianal disease increase this risk [106]. Evidence of increased incidence of congenital anomalies for infants of patients with CD is inconclusive [106].

The impact of active disease and flares on pregnancy outcomes highlights the importance of evaluation of remission prior to conception and close disease monitoring throughout pregnancy, with therapy adjustments as needed. The presence of active IBD at conception and a personal history of disease flare during a prior pregnancy have been found to be associated with disease flare during the current pregnancy, and those who have flares have higher rates of hospitalization, preterm delivery, and low birthweight compared to patients with IBD who stay in remission [127, 129]. Active disease itself confers higher risk of stillbirth, SGA, and 5-minute Apgar score <7 [106]. Regarding disease monitoring, while many biomarkers are rendered less useful during pregnancy, but fecal calprotectin has been shown to maintain its correlation with disease activity [106]. Endoscopy is generally considered to be safe during pregnancy, without evidence of adverse pregnancy outcomes, and should be limited to evaluations that are likely to change management [106]. Additionally, as radiation should be avoided during pregnancy when possible, non-contrast MRI and IUS may be useful tools for disease evaluation during pregnancy [106].

Pre-Conception Planning

Prenatal counselling is instrumental to optimizing outcomes. First and foremost, inducing remission prior to conception should be a priority, given the association of active disease and flares with poor pregnancy outcomes [127, 129]. Preconception counseling has been associated with decreased disease activity during pregnancy [130]. Referral to IBD prenatal clinics has been shown to reduce rates of pregnancy complications, LBW infants, and c-sections to approximately those of the general population; while these specialized clinics may not be widely available, the engagement of multidisciplinary care during the prenatal and throughout pregnancy is recommended [106]. The risks and benefits associated with each patient's medical regimen must be discussed prior to attempting conception. Most medications are considered to be safe during pregnancy, and often the risk of active disease or disease flares outweighs the risk conferred by the medications. Notable exceptions include methotrexate, which should be discontinued 6 months prior to conception, and dibutyl phthalate-containing 5-

aminosalicylates, which should be switched to a safer alternative formulation. Achieving remission prior to conception and minimizing steroid use during pregnancy for flares is advised. More detail on medication management during and after pregnancy can be found below.

Preconception counseling provides an opportunity to optimize many facets of pregnancy that are affected by CD. Preconception counseling been associated with smoking cessation and improved folate intake, which is recommended to be higher than the general population (2mg per day) for CD patients with ileal involvement, on certain medications, or on low residue diets [130, 131]. Patients should be made aware prenatally of the complications for which they are at higher risk. CD patients are at increased risk for iron and vitamin B12 deficiency; checking these levels during the first trimester and supplementing as needed is appropriate [131]. Approximately a quarter of IBD patients with stomas at conception have been demonstrated to have stoma-related complications during pregnancy (e.g., stoma prolapse, parastomal hernias, and obstruction), many of which require surgical intervention [132]. Patients with CD are also at a higher risk than the general population for venous thromboembolic events during pregnancy; individual risk assessments should be completed prenatally and during pregnancy for these patients, and low molecular weight heparin should be initiated when indicated [106]. Patients should be made aware of these risks and monitored for these complications appropriately.

Delivery

Many patients with CD undergo successful vaginal delivery, including those with ostomies. Mode of delivery should generally be driven by obstetric considerations rather than CD. Relative contraindications to vaginal delivery include active perianal disease, history of rectovaginal fistula, or IPAA due to the risk of perineal trauma during delivery [106, 133]; this decision should be multidisciplinary and include the patient, the obstetrician, the gastroenterologist, and the colorectal surgeon. Vaginal delivery may be undertaken in patients with CD without these relative contraindications, and is not associated with development of new perianal disease, relapse of inactive perianal disease, or fistula development (even with consideration of episiotomy or second-degree tear) compared to c-section [134, 135]. Compared to the general population, patients with CD may have higher rates of fecal incontinence following vaginal delivery compared to the general population, but evidence is limited and mitigating this potential risk alone is not currently considered an indication for c-section [136].

Postpartum Considerations

Breastfeeding does not impact IBD activity. Interestingly, 56% of women with IBD do not breastfeed their children due to physician recommendation, fear of medication interactions, or personal choice [137]. Regarding the safety of CD medication regimens during breastfeeding, in brief, aminosalicylates and anti-TNF medications can be continued during breastfeeding, thiopurines can be continued but breastfeeding should be avoided in the four hours following drug ingestion, and methotrexate is contraindicated [138, 139]. More detail is provided below. Regarding medications that may be administered perioperatively for surgical CD treatment, sedatives midazolam, fentanyl, and propofol can be used but are excreted in breast milk. The half-life of midazolam in breast milk is about an hour; therefore, pumping prior to the procedure and dumping the milk is a reasonable approach. While most medications used to treat IBD are low risk, appropriate counseling should be provided to patients so they are aware of any risks associated with breastfeeding while on medical therapy [57, 140].

There are several other postpartum considerations specific to patients with CD. There does not appear to be an increase in risk of relapse in postpartum patients with CD compared to non-postpartum patients with CD, but patients who discontinued therapy during pregnancy should be promptly reinitiated on therapy to mitigate flare development [141]. Venous thromboembolism risk does not appear to remain increased in CD patients postpartum as it does in UC patients [142]. CD patients are at a higher risk than the general population for the development of mental health disorders postpartum, which warrants close follow-up [143].

Medications

The peripartum use of immunosuppressive therapy, including thiopurines and biologic agents, is a topic of significant concern for patients as well as many providers. Most medications used for the treatment of CD are not associated with adverse outcomes during pregnancy or breastfeeding. Maintaining remission is critical in these patients, and an understanding of how to safely maintain appropriate medical therapy throughout pregnancy and post-partum period is imperative to achieving this goal [108].

Aminosalicylates

5-aminosalicylates are considered safe to continue during pregnancy and while breastfeeding; some studies report higher rates of premature birth, LBW, and stillbirth, but these are confounded by disease severity [106]. Physicians should advise patients receiving sulfasalazine to take at least 2 mg of folic acid due to the antifolate effects of this drug. Rarely, diarrhea has occurred in the infant in a mother receiving aminosalicylate therapy. If diarrhea develops breastfeeding should be discontinued [108]. In addition, Asacol, a specific mesalamine formulation, contains dibutyl phthalate in the coating of the drug, which was linked to malformations of the male urogenital tract of rats when given at extremely high doses [144–146]. Patients using formulations with dibutyl phthalate should switch to a different formulation.

Corticosteroids

All corticosteroids cross the placental barrier to the fetus, but are rapidly converted by placental 11 beta-hydroxysteroid dehydrogenase to less active metabolites, resulting in overall low fetal blood concentrations. Prednisone, prednisolone, and methylprednisolone are short-acting and are more rapidly metabolized, resulting in lower fetal concentrations than longer-acting corticosteroids such as dexamethasone [147]. Two small case-control studies demonstrated an association with corticosteroids and fetal cleft palate development, but this finding is now thought to be erroneous following larger meta-analyses [106, 148, 149].

Fetal low birth weight, preterm birth, neonatal intensive care unit administration, adrenal suppression, and severe postnatal infections have also been associated with exposure to glucocorticoids, though the evidence for the latter 2 is limited to low quality studies.

Glucocorticoids also increase the risk of hypertension, gestational diabetes, and preeclampsia [150, 151]. In general, corticosteroid therapy is felt to be associated with minimal risk in pregnant patients with IBD, but non-steroidal strategies are preferred when possible [106].

Corticosteroids are considered safe to continue during pregnancy, as they are secreted into breastmilk at low levels because of their protein-binding in the serum [152]. Secretion into milk is dose-dependent, therefore breastfeeding mothers requiring high doses of steroids may preferentially be given a steroid that reaches lower serum & milk levels such as prednisolone. Even still, no adverse effects have been reported in the infants of breastfeeding mothers taking prednisone.

Thiopurines

While cleft palate, skeletal anomalies, and urogenital malformations have been noted in animal studies of thiopurine exposure during pregnancy [153], these risks have not been replicated in human studies. Across multiple studies, AZA and 6MP use during pregnancy have not been associated with a higher risk of pregnancy adverse events or congenital anomalies, compared to pregnant patients with IBD who are not taking these medications [106]. Metabolites of these drugs do cross the placenta. While there is a theoretical risk of fetal immunosuppression due to these medications, prospective studies have not demonstrated immunological abnormalities (though newborns may have higher rates of transient anemia at birth) [154, 155]. Based on the above, these medications are typically continued throughout pregnancy in order to keep the mother in remission [108]. Peak excretion of AZA/6MP occurs within 4 hours of drug ingestion; therefore, breastfeeding women should be counseled to avoid feeding until at least 4 hours after drug ingestion [138].

Methotrexate

Exposure to MTX has been associated with miscarriage, growth retardation, fetal loss, and congenital malformations [156]. Patients should use at least two forms of contraception while on therapy. The FDA recommends that patients taking methotrexate wait to conceive for 6 and 3 months following cessation of MTX therapy for females and males, respectively [157].

TNF Antagonists

Infliximab and adalimumab are IgG1 antibodies that can cross the placental barrier. Across multiple large studies, TNF antagonists have not been linked to an increased risk of birth defects or adverse pregnancy outcomes [158–162]. In general, continuation of biologic therapy throughout pregnancy is recommended for patients with active disease at conception or high risk of relapse, in which the last the latest third trimester dose should be timed with the expected due date [106]. For patients in remission, continuation is still recommended to mitigate relapse, but for patients who prefer to stop their biologic therapy during pregnancy, the therapy should be initiated as soon as possible after delivery [106].

Both infliximab and adalimumab are considered to be safe to continue during breastfeeding. As these agents are made predominantly of IgG immunoglobulins, secretion is limited since IgA is the predominant immunoglobulin in human breast milk. Additional, large protein molecules (i.e., biologics) are likely inactivated by digestive enzymes. Small cohorts show overall safety of TNF antagonists in breastfeeding due to low or undetectable levels of infliximab and adalimumab, respectively, in infant serum [139]. Neither medication has been associated with adverse outcomes for nursing infants [163, 164]. However, infants who have maternal biologic exposure during pregnancy should not receive live vaccines until 1 year of life, or until serum drug levels are undetectable in the infant [106].

Certolizumab pegol is a PEGylated Fab fragment of a humanized anti-TNF monoclonal antibody. Fab fragments cross the placental barrier by passive diffusion, unlike infliximab and adalimumab which are actively transported. Accordingly, there is none or minimal placental transfer of certolizumab pegol to the fetus during pregnancy. A study of ten women exposed to CZP during pregnancy demonstrated very low to undetectable levels in cord blood and undetectable levels in breast milk [161].

Other Biologics

Data for the integrin inhibitors vedolizumab and natalizumab, and the interleukin inhibitor ustekinumab continues to emerge. Vedolizumab use during pregnancy has been evaluated across a mix of retrospective and prospective trials, and no adverse maternal or fetal outcomes were identified [165–168]. Infants have been found to have detectable vedolizumab levels at birth, with universal clearance by 6 months of age; in this small series, no infectious complications occurred and no developmental milestones were delayed during the follow-up period up to the first year of life [167]. Breastfeeding did not appear to affect clearance of vedolizumab from infants, nor did infants of breastfeeding moms have a higher risk of infection during the first year of life, but numbers are small [167]. Data on the safety of natalizumab in pregnancy for CD patients is very limited, but studies in pregnant patients with multiple sclerosis demonstrate a low adverse event rate [169].

Across several studies, ustekinumab use during pregnancy has not been shown to be associated with negative maternal or fetal complications, including infections or developmental delay in the first year of life [165, 168, 170, 171]. Ustekinumab may clear more slowly than vedolizumab from infants, with a median clearance estimated to be ~6.7 months [170]. For breastfeeding mothers on ustekinumab therapy, no increase in infection outcomes was seen in the first year of life, but data is limited [170].

Surgery

Indications for surgery in pregnant women with CD do not differ from those for non-pregnant patients. For patients who are very ill, ongoing illness is often a greater risk to the fetus than surgical intervention [172]. Most reports of CD surgery during pregnancy demonstrate a predominance of operations during the 1st or 2nd trimesters (73-92%) [173, 174]. Surgery during pregnancy is most often pursued for complicated stricturing or perforating disease, or severe disease flare; 77% of procedures in a recent case series were emergency surgeries [173]. While rates of minimally invasive approaches have improved over the last several decades, still less than half of these procedures are completed laparoscopically [173]. The majority of procedures involve bowel resection (small intestine / ileocecal more common than colon), more than half include ostomy creation, most of which are temporary [173]. Creation of a temporary ileostomy is generally recommended to mitigate postoperative complications after primary anastomosis and avoid exposure to pelvic organs, but as the stoma-related complication rate during pregnancy is estimated to be approximately 25%, the necessity of diversion should be carefully considered [132, 175]. Less than a quarter of procedures performed during pregnancy are for perianal disease [173, 174, 176]. The rate of surgical complications varies widely; in one case series, complications occurred in approximately a quarter of patients and were largely infectious in nature [173], while an earlier series reported complication rates closer to two-thirds and included fistula development, adhesive bowel obstruction, and stoma prolapse [174]. Maternal surgical mortality rate ranges from 0% (0/44 and 0/20 in two case series) to 6.7% (1/15 in small case series 1992-2015) [173, 174, 176].

Surgical procedures during pregnancy are associated with higher fetal risks, though it remains unclear whether this increased risk is driven by the acute surgery-necessitating illness vs the operation itself, or if there are substantial differences driven by surgical indication (CD vs other acute surgical disease). Undergoing any non-obstetric abdominal surgical procedure (e.g., appendectomy, cholecystectomy) during pregnancy carriers an increased risk of miscarriage (particularly during the first trimester and during the first 2 weeks after the procedure), an increased risk of preterm and very preterm birth, and an higher prevalence of small for gestational age pregnancies [177]. There may be additional risk conferred by the surgical indication being CD, though no direct comparisons have been made to date. Compared to reports for non-CD non-obstetric abdominal surgery during pregnancy, CD operations most recently have been associated with rates of 61% for premature delivery (vs 10%), 47% for low birth weight, 22% for small for gestational age (vs 3.4%), and 11% for fetal loss (vs 8%); these rates are lower than those previously reported in older case series, in which few or no patients utilized biologic therapy [173, 174, 176, 177]. Previous case series reported preterm delivery following all 3rd trimester operations, including frequent utilization of concomitant cesarean section during the CD procedure, but a more recent case series cited rates closer to 60% [173, 174, 176]. Among the patients who underwent a surgical CD procedure during their pregnancy, 42% of their newborns required hospitalization and three quarters of these required intensive care [173].

References

[1] Lewis JD, Parlett LE, Jonsson Funk ML, Brensinger C, Pate V, Wu Q, et al. Incidence, Prevalence, and Racial and Ethnic Distribution of Inflammatory Bowel Disease in the United States. *Gastroenterology*. 2023 Nov 1;165(5):1197-1205.e2.

[2] Kuenzig ME, Fung SG, Marderfeld L, Mak JWY, Kaplan GG, Ng SC, et al. Twenty-first Century Trends in the Global Epidemiology of Pediatric-Onset Inflammatory Bowel Disease: Systematic Review. *Gastroenterology*. 2022 Apr 1;162(4):1147-1159.e4.

[3] Heyman MB, Kirschner BS, Gold BD, Ferry G, Baldassano R, Cohen SA, et al. Children with early-onset inflammatory bowel disease (IBD): Analysis of a pediatric IBD consortium registry. *J Pediatr*. 2005 Jan;146(1):35–40.

[4] Ouahed J, Spencer E, Kotlarz D, Shouval DS, Kowalik M, Peng K, et al. Very early onset inflammatory bowel disease: A clinical approach with a focus on the role of genetics and underlying immune deficiencies. *Inflamm Bowel Dis*. 2020 May 12;26(6):820–42.

[5] Benchimol EI, Bernstein CN, Bitton A, Carroll MW, Singh H, Otley AR, et al. Trends in epidemiology of pediatric inflammatory bowel disease in Canada: Distributed network analysis of multiple population-based provincial health administrative databases. *Am J Gastroenterol*. 2017 Apr 18;112(7): 1120–34.

[6] Vernier-Massouille G, Balde M, Salleron J, Turck D, Dupas JL, Mouterde O, et al. Natural history of pediatric Crohn's disease: a population-based cohort study. *Gastroenterology*. 2008 Oct;135(4):1106–13.

[7] de Bie CI, Paerregaard A, Kolacek S, Ruemmele FM, Koletzko S, Fell JME, et al. Disease phenotype at diagnosis in pediatric Crohn's disease: 5-year analyses of the EUROKIDS Registry. *Inflamm Bowel Dis*. 2013 Feb;19(2):378–85.

[8] Gupta N, Bostrom AG, Kirschner BS, Ferry GD, Gold BD, Cohen SA, et al. Incidence of stricturing and penetrating complications of Crohn's disease diagnosed in pediatric patients. *Inflamm Bowel Dis*. 2010 Apr;16(4):638–44.

[9] Charbit-Henrion F, Parlato M, Hanein S, Duclaux-Loras R, Nowak J, Begue B, et al. Diagnostic yield of next-generation sequencing in very early-onset inflammatory bowel diseases: A multicentre study. *J Crohns Colitis*. 2018 Aug 29;12(9):1104–12.

[10] Halme L, Paavola-Sakki P, Turunen U, Lappalainen M, Färkkilä M, Kontula K, et al. Family and twin studies in inflammatory bowel disease. 2006; Available from: http://www.wjgnet.com/1007-9327/12/3668.asp.

[11] Weidner J, Glauche I, Manuwald U, Kern I, Reinecke I, Bathelt F, et al. Correlation of Socioeconomic and Environmental Factors With Incidence of Crohn Disease in Children and Adolescents: Systematic Review and Meta-Regression. *JMIR Public Health Surveill* [Internet]. 2024 Mar 25;10(12):e48682. Available from: https://publichealth.jmir.org/2024/1/e48682.

[12] Gupta N, Bostrom AG, Kirschner BS, Cohen SA, Abramson O, Ferry GD, et al. Presentation and Disease Course in Early- Compared to Later-Onset Pediatric Crohn's Disease. *Am J Gastroenterol*. 2008 Aug;103(8):2092–8.

[13] Sawczenko A, Sandhu B. Presenting features of inflammatory bowel disease in Great Britain and Ireland. *Arch Dis Child*. 2003 Nov 1;88(11):995–1000.

[14] North American Society for Pediatric Gastroenterology H and N, Colitis Foundation of America, Bousvaros A, Antonioli DA, Colletti RB, Dubinsky MC, et al. Differentiating ulcerative colitis from Crohn disease in children and young adults: report of a working group of the North American Society for Pediatric Gastroenterology, Hepatology, and Nutrition and the Crohn's and Colitis Foundation of America. *J Pediatr Gastroenterol Nutr*. 2007 May;44(5):653–74.

[15] Ishige T. Growth failure in pediatric onset inflammatory bowel disease: Mechanisms, epidemiology, and management. *Transl Pediatr*. 2019 Jan 1;8(1):16–22.

[16] Motil K, Grand R, Davis-Kraft L, Ferlic L, Smith E. Growth failure in children with inflammatory bowel disease: a prospective study. *Gastroenterology*. 1993 Sep;105(3):681–91.

[17] Kanof M, Lake A, Bayless T. Decreased height velocity in children and adolescents before the diagnosis of Crohn's disease. *Gastroenterology*. 1988 Dec;95(6):1523–7.

[18] Levine A, Koletzko S, Turner D, Escher JC, Cucchiara S, De Ridder L, et al. ESPGHAN revised porto criteria for the diagnosis of inflammatory bowel disease in children and adolescents. *J Pediatr Gastroenterol Nutr*. 2014;58(6):795–806.

[19] Levine A, Griffiths A, Markowitz J, Wilson DC, Turner D, Russell RK, et al. Pediatric modification of the Montreal classification for inflammatory bowel disease: The Paris classification. *Inflamm Bowel Dis*. 2011 Jun;17(6):1314–21.

[20] Satsangi J, Silverberg MS, Vermeire S, Colombel JF. The Montreal classification of inflammatory bowel disease: Controversies, consensus, and implications. *Gut*. 2006 Jun;55(6):749–53.

[21] Maaser C, Sturm A, Vavricka SR, Kucharzik T, Fiorino G, Annese V, et al. ECCO-ESGAR Guideline for Diagnostic Assessment in IBD Part 1: Initial diagnosis, monitoring of known IBD, detection of complications. *J Crohns Colitis*. 2019 Feb 1;13(2):144-164K.

[22] Reese GE, Constantinides VA, Simillis C, Darzi AW, Orchard TR, Fazio VW, et al. Diagnostic precision of anti-Saccharomyces cerevisiae antibodies and perinuclear antineutrophil cytoplasmic antibodies in inflammatory bowel disease. *Am J Gastroenterol*. 2006 Oct;101(10):2410–22.

[23] Lichtenstein GR, Loftus E V, Isaacs KL, Regueiro MD, Gerson LB, Sands BE. ACG Clinical Guideline: Management of Crohn's Disease in Adults. *Am J Gastroenterol*. 2018 Apr;113(4):481–517.

[24] Ungaro RC, Hu L, Ji J, Nayar S, Kugathasan S, Denson LA, et al. Machine learning identifies novel blood protein predictors of penetrating and stricturing complications in newly diagnosed paediatric Crohn's disease. *Aliment Pharmacol Ther*. 2021 Jan 1;53(2):281–90.

[25] Estay C, Simian D, Lubascher J, Figueroa C, O'Brien A, Quera R. Ionizing radiation exposure in patients with inflammatory bowel disease: are we overexposing our patients? *J Dig Dis*. 2015 Feb;16(2):83–9.

[26] Kellar A, Dolinger M, Novak KL, Chavannes M, Dubinsky M, Huynh H. Intestinal Ultrasound for the Pediatric Gastroenterologist: A Guide for Inflammatory Bowel Disease Monitoring in Children: Expert Consensus on Behalf of the International Bowel Ultrasound Group (IBUS) Pediatric Committee. *J Pediatr Gastroenterol Nutr*. 2023 Feb 1;76(2):142–8.

[27] Calabrese E, Maaser C, Zorzi F, Kannengiesser K, Hanauer SB, Bruining DH, et al. Bowel ultrasonography in the management of Crohn's disease. A review with recommendations of an international panel of experts. *Inflamm Bowel Dis*. 2016 May 1;22(5):1168–83.

[28] Liao Z, Gao R, Xu C, Li ZS. Indications and detection, completion, and retention rates of small-bowel capsule endoscopy: a systematic review. *Gastrointest Endosc*. 2010 Feb;71(2):280–6.

[29] Van Weyenberg SJB, Van Turenhout ST, Bouma G, Van Waesberghe JHTM, Van der Peet DL, Mulder CJJ, et al. Double-balloon endoscopy as the primary method for small-bowel video capsule endoscope retrieval. *Gastrointest Endosc*. 2010 Mar;71(3):535–41.

[30] Castiglione F, Mainenti PP, De Palma GD, Testa A, Bucci L, Pesce G, et al. Noninvasive diagnosis of small bowel Crohn's disease: Direct comparison of bowel sonography and magnetic resonance enterography. *Inflamm Bowel Dis*. 2013 Mar;19(4):991–8.

[31] Taylor SA, Mallett S, Bhatnagar G, Baldwin-Cleland R, Bloom S, Gupta A, et al. Diagnostic accuracy of magnetic resonance enterography and small bowel ultrasound for the extent and activity of newly diagnosed and relapsed Crohn's disease (METRIC): a multicentre trial. *Lancet Gastroenterol Hepatol*. 2018 Aug 1;3(8):548–58.

[32] Choi M, Lim S, Choi MG, Shim KN, Lee SH. Effectiveness of Capsule Endoscopy Compared with Other Diagnostic Modalities in Patients with Small Bowel Crohn's Disease: A Meta-Analysis. *Gut Liver*. 2017 Jan 15;11(1):62–72.

[33] Thakkar K, El-Serag HB, Mattek N, Gilger M. Complications of pediatric colonoscopy: a five-year multicenter experience. *Clin Gastroenterol Hepatol*. 2008 May;6(5):515–20.

[34] Baert F, Moortgat L, Van Assche G, Caenepeel P, Vergauwe P, De Vos M, et al. Mucosal healing predicts sustained clinical remission in patients with early-stage Crohn's disease. *Gastroenterology*. 2010 Feb;138(2):463–8; quiz e10-1.

[35] Neurath MF, Travis SPL. Mucosal healing in inflammatory bowel diseases: a systematic review. *Gut*. 2012 Nov;61(11):1619–35.

[36] Rubin DT, Uluscu O, Sederman R. Response to biologic therapy in Crohn's disease is improved with early treatment: An analysis of health claims data. *Inflamm Bowel Dis*. 2012 Dec;18(12):2225–31.

[37] Van Rheenen PF, Aloi M, Assa A, Bronsky J, Escher JC, Fagerberg UL, et al. The Medical Management of Paediatric Crohn's Disease: An ECCO-ESPGHAN Guideline Update. *J Crohns Colitis*. 2021 Feb 1;15(2):171–94.

[38] Gisbert JP, Bermejo F, Pérez-Calle JL, Taxonera C, Vera I, McNicholl AG, et al. Fecal calprotectin and lactoferrin for the prediction of inflammatory bowel disease relapse. *Inflamm Bowel Dis*. 2009 Aug;15(8):1190–8.

[39] Romero-Mascarell C, Fernández-Esparrach G, Rodríguez-De Miguel C, Masamunt MC, Rodríguez S, Rimola J, et al. Fecal Calprotectin for Small Bowel Crohn's Disease: Is It a Cutoff Issue? *Diagnostics* (Basel). 2022 Sep 15;12(9).

[40] Hyams J, Markowitz J, Otley A, Rosh J, Mack D, Bousvaros A, et al. Evaluation of the pediatric crohn disease activity index: a prospective multicenter experience. *J Pediatr Gastroenterol Nutr*. 2005 Oct;41(4):416–21.

[41] Focht G, Cytter-Kuint R, Greer MLC, Pratt LT, Castro DA, Church PC, et al. Development, Validation, and Evaluation of the Pediatric Inflammatory Crohn's Magnetic Resonance Enterography Index From the ImageKids Study. *Gastroenterology*. 2022 Nov 1;163(5):1306–20.

[42] Ruemmele FM, Veres G, Kolho KL, Griffiths A, Levine A, Escher JC, et al. Consensus guidelines of ECCO/ESPGHAN on the medical management of pediatric Crohn's disease. *J Crohns Colitis*. 2014 Oct;8(10):1179–207.

[43] Rufo PA, Denson LA, Sylvester FA, Szigethy E, Sathya P, Lu Y, et al. Health supervision in the management of children and adolescents with IBD: NASPGHAN recommendations. *J Pediatr Gastroenterol Nutr*. 2012 Jul;55(1):93–108.

[44] Svolos V, Hansen R, Nichols B, Quince C, Ijaz UZ, Papadopoulou RT, et al. Treatment of Active Crohn's Disease With an Ordinary Food-based Diet That Replicates Exclusive Enteral Nutrition. *Gastroenterology*. 2019 Apr 1;156(5):1354-1367.e6.

[45] Levine A, Wine E, Assa A, Sigall Boneh R, Shaoul R, Kori M, et al. Crohn's Disease Exclusion Diet Plus Partial Enteral Nutrition Induces Sustained Remission in a Randomized Controlled Trial. *Gastroenterology*. 2019 Aug 1;157(2):440-450.e8.

[46] Levine A, Broide E, Stein M, Bujanover Y, Weizman Z, Dinari G, et al. Evaluation of oral budesonide for treatment of mild and moderate exacerbations of Crohn's disease in children. *J Pediatr*. 2002 Jan;140(1):75–80.

[47] Faubion WA, Loftus E V, Harmsen WS, Zinsmeister AR, Sandborn WJ. The natural history of corticosteroid therapy for inflammatory bowel disease: a population-based study. *Gastroenterology*. 2001 Aug;121(2):255–60.

[48] Hyams J, Crandall W, Kugathasan S, Griffiths A, Olson A, Johanns J, et al. Induction and maintenance infliximab therapy for the treatment of moderate-to-severe Crohn's disease in children. *Gastroenterology*. 2007 Mar;132(3):863–73; quiz 1165–6.

[49] Ruemmele FM, Lachaux A, Cézard JP, Morali A, Maurage C, Giniès JL, et al. Efficacy of infliximab in pediatric Crohn's disease: a randomized multicenter open-label trial comparing scheduled to on demand maintenance therapy. *Inflamm Bowel Dis*. 2009 Mar;15(3):388–94.

[50] Patel P, Kaplan J, Moses J, Pasternak B, Samson C, Suskind D, et al. Aminosalicylate Use in Pediatric Patients with Crohn's Disease. *Inflamm Bowel Dis*. 2023 Jan 26;29(Supplement_1):S33–S33.

[51] Deepak P, Sifuentes H, Sherid M, Stobaugh D, Sadozai Y, Ehrenpreis ED. T-cell non-Hodgkin's lymphomas reported to the FDA AERS with tumor necrosis factor-alpha (TNF-α) inhibitors: results of the REFURBISH study. *Am J Gastroenterol*. 2013 Jan;108(1):99–105.

[52] Colombel JF, Sandborn WJ, Reinisch W, Mantzaris GJ, Kornbluth A, Rachmilewitz D, et al. Infliximab, Azathioprine, or Combination Therapy for Crohn's Disease. *New Engl J Med*. 2010 Apr 15;362(15):1383–95.

[53] Markowitz J, Grancher K, Kohn N, Lesser M, Daum F. A multicenter trial of 6-mercaptopurine and prednisone in children with newly diagnosed Crohn's disease. *Gastroenterology*. 2000 Oct;119(4):895–902.

[54] Lemaitre M, Kirchgesner J, Rudnichi A, Carrat F, Zureik M, Carbonnel F, et al. Association Between Use of Thiopurines or Tumor Necrosis Factor Antagonists Alone or in Combination and Risk of Lymphoma in Patients With Inflammatory Bowel Disease. *JAMA*. 2017 Nov 7;318(17):1679–86.

[55] Joosse ME, Aardoom MA, Kemos P, Turner D, Wilson DC, Koletzko S, et al. Malignancy and mortality in paediatric-onset inflammatory bowel disease: a 3-year prospective, multinational study from the paediatric IBD Porto group of ESPGHAN. *Aliment Pharmacol Ther*. 2018 Sep 1;48(5):523–37.

[56] Hyams JS, Dubinsky MC, Baldassano RN, Colletti RB, Cucchiara S, Escher J, et al. Infliximab Is Not Associated With Increased Risk of Malignancy or Hemophagocytic Lymphohistiocytosis in Pediatric Patients With Inflammatory Bowel Disease. *Gastroenterology*. 2017 Jun 1;152(8):1901-1914.e3.

[57] McLean LP, Cross RK. Adverse events in IBD: to stop or continue immune suppressant and biologic treatment. *Expert Rev Gastroenterol Hepatol*. 2014 Mar;8(3):223–40.

[58] Hyams JS, Griffiths A, Markowitz J, Baldassano RN, Faubion WA, Colletti RB, et al. Safety and efficacy of adalimumab for moderate to severe Crohn's disease in children. *Gastroenterology*. 2012 Aug;143(2):365-74.e2.

[59] Atia O, Friss C, Focht G, Magen Rimon R, Ledderman N, Ben-Tov A, et al. Durability of Adalimumab and Infliximab in Children with Crohn's Disease: A Nationwide Comparison From the epi-IIRN Cohort. *Inflamm Bowel Dis*. 2024 Nov 4;30(11):2097–104.

[60] Penagini F, Cococcioni L, Pozzi E, Dilillo D, Rendo G, Mantegazza C, et al. Biological therapy in pediatric age. *Pharmacol Res*. 2020 Nov 1;161.

[61] Colombel JF, Adedokun OJ, Gasink C, Gao LL, Cornillie FJ, D'Haens GR, et al. Combination Therapy With Infliximab and Azathioprine Improves Infliximab Pharmacokinetic Features and Efficacy: A Post Hoc Analysis. *Clin Gastroenterol Hepatol*. 2019 Jul 1;17(8):1525-1532.e1.

[62] Hyams JS, Dubinsky M, Rosh J, Ruemmele FM, Eichner SF, Maa J, et al. The effects of concomitant immunomodulators on the pharmacokinetics, efficacy and safety of adalimumab in paediatric patients with Crohn's disease: a post hoc analysis. *Aliment Pharmacol Ther*. 2019 Jan 2;49(2):155–64.

[63] Matsumoto T, Motoya S, Watanabe K, Hisamatsu T, Nakase H, Yoshimura N, et al. Adalimumab Monotherapy and a Combination with Azathioprine for Crohn's Disease: A Prospective, Randomized Trial. *J Crohns Colitis*. 2016 Nov;10(11):1259–66.

[64] Merras-Salmio L, Kolho K. Golimumab Therapy in Six Patients With Severe Pediatric Onset Crohn Disease. *J Pediatr Gastroenterol Nutr*. 2016 Sep;63(3):344–7.

[65] Dayan JR, Dolinger M, Benkov K, Dunkin D, Jossen J, Lai J, et al. Real World Experience with Ustekinumab in Children and Young Adults at a Tertiary Care Pediatric Inflammatory Bowel Disease Center. *J Pediatr Gastroenterol Nutr*. 2019 Jul 1;69(1):61–7.

[66] Chavannes M, Martinez-Vinson C, Hart L, Kaniki N, Chao CY, Lawrence S, et al. Management of Paediatric Patients with Medically Refractory Crohn's Disease Using Ustekinumab: A Multi-Centred Cohort Study. *J Crohns Colitis*. 2019 Apr 26;13(5):578–84.

[67] Shah P, McDonald D. Vedolizumab: An Emerging Treatment Option for Pediatric Inflammatory Bowel Disease. *J Pediatric Pharm Ther*. 2021 Dec 1;26(8):795–801.

[68] Zimmerman LA, Zalieckas JM, Shamberger RC, Bousvaros A. Postoperative complications of pediatric patients with inflammatory bowel disease treated with vedolizumab. *J Pediatr Surg*. 2018 Jul 1;53(7):1330–3.

[69] Singh N, Deshpande R, Rabizadeh S, Dubinsky M. Real World Experience With Natalizumab at a Tertiary Care Pediatric IBD Center. *J Pediatr Gastroenterol Nutr*. 2016 Jun;62(6):863–6.

[70] Warnke C, Menge T, Hartung HP, Racke MK, Cravens PD, Bennett JL, et al. Natalizumab and Progressive Multifocal Leukoencephalopathy. *Arch Neurol*. 2010 Aug 1;67(8).

[71] Prantera C, Zannoni F, Scribano ML, Berto E, Andreoli A, Kohn A, et al. An antibiotic regimen for the treatment of active Crohn's disease: a randomized, controlled clinical trial of metronidazole plus ciprofloxacin. *Am J Gastroenterol*. 1996 Feb;91(2):328–32.

[72] Caro-Patón T, Carvajal A, Martin de Diego I, Martin-Arias LH, Alvarez Requejo A, Rodríguez Pinilla E. Is metronidazole teratogenic? A meta-analysis. *Br J Clin Pharmacol*. 1997 Aug;44(2):179–82.

[73] Czeizel AE, Rockenbauer M. A population based case-control teratologic study of oral metronidazole treatment during pregnancy. *Br J Obstet Gynaecol*. 1998 Mar;105(3):322–7.

[74] Falagas ME, Walker AM, Jick H, Ruthazer R, Griffith J, Snydman DR. Late incidence of cancer after metronidazole use: a matched metronidazole user/nonuser study. *Clin Infect Dis*. 1998 Feb;26(2):384–8.

[75] Singh Ranger G, Lamparelli MJ, Aldridge A, Chong SK, Mitton SG, Albanese A, et al. Surgery results in significant improvement in growth in children with Crohn's disease refractory to medical therapy. *Pediatr Surg Int*. 2006 Apr;22(4):347–52.

[76] Sharf T, O'Guinn ML, Keane OA, Gayer CP. Biologics and the timing of operative management of pediatric inflammatory bowel disease. *J Pediatr Surg Open*. 2023 Dec;4:100084.

[77] Carter M, Lim IIP. Surgical management of pediatric Crohn's disease. *Semin Pediatr Surg*. 2024 Apr 1;33(2).

[78] Blackburn SC, Wiskin AE, Barnes C, Dick K, Afzal NA, Griffiths DM, et al. Surgery for children with Crohn's disease: indications, complications and outcome. *Arch Dis Child*. 2014 May;99(5):420–6.

[79] Hassan C, Zullo A, De Francesco V, Ierardi E, Giustini M, Pitidis A, et al. Systematic review: Endoscopic dilatation in Crohn's disease. *Aliment Pharmacol Ther*. 2007 Dec;26(11–12):1457–64.

[80] Kolho KL, Nikkonen A, Merras-Salmio L, Molander P. The need for surgery in pediatric patients with inflammatory bowel disease treated with biologicals. *Int J Colorectal Dis*. 2024 Apr 25;39(1):58.

[81] Ungaro RC, Yzet C, Bossuyt P, Baert FJ, Vanasek T, D'Haens GR, et al. Deep Remission at 1 Year Prevents Progression of Early Crohn's Disease. *Gastroenterology*. 2020 Jul;159(1):139–47.

[82] Mueller JL, Kaplan AJ, Kaplan JL, Griggs CL. Characteristics Associated With Early Ileocolonic Resection in Pediatric Crohn's Disease. *J Surg Res*. 2025 Jan 2;306:94–100.

[83] Rumenova Shentova-Eneva R, Kofinova D, Hadzhiyski P, Ivanova-Todorova E, Yaneva P, Lazarova E, et al. Risk Factors for Surgery in Pediatric Patients with Crohn's Disease. *Medical Principles and Practice*. 2022 May 27;31(2):195–200.

[84] Stokes AL, Kulaylat AN, Rocourt D V., Hollenbeak CS, Koltun W, Falaiye T. Rates and trends for inpatient surgeries in pediatric Crohn's disease in the United States from 2003 to 2012. *J Pediatr Surg*. 2018 Jul 1;53(7):1334–8.

[85] Pacilli M, Eaton S, Fell JM, Rawat D, Clarke S, Haddad MJ. Surgery in Children With Crohn Disease Refractory to Medical Therapy. *J Pediatr Gastroenterol Nutr*. 2011 Mar;52(3):286–90.

[86] Turunen P, Ashorn M, Auvinen A, Iltanen S, Huhtala H, Kolho KL. Long-term health outcomes in pediatric inflammatory bowel disease: A population-based study. *Inflamm Bowel Dis*. 2009 Jan;15(1):56–62.

[87] Kelay A, Tullie L, Stanton M. Surgery and paediatric inflammatory bowel disease. *Transl Pediatr*. 2019 Dec;8(5):436–48.

[88] Gupta N, Cohen SA, Bostrom AG, Kirschner BS, Baldassano RN, Winter HS, et al. Risk Factors for Initial Surgery in Pediatric Patients With Crohn's Disease. *Gastroenterology*. 2006;130(4):1069–77.

[89] Boualit M, Salleron J, Turck D, Fumery M, Savoye G, Dupas JL, et al. Long-term outcome after first intestinal resection in pediatric-onset Crohn's disease: a population-based study. *Inflamm Bowel Dis*. 2013 Jan;19(1):7–14.

[90] Sharlin C, Patel A, Fernando S, Carroll J, Procopio B, McOmber M, et al. Use of Lumen-Apposing Metal Stents for Inflammatory Bowel Disease-Related Strictures at a Pediatric Center: A Case Series. *JPGN Rep*. 2021 May;2(2):e055.

[91] Ba'ath ME, Mahmalat MW, Kapur P, Smith NP, Dalzell AM, Casson DH, et al. Surgical management of inflammatory bowel disease. *Arch Dis Child*. 2007 Apr 1;92(4):312–6.

[92] Yamaguchi A, Matsui T, Sakurai T, Ueki T, Nakabayashi S, Yao T, et al. The clinical characteristics and outcome of intraabdominal abscess in Crohn's disease. *J Gastroenterol*. 2004;39(5):441–8.

[93] Bell SJ, Williams AB, Wiesel P, Wilkinson K, Cohen RCG, Kamm MA. The clinical course of fistulizing Crohn's disease. *Aliment Pharmacol Ther*. 2003 May 1;17(9):1145–51.

[94] Lunniss PJ, Kamm MA, Phillips RK. Factors affecting continence after surgery for anal fistula. *Br J Surg*. 1994 Sep;81(9):1382–5.

[95] Thornton M, Solomon MJ. Long-term indwelling seton for complex anal fistulas in Crohn's disease. *Dis Colon Rectum*. 2005 Mar;48(3):459–63.

[96] Seemann NM, King SK, Elkadri A, Walters T, Fish J, Langer JC. The operative management of children with complex perianal Crohn's disease. *J Pediatr Surg*. 2016 Dec;51(12):1993–7.

[97] Johnston WR, Hwang R, Mattei P. Ostomy Management for Pediatric Perianal Crohn's Disease. *J Pediatr Surg*. 2024 Jun 1;59(6):1108–12.

[98] Lightner AL, McKenna NP, Alsughayer A, Loftus E V., Raffals LE, Faubion WA, et al. Anti-TNF biologic therapy does not increase postoperative morbidity in pediatric Crohn's patients. *J Pediatr Surg*. 2019 Oct 1;54(10):2162–5.

[99] Cohen BL, Fleshner P, Kane S V, Herfarth HH, Palekar N, Farraye FA, et al. Prospective Cohort Study to Investigate the Safety of Preoperative Tumor Necrosis Factor Inhibitor Exposure in Patients With Inflammatory Bowel Disease Undergoing Intra-abdominal Surgery. *Gastroenterology*. 2022 Jul;163(1):204–21.

[100] Brand MI, Dujovny N. Preoperative considerations and creation of normal ostomies. *Clin Colon Rectal Surg*. 2008 Feb;21(1):5–16.

[101] Baldassano RN, Han PD, Jeshion WC, Berlin JA, Piccoli DA, Lautenbach E, et al. Pediatric Crohn's disease: risk factors for postoperative recurrence. *Am J Gastroenterol*. 2001 Jul;96(7):2169–76.

[102] Piekkala M, Pakarinen M, Ashorn M, Rintala R, Kolho KL. Long-term outcomes after surgery on pediatric patients with Crohn disease. *J Pediatr Gastroenterol Nutr*. 2013 Mar;56(3):271–6.

[103] Regueiro M, Schraut W, Baidoo L, Kip KE, Sepulveda AR, Pesci M, et al. Infliximab Prevents Crohn's Disease Recurrence After Ileal Resection. *Gastroenterology*. 2009;136(2).

[104] De Cruz P, Kamm MA, Hamilton AL, Ritchie KJ, Krejany EO, Gorelik A, et al. Efficacy of thiopurines and adalimumab in preventing Crohn's disease recurrence in high-risk patients - A POCER study analysis. *Aliment Pharmacol Ther*. 2015 Oct 1;42(7):867–79.

[105] Hanauer SB. Inflammatory bowel disease: Epidemiology, pathogenesis, and therapeutic opportunities. *Inflamm Bowel Dis*. 2006 Jan;12:S3–9.

[106] Torres J, Chaparro M, Julsgaard M, Katsanos K, Zelinkova Z, Agrawal M, et al. European Crohn's and Colitis Guidelines on Sexuality, Fertility, Pregnancy, and Lactation. *J Crohns Colitis*. 2023 Jan 1;17(1):1–27.

[107] Ban L, Tata LJ, Humes DJ, Fiaschi L, Card T. Decreased fertility rates in 9639 women diagnosed with inflammatory bowel disease: A United Kingdom population-based cohort study. *Aliment Pharmacol Ther*. 2015 Oct 1;42(7):855–66.

[108] Mahadevan U. Fertility and pregnancy in the patient with inflammatory bowel disease. *Gut*. 2006 Aug;55(8):1198–206.

[109] Cornish JA, Tan E, Teare J, Teoh TG, Rai R, Darzi AW, et al. The effect of restorative proctocolectomy on sexual function, urinary function, fertility, pregnancy and delivery: a systematic review. *Dis Colon Rectum*. 2007 Aug;50(8):1128–38.

[110] Waljee A, Waljee J, Morris AM, Higgins PDR. Threefold increased risk of infertility: a meta-analysis of infertility after ileal pouch anal anastomosis in ulcerative colitis. *Gut*. 2006 Nov;55(11):1575–80.

[111] Bartels SAL, D'Hoore A, Cuesta MA, Bensdorp AJ, Lucas C, Bemelman WA. Significantly increased pregnancy rates after laparoscopic restorative proctocolectomy: a cross-sectional study. *Ann Surg*. 2012 Dec;256(6):1045–8.

[112] Beyer-Berjot L, Maggiori L, Birnbaum D, Lefevre JH, Berdah S, Panis Y. A total laparoscopic approach reduces the infertility rate after ileal pouch-anal anastomosis: a 2-center study. *Ann Surg*. 2013 Aug;258(2):275–82.

[113] Pabby V, Oza SS, Dodge LE, Hacker MR, Moragianni VA, Correia K, et al. In Vitro Fertilization Is Successful in Women With Ulcerative Colitis and Ileal Pouch Anal Anastomosis. *Am J Gastroenterol*. 2015 Jun;110(6):792–7.

[114] Pachler FR, Toft G, Bisgaard T, Laurberg S. Use and Success of in Vitro Fertilisation following Restorative Proctocolectomy and Ileal Pouch-anal Anastomosis. A Nationwide 17-year Cohort Study. *J Crohns Colitis*. 2019 Sep 27;13(10):1283–6.

[115] Ananthakrishnan AN, Martin C, Kane S, Sandler RS, Long MD. Paternal Disease Activity Is Associated With Difficulty in Conception Among Men With Inflammatory Bowel Diseases. *Clin Gastroenterol Hepatol*. 2019 Jan 1;17(1):203–4.

[116] Grosen A, Bungum M, Christensen LA, Cordelli E, Larsen OH, Leter G, et al. Semen Quality and Sperm DNA Integrity in Patients with Severe Active Inflammatory Bowel Disease and Effects of Tumour Necrosis Factor-alpha Inhibitors. *J Crohns Colitis*. 2019 Apr 26;13(5):564–71.

[117] Banerjee A, Scarpa M, Pathak S, Burra P, Sturniolo GC, Russo FP, et al. Inflammatory Bowel Disease Therapies Adversely Affect Fertility in Men- A Systematic Review and Meta-analysis. *Endocr Metab Immune Disord Drug Targets* [Internet]. 2019;19(7):959–74. Available from: http://www.eurekaselect.com/170675/article.

[118] Nassan FL, Coull BA, Skakkebaek NE, Williams MA, Dadd R, Mínguez-Alarcón L, et al. A crossover–crossback prospective study of dibutyl-phthalate exposure from mesalamine medications and semen quality in men with inflammatory bowel disease. *Environ Int*. 2016 Oct 1;95:120–30.

[119] Carini F, Mazzola M, Gagliardo C, Scaglione M, Giammanco M, Tomasello G. Inflammatory bowel disease and infertility: Analysis of literature and future perspectives. *Acta Biomedica*. 2021 Nov 3;92(5).

[120] Jensen NB, Justesen SD, Larsen A, Ernst E, Pedersen LH. A systematic overview of the spermatotoxic and genotoxic effects of methotrexate, ganciclovir and mycophenolate mofetil. *Acta Obstet Gynecol Scand*. 2021 Sep 1;100(9):1557–80.

[121] Eck LK, Jensen TB, Mastrogiannis Di, Torp-Pedersen A, Askaa B, Nielsen TK, et al. Risk of adverse pregnancy outcome after paternal exposure to methotrexate within 90 days before pregnancy. *Obstet Gynecol*. 2017;129(4):707–14.

[122] Beghin D, Cournot MP, Vauzelle C, Elefant E. Paternal exposure to methotrexate and pregnancy outcomes. *J Rheumatol*. 2011 Apr;38(4):628–32.

[123] Puchner R, Danninger K, Puchner A, Pieringer H. Impact of TNF-blocking agents on male sperm characteristics and pregnancy outcomes in fathers exposed to TNF-blocking agents at time of conception. *Clin Exp Rheumatol*. 2012;30(5):765–7.

[124] Scarberry K, Brady JT, Scarberry K, Stein SL, Steinhagen E. Surgery for Crohn's Disease Affects Male Sexual Function. *Ann Colorect Res*. 2019 Mar 3;In Press(In Press).

[125] Shmidt E, Suárez-Fariñas M, Mallette M, Moniz H, Bright R, Shah SA, et al. Erectile dysfunction is highly prevalent in men with newly diagnosed inflammatory bowel disease. *Inflamm Bowel Dis*. 2019 Jul 17;25(8):1408–16.

[126] de Silva PS, Hansen HH, Wehberg S, Friedman S, Nørgård BM. Risk of Ectopic Pregnancy in Women With Inflammatory Bowel Disease: A 22-Year Nationwide Cohort Study. *Clin Gastroenterol Hepatol*. 2018 Jan;16(1):83-89.e1.

[127] Tandon P, Govardhanam V, Leung K, Maxwell C, Huang V. Systematic review with meta-analysis: risk of adverse pregnancy-related outcomes in inflammatory bowel disease. *Aliment Pharmacol Ther*. 2020 Feb 1;51(3):320–33.

[128] Boyd HA, Basit S, Harpsøe MC, Wohlfahrt J, Jess T. Inflammatory bowel disease and risk of adverse pregnancy outcomes. *PLoS One*. 2015 Jun 17;10(6).

[129] Rottenstreich A, Fridman Lev S, Rotem R, Mishael T, Grisaru Granovsky S, Koslowsky B, et al. Disease flare at prior pregnancy and disease activity at conception are important determinants of disease relapse at subsequent pregnancy in women with inflammatory bowel diseases. *Arch Gynecol Obstet*. 2020 Jun 6;301(6):1449–54.

[130] de Lima A, Zelinkova Z, van der Ent C, van der Woude CJ. Anti-TNF is Safe to Stop in the Second Trimester of Pregnancy in IBD Women in Remission. *Gastroenterology*. 2014 May;146(5):S-78.

[131] Mahadevan U, Robinson C, Bernasko N, Boland B, Chambers C, Dubinsky M, et al. Inflammatory Bowel Disease in Pregnancy Clinical Care Pathway: A Report From the American Gastroenterological Association IBD Parenthood Project Working Group. *Gastroenterology*. 2019 Apr 1;156(5):1508–24.

[132] Blackwell S, Selinger C, Brookes M, Fearnhead N, PAPooSE SG, PAPooSE C. PMO-32 Pregnancy outcomes after stoma surgery for IBD: the results of a multi-centre retrospective audit. In: Posters [Internet]. BMJ Publishing Group Ltd and British Society of Gastroenterology; 2021. p. A93.2-A93. Available from: https://gut.bmj.com/lookup/doi/10.1136/gutjnl-2021-BSG.171.

[133] Juhasz ES, Fozard B, Dozois RR, Ilstrup DM, Nelson H. Ileal pouch-anal anastomosis function following childbirth. An extended evaluation. *Dis Colon Rectum*. 1995 Feb;38(2):159–65.

[134] Foulon A, Dupas JL, Sabbagh C, Chevreau J, Rebibo L, Brazier F, et al. Defining the Most Appropriate Delivery Mode in Women with Inflammatory Bowel Disease: A Systematic Review. *Inflamm Bowel Dis*. 2017 May 1;23(5):712–20.

[135] Smink M, Lotgering FK, Albers L, de Jong DJ. Effect of childbirth on the course of Crohn's disease; results from a retrospective cohort study in the Netherlands. *BMC Gastroenterol*. 2011 Jan 26;11.

[136] Ong JPL, Edwards GJ, Allison MC. Mode of delivery and risk of fecal incontinence in women with or without inflammatory bowel disease: Questionnaire survey. *Inflamm Bowel Dis*. 2007 Nov;13(11):1391–4.

[137] Kane S, Lemieux N. The role of breastfeeding in postpartum disease activity in women with inflammatory bowel disease. *Am J Gastroenterol*. 2005 Jan;100(1):102–5.

[138] Christensen LA, Dahlerup JF, Nielsen MJ, Fallingborg JF, Schmiegelow K. Azathioprine treatment during lactation. *Aliment Pharmacol Ther*. 2008 Nov 15;28(10):1209–13.

[139] Gisbert JP, Chaparro M. Safety of anti-TNF agents during pregnancy and breastfeeding in women with inflammatory bowel disease. *Am J Gastroenterol*. 2013 Sep;108(9):1426–38.

[140] Yarur A, Kane S V. Update on pregnancy and breastfeeding in the era of biologics. *Dig Liver Dis*. 2013 Oct;45(10):787–94.

[141] Pedersen N, Bortoli A, Duricova D, D Inca R, Panelli MR, Gisbert JP, et al. The course of inflammatory bowel disease during pregnancy and postpartum: a prospective European ECCO-EpiCom Study of 209 pregnant women. *Aliment Pharmacol Ther*. 2013 Sep;38(5):501–12.

[142] Kim YH, Pfaller B, Marson A, Yim HW, Huang V, Ito S, et al. The risk of venous thromboembolism in women with inflammatory bowel disease during pregnancy and the postpartum period: A systematic review and meta-analysis. *Medicine* (United States). 2019 Sep 1;98(38).

[143] Vigod SN, Kurdyak P, Brown HK, Nguyen GC, Targownik LE, Seow CH, et al. Inflammatory bowel disease and new-onset psychiatric disorders in pregnancy and post partum: a population-based cohort study. *Gut.* 2019 Sep;68(9):1597–605.

[144] Vo TTB, Jung EM, Dang VH, Yoo YM, Choi KC, Yu FH, et al. Di-(2 ethylhexyl) phthalate and flutamide alter gene expression in the testis of immature male rats. *Reprod Biol Endocrinol.* 2009 Sep 26;7:104.

[145] Gray LE, Ostby J, Furr J, Price M, Veeramachaneni DN, Parks L. Perinatal exposure to the phthalates DEHP, BBP, and DINP, but not DEP, DMP, or DOTP, alters sexual differentiation of the male rat. *Toxicol Sci.* 2000 Dec;58(2):350–65.

[146] Parks LG, Ostby JS, Lambright CR, Abbott BD, Klinefelter GR, Barlow NJ, et al. The plasticizer diethylhexyl phthalate induces malformations by decreasing fetal testosterone synthesis during sexual differentiation in the male rat. Toxicol Sci. 2000 Dec;58(2):339–49.

[147] van der Woude CJ, Ardizzone S, Bengtson MB, Fiorino G, Fraser G, Katsanos K, et al. The Second European Evidenced-Based Consensus on Reproduction and Pregnancy in Inflammatory Bowel Disease. *J Crohns Colitis.* 2015 Feb;9(2):107–24.

[148] Carmichael SL, Shaw GM. Maternal corticosteroid use and risk of selected congenital anomalies. *Am J Med Genet.* 1999 Sep 17;86(3):242–4.

[149] Rodríguez-Pinilla E, Martínez-Frías ML. Corticosteroids during pregnancy and oral clefts: a case-control study. *Teratology.* 1998 Jul;58(1):2–5.

[150] Reinisch JM, Simon NG, Karow WG, Gandelman R. Prenatal exposure to prednisone in humans and animals retards intrauterine growth. *Science* (1979). 1978 Oct 27;202(4366):436–8.

[151] Homar V, Grosek S, Battelino T. High-dose methylprednisolone in a pregnant woman with Crohn's disease and adrenal suppression in her newborn. *Neonatology.* 2008;94(4):306–9.

[152] Laube R, Paramsothy S, Leong RW. Use of medications during pregnancy and breastfeeding for Crohn's disease and ulcerative colitis. *Exp Opin Drug Saf.* 2021;20(3):275–92.

[153] Polifka JE, Friedman JM. Teratogen update: azathioprine and 6-mercaptopurine. *Teratology.* 2002 May;65(5):240–61.

[154] de Meij TGJ, Jharap B, Kneepkens CMF, van Bodegraven AA, de Boer NKH. Long-term follow-up of children exposed intrauterine to maternal thiopurine therapy during pregnancy in females with inflammatory bowel disease. *Aliment Pharmacol Ther.* 2013 Jul 16;38(1):38–43.

[155] Jharap B, de Boer NKH, Stokkers P, Hommes DW, Oldenburg B, Dijkstra G, et al. Intrauterine exposure and pharmacology of conventional thiopurine therapy in pregnant patients with inflammatory bowel disease. *Gut.* 2014 Mar;63(3):451–7.

[156] Kozlowski RD, Steinbrunner J V, MacKenzie AH, Clough JD, Wilke WS, Segal AM. Outcome of first-trimester exposure to low-dose methotrexate in eight patients with rheumatic disease. *Am J Med.* 1990 Jun;88(6):589–92.

[157] U.S. Food & Drug Administration. Labeling-Package Insert: Methotrexate [Internet]. 2024. Available from: www.fda.gov/medwatch.

[158] Nielsen OH, Loftus Jr E V, Jess T. Safety of TNF-α inhibitors during IBD pregnancy: a systematic review. *BMC Med.* 2013 Jul 31;11(1):174.

[159] Schnitzler F, Fidder H, Ferrante M, Ballet V, Noman M, Van Assche G, et al. Outcome of pregnancy in women with inflammatory bowel disease treated with antitumor necrosis factor therapy. *Inflamm Bowel Dis.* 2011 Sep;17(9):1846–54.

[160] Seirafi M, de Vroey B, Amiot A, Seksik P, Roblin X, Allez M, et al. Factors associated with pregnancy outcome in anti-TNF treated women with inflammatory bowel disease. *Aliment Pharmacol Ther.* 2014 Aug;40(4):363–73.

[161] Mahadevan U, Wolf DC, Dubinsky M, Cortot A, Lee SD, Siegel CA, et al. Placental transfer of anti-tumor necrosis factor agents in pregnant patients with inflammatory bowel disease. *Clin Gastroenterol Hepatol.* 2013 Mar;11(3):286–92; quiz e24.

[162] Mahadevan U, Long MD, Kane S V., Roy A, Dubinsky MC, Sands BE, et al. Pregnancy and Neonatal Outcomes After Fetal Exposure to Biologics and Thiopurines Among Women With Inflammatory Bowel Disease. *Gastroenterology.* 2021 Mar 1;160(4):1131–9.

[163] Barrau M, Roblin X, Andromaque L, Rozieres A, Faure M, Paul S, et al. What Should We Know about Drug Levels and Therapeutic Drug Monitoring during Pregnancy and Breastfeeding in Inflammatory Bowel Disease under Biologic Therapy? *J Clin Med.* 2023 Dec 1;12(23).

[164] Ben-Horin S, Yavzori M, Katz L, Picard O, Fudim E, Chowers Y, et al. Adalimumab level in breast milk of a nursing mother. *Clin Gastroenterol Hepatol.* 2010 May;8(5):475–6.

[165] Wils P, Seksik P, Stefanescu C, Nancey S, Allez M, Pineton de Chambrun G, et al. Safety of ustekinumab or vedolizumab in pregnant inflammatory bowel disease patients: a multicentre cohort study. *Aliment Pharmacol Ther.* 2021 Feb;53(4):460–70.

[166] Moens A, van der Woude CJ, Julsgaard M, Humblet E, Sheridan J, Baumgart DC, et al. Pregnancy outcomes in inflammatory bowel disease patients treated with vedolizumab, anti-TNF or conventional therapy: results of the European CONCEIVE study. *Aliment Pharmacol Ther.* 2020 Jan 1;51(1):129–38.

[167] Julsgaard M, Baumgart DC, Baunwall SMD, Hansen MM, Grosen A, Bibby BM, et al. Vedolizumab clearance in neonates, susceptibility to infections and developmental milestones: a prospective multicentre population-based cohort study. *Aliment Pharmacol Ther.* 2021 Nov 1;54(10):1320–9.

[168] Chugh R, Long MD, Jiang Y, Weaver KN, Beaulieu DB, Scherl EJ, et al. Maternal and Neonatal Outcomes in Vedolizumab- and Ustekinumab-Exposed Pregnancies: Results From the PIANO Registry. *Am J Gastroenterol.* 2024 Mar 1;119(3):468–76.

[169] Chowdhury R, Kane S V. Pregnancy and Crohn's disease: Concerns and assurance of medical therapy. *Gastroenterol Rep (Oxf).* 2022;10.

[170] Julsgaard M, Wieringa JW, Baunwall SMD, Bibby BM, Driessen GJA, Kievit L, et al. Infant Ustekinumab Clearance, Risk of Infection, and Development After Exposure During Pregnancy. *Clin Gastroenterol Hepatol.* 2024 Jan 1.

[171] Abraham BP, Ott E, Busse C, Murphy C, Miller L, Baumgart DC, et al. Ustekinumab Exposure in Pregnant Women from Inflammatory Bowel Disease Clinical Trials: Pregnancy Outcomes Through Up to 5 Years in Crohn's Disease and 2 Years in Ulcerative Colitis. *Crohns Colitis 360.* 2022 Jul 1;4(3).

[172] Hill J, Clark A, Scott NA. Surgical treatment of acute manifestations of Crohn's disease during pregnancy. *J Roy Soc Med.* 1997 Feb;90(2):64–6.

[173] Chaparro M, Kunovský L, Aguas M, Livne M, Rivière P, Bar-Gil Shitrit A, et al. Surgery due to Inflammatory Bowel Disease During Pregnancy: Mothers and Offspring Outcomes From an ECCO Confer Multicentre Case Series [Scar Study]. *J Crohns Colitis.* 2022 Sep 1;16(9):1428–35.

[174] Germain A, Chateau T, Beyer-Berjot L, Zerbib P, Lakkis Z, Amiot A, et al. Surgery for Crohn's disease during pregnancy: A nationwide survey. *United Eur Gastroenterol J.* 2020 Jul 1;8(6):736–40.

[175] Visser BC, Glasgow RE, Mulvihill KK, Mulvihill SJ. Safety and timing of nonobstetric abdominal surgery in pregnancy. *Dig Surg.* 2001;18(5):409–17.

[176] Killeen S, Gunn J, Hartley J. Surgical management of complicated and medically refractory inflammatory bowel disease during pregnancy. *Colorect Dis.* 2017 Feb 1;19(2):123–38.

[177] Rasmussen AS, Christiansen CF, Ulrichsen SP, Uldbjerg N, Nørgaard M. Non-obstetric abdominal surgery during pregnancy and birth outcomes: A Danish registry-based cohort study. *Acta Obstet Gynecol Scand.* 2020 Apr 1;99(4):469–76.

Section III. Postoperative Considerations

Chapter 13

Complications of Surgery

Matthew Cahn[1], MD
Leah Sukri[1], MD
and Stephen M. Kavic[2,*], MD, MSHPE
[1]University of Maryland Medical Center, Baltimore, Maryland, USA
[2]University of Maryland School of Medicine, Baltimore, Maryland, USA

Abstract

The majority of patients with Crohn's disease eventually require surgery within ten years of diagnosis, most often due to failure of medical therapy or obstruction secondary to ileocolic stenosis. Due to the transmural, chronic, inflammatory nature of the disease, as well as the inherent characteristics of the Crohn's patient population, there are a number of common and often difficult to treat complications associated with surgery for Crohn's disease. These include surgical site infection, intra-abdominal septic complications, anastomotic complications (e.g., stenosis or leak), enterocutaneous fistulas, surgical recurrence, and development of venous thromboembolism. Patients with septic complications, penetrating disease phenotype, and multiple other risk factors to be discussed, tend to require multiple reoperations and intestinal resections, increasing the risk for short gut syndrome and ultimately, intestinal failure. Surgeons must be able to identify high-risk patients and be aware of the current diagnostic and management principles of Crohn's disease complications in order to have appropriate and complete pre-operative discussions and to minimize patient morbidity and mortality post-operatively.

Introduction

Surgical management of Crohn's Disease (CD) is not curative and is reserved for specific indications, including intractable disease despite medical optimization, bowel perforation, bowel obstruction, uncontrolled hemorrhage, dysplasia, cancer, and abdominal collections not amenable to percutaneous intervention [1]. Despite improved medical management strategies, the need for surgery remains high for patients with CD, and between 66-80% of patients requiring surgery at some point in their life [1, 2]. Various studies have investigated the rate of need for surgery following a diagnosis of CD, citing 16.3%-44% at 1-year, 33.3-61% at 5-years, and 46.6-71% at 10-years following diagnosis [3].

---

* Corresponding Author's Email: Skavic@som.umaryland.edu

In: Surgery for Crohn's Disease. Second Edition
Editors: Stephen M. Kavic, Rebecca Brown and Kerri Lopez
ISBN: 979-8-89530-676-5

Additionally, many patients will require multiple surgical interventions. The incidence of clinical recurrence (i.e., a return of CD symptoms after surgery) is between 17-55% at 5 years, 32-76% at 10-years, and 72-73% at 20-years [4]. Globally, about half of surgical patients with CD will require a repeat surgical procedure after their index surgery [5]. The incidence of surgical recurrence (i.e., the need for reoperation due to CD) varies, and is estimated at 11-32% at 5-years, 20-44% at 10-years, and 46-55% at 20 years [4]. The high frequency of surgical intervention underscores the importance of understanding the implications of post-operative complications when treating patients with CD.

Despite the relatively younger age and fewer comorbidities of surgical patients with CD compared to typical surgical populations, patients with CD experience more post-operative complications [6, 7]. Studies have demonstrated an overall morbidity rate of 25.5-37% following bowel resection for CD with 4.5-13.4% of patients experiencing a major complication [8-10]. In comparison, the morbidity rate of emergency abdominal surgery in a general population has been reported to be around 14% [11]. Patients with CD are commonly immunosuppressed, have poor nutritional status, or have hostile intra-abdominal conditions (e.g., adhesions, distorted anatomy, shortened and friable mesentery, or the presence of intra-abdominal abscesses and fistulas), all of which increase the risk of post-operative complications [12, 13]. Specifically, patients with CD have an increased incidence of intra-abdominal septic complications (IASCs), which is the term that encompasses anastomotic leak, enterocutaneous fistulas, and intra-abdominal abscesses. These post-operative complications are associated with decreased quality of life, disease recurrence, as well as significant morbidity and mortality [14-16].

Due to the complexity and morbidity inherent in the surgical management of CD, one must understand the epidemiology, risk factors, pathogenesis, presentation, diagnosis, and management of post-operative complications for the CD. Complications discussed in this chapter include infection (surgical site infections and intra-abdominal sepsis), anastomotic complications, bleeding, venous thromboembolism (VTE), disease recurrence, and fistulas. Many of these – such as anastomotic leak, enterocutaneous fistula (ECF), and infection – overlap, and can subject the patient to a cycle of readmissions and repeat interventions. Short gut syndrome and intestinal failure are chronic complications of large resections, repeated resections, recurrent complications, and severe, unremitting disease activity.

Surgical Site Infections

Surgical site infections (SSIs) are the most common post-operative complication for CD patients. They can occur in the superficial (or incisional) space, deep space, or organ space within 30-days of surgery [17]. Treatment of SSI in CD patients is similar to the general population. Antibiotics are administered and source control is obtained with either local wound care, drain placement, or washout, either at bedside or in the operating room.

SSIs are associated with more post-operative pain, increased patient dissatisfaction, increased inpatient hospital costs as well as increased healthcare utilization following discharge [17-19]. Patients with CD have significantly increased risk for all SSIs (17.8%) compared to patients undergoing colorectal procedures for benign pathologies, such as diverticulitis (12.8%) and oncologic resections for colorectal cancer (12.0%) [20]. The increased infectious risk may be due to the natural history of CD, patient characteristics that are unique to the CD population, as well as the high prevalence of immunosuppressive treatments for CD. Figure 13.1 lists risk factors associated with SSIs for CD patients. A more comprehensive review of these risk factors is reserved for later in the chapter.

Complication	Incidence	Risk Factors
Wound Dehiscence	1-3%	Hypoalbuminemia
Surgical Site Infection	9-27%	Hypoprealbuminemia, hypoalbuminemia, preoperative weight loss, elevated intra-operative lactate, extended OR time, colonic surgery, proctectomy, stoma formation
Superficial Surgical Site Infection	8-22%	Anemia, blood transfusion, preoperative leukocytosis, preoperative neutrophilia, penetrating disease, hypoalbuminemia, elevated CRP, pre-operative fistula, ostomy formation, proctectomy
Deep Surgical Site Infection	2-7%	Hypoalbuminemia, blood transfusion
Organ space SSI	6-10%	Hypoalbuminemia, preoperative weight loss, blood loss, extended OR time, wound contamination, stoma formation, proctectomy
Intra-abdominal septic complication	3-12%	Hypoalbuminemia, low BMI, preoperative steroid use, prior intestinal resection, penetrating disease, intra-abdominal abscess, preoperative fistula, extended OR time, Less common: positive proximal margin, perianal disease, disease duration > 10 years, thiopurine therapy, smoking
Anastomotic Leak	2-9%	Hypoalbuminemia, preoperative weight loss, smoking, male sex, preoperative abscess, preoperative steroid use, repeat intestinal resection, extended OR time, emergency surgery
Enterocutaneous Fistula	2-15%	Recurrent disease, disease activity, Extensive lysis of adhesions, anastomotic leak, open surgery
Anastomotic Stricture	40%	Ischemia of anastomosis, anastomotic leak, recurrent disease,
Hemorrhage	0.5-4.2%	Hypoalbuminemia, NSAID use, antiplatelet medication, severe disease activity, thickened/ friable mesentery
Surgical Recurrence	30% at 5 years 40% at 10 years 55% at 20 years	Smoking, abscess or fistula at surgery, penetrating disease, conservative resection, postoperative IASC no endoscopic follow-up, no prophylaxis,
Venous Thromboembolism	1-3%	Steroid use, smoking, open surgery, ostomy creation, emergency surgery
Short Bowel Syndrome	5-10%	Earlier age at diagnosis, early age at first surgery, misdiagnosed patients, delay in diagnosis, penetrating disease, postoperative IASC, repeated bowel resections

Figure 13.1. Complications of surgery for Crohn's disease, along with incidence and risk factors.

Intra-Abdominal Septic Complications

Intra-abdominal septic complications (IASCs) encompass the most severe complications for CD patients. Specifically, these complications include anastomotic leaks, intra-abdominal abscesses, and enterocutaneous fistulas (ECF). The incidence of post-operative IASCs exceeds that for other benign diseases and is estimated to occur in 2 – 16% of CD patients after surgery [21]. IASCs prolong hospital stay, affect quality of life, and increase the risk for surgical recurrence [14]. More importantly, IASCs account for about half of postoperative deaths in CD [22].

Abscesses

Abdominal and/or pelvic abscesses develop as a natural progression of CD itself, or as a complication of surgery. In surgical patients, abscesses develop post-operatively in up to 9% of CD patients within ten years, especially in those with anastomotic leaks or postoperative fistula [23]. Those with penetrating disease behavior are more likely to develop abscesses than those with stricturing or non-stricturing non-penetrating disease [24]. Most abscesses develop near the anastomotic site, however abscesses can develop in almost any location, including the abdominal wall, peritoneal cavity, retroperitoneum, iliopsoas, and subphrenic regions [23]. Anastomotic technique (stapled or hand-sewn) does not affect the incidence of postoperative abscess [25].

There are three general approaches to treating an abscess: medical management with antibiotics, percutaneous drainage, or surgical drainage, with or without resection of the involved segments. About 25% of abscesses will recur after treatment, although this rate is lower with surgical drainage compared to those treated medically or with percutaneous drainage [23]. However, medical management or percutaneous drainage can be used to delay or prevent re-operation if appropriate for the patient's clinical condition. Regardless of approach, earlier intervention to drain abdominal or pelvic abscesses is associated with shorter time to resolution compared to patients treated solely with antibiotics [26].

Enterocutaneous Fistula

After a colorectal resection in patients with CD, the most common causes of ECF are anastomotic leak and failure to recognize an inadvertent enterotomy. CD is a significant risk factor for development of an early postoperative ECF, 4.7 times higher than other causes; development of an ECF is also associated with a 2.5 fold increase of in-hospital mortality compared to patients without postoperative ECF [27]. The same study identified lysis of adhesions as another risk factor for postoperative ECF, and laparoscopic surgery is associated with an overall lower rate of ECF. However, the patient population for this study included both benign and malignant pathologies and was not specific to patients with CD.

Typically, ECF present clinically around postoperative days 5-10 with fevers and protracted ileus. Sometimes a superficial abscess may appear, which when subsequently drained reveals enteric content. In other patients, enteric contents may be seen spontaneously draining from the wound dressings [28].

Management of ECFs in this setting is complex, multidisciplinary, and depends on surgeon experience and judgment. Along with initial resuscitation and treatment of any associated sepsis with antibiotics, drainage should be contained to minimize skin irritation and further wound contamination. It is important to identify the fistula either clinically or radiologically with either CT scan or fistulogram to determine the location of the fistula and whether it arises spontaneously from healthy bowel, diseased bowel, or from an anastomotic breakdown.

In patients with an ECF, it is important to correct electrolyte derangements, especially common in high-output fistulas, and provide supplementation of nutrients, vitamins, and trace minerals necessary for immune function and wound healing [29]. Enteral nutrition helps maintain the natural gut immune barrier and has been associated with higher rates of ECF closure, as long as a distal obstruction is not present [30]. However, parenteral nutrition may be required alone or in combination for patients with high output fistulas to meet nutritional demands [31]. More recently, exclusive enteral nutrition (EEN), a completely liquid diet administered via a nasogastric tube or taken orally, has been proposed as a strategy to treat ECF in CD patients. It is proposed to provide benefit by reducing the proinflammatory response to antigens in whole foods, improving nutrient deficiencies, and correcting microbiota disturbances [32]. Multiple observational studies have found an increased rate of spontaneous closure of ECF in CD patients on EEN therapy, although further investigation is required [33-35].

Though not always possible, ECFs are best repaired when inflammation has subsided and the abdominal wall has become soft [36]. If a fistula is to close spontaneously, about 90% will do so within 4-6 weeks of diagnosis, but spontaneous closure occurs in only 30% of fistulas overall [37]. Therefore, most surgeons recommend 4 weeks of conservative management, which includes wound management, nutritional support, and control of sepsis, while observing for spontaneous closure.

The principles of fistula repair include transection of the fistulous tract, resection of the diseased bowel segment, and primary closure of the fistulous opening at the target organ [38]. To achieve these goals, one typically utilizes an incision site distinct from the fistula tract as the chronic inflammatory nature of these tracts makes dissection difficult and avoids wound healing complications inherent with scar and inflamed tissue [36]. A laparoscopic approach for fistulous complications is not only safe and feasible, but is also associated with decreased length of stay and postoperative mortality with an observed 20% conversion rate to open procedures [39].

Anastomotic Leak

Anastomotic leaks (ALs) are perhaps the most feared complication of CD surgery, as they can lead to intra-abdominal sepsis, enterocutaneous fistulas, and intestinal failure [40]. ALs usually manifest clinically between postoperative days five and seven, although up to 12 percent occur after postoperative day 30 [41]. Intraperitoneal leaks, leading to contamination of the peritoneal cavity, are more likely to be associated with septic peritonitis and resulting pain, fever, and tachycardia [42], in contrast to extraperitoneal leaks, which can be more subtle in presentation, with pain, fistulas, or rectal drainage [43].

If a stable patient shows signs of a clinical leak, and low-grade sepsis, management begins with timely initiation of supportive care, to include fluid resuscitation and broad-spectrum antibiotics. Although a CT scan with oral and intravenous contrast is the standard diagnostic imaging, leakage of intraluminal contrast is only seen in 10% of patients. Instead, secondary signs of leakage such as free air more than 7 days from surgery, fluid collections, or perianastomotic extraluminal air is more commonly reported [44, 45].

Asymptomatic patients with a subclinical leak discovered incidentally on imaging, can be managed with observation. If the patient is stable with small (<3 cm), contained abscesses on imaging, the patient can be treated conservatively with bowel rest and broad-spectrum antibiotics. Larger abscesses (>3 cm) should be drained percutaneously if feasible, with surgery reserved for abscesses not amenable to drainage or if patient's clinical condition does not improve. Intraoperatively, if the primary finding is an inoperable phlegmon, drains can be placed by the anastomosis and a proximal loop ileostomy or colostomy created for temporary fecal diversion. A small anastomotic defect may be repaired primarily with placement of drains and proximal diversion. An anastomotic defect >1 cm or greater than 1/3 of the circumference of the bowel wall can be resected with creation of a stoma, re-anastomosis and proximal diversion, or exteriorization of both ends of the stoma. Unstable patients with generalized peritonitis or high-grade sepsis, should immediately undergo emergent exploratory laparotomy.

Rates of ALs can vary widely based on facility but have been reported to range from 1 – 30% [46]. Unsurprisingly, ALs are associated with increased morbidity, mortality, prolonged hospital stay, as well as increased healthcare costs [47]. The risk of AL for CD patients seems to increase with more distal anastomoses. The reported leak rate for an ileocolic anastomosis is between 1-10% and is associated with 14% 60-day mortality, compared to a 2.3% mortality in similar patients who do not experience an anastomotic leak [48, 49]. Extraperitoneal anastomoses, including a low anterior resection or ultralow anterior resection are at higher risk for leak compared to more proximal, intraperitoneal anastomoses [50]. The risk seems to be inversely correlated with distance of the anastomosis from the anal verge and likely the corresponding decrease in blood flow to the anastomotic site. Furthermore, male sex and increased BMI also seem to uniquely increase the risk for AL in more distal anastomoses, likely due to the technical difficulties encountered in the narrower, deeper pelvis [51].

Many studies investigating anastomotic technique and their influence on postoperative outcomes are observational and retrospective in nature, thus there lacks a clear consensus on the optimal surgical strategy [52]. Two meta-analysis found that end-to-end anastomoses were associated with increased risk for post-operative AL compared to side-to-side anastomoses [53, 54], although another meta-analysis failed to replicate this finding [55]. When comparing the incidence of AL with stapled versus hand-sewn anastomoses, the results for CD patients are variable. One study from 2005 noted a 7-fold reduction in anastomotic complications when utilizing stapled techniques instead of hand-sewn anastomoses [56]. On the other hand, another group demonstrated intestinal complications and the need for early reoperation were significantly reduced by the use of a hand-sewn anastomosis [57].

To avoid complications, one should keep in mind the following standard requirements of an intestinal anastomosis: maintenance of adequate blood flow, freedom from tension, and the presence of minimal to no contamination in the abdomen. The decision to avoid anastomosis and resort to an ostomy in CD surgery should also consider factors previously discussed including the degree of malnutrition, dose of steroids, and severity of co-existing septic issues.

Anastomotic Stricture

Anastomotic strictures are another common and unfortunate complication of CD surgery. Colorectal strictures are defined as the inability to pass a scope at least 12mm in diameter through the area of stenosis. Clinically, patients may be asymptomatic or present with partial or complete bowel obstruction. Recurrent disease at the site of anastomosis eventually causes transmural inflammatory edema and fibrosis, with approximately 30% of patients requiring a second surgery within 10 years of primary ileocolonic resection with over 40% of patients experiencing obstructive symptoms within 4 years [54, 58].

If presenting with symptomatic obstruction, strictures in CD should first be treated conservatively with intravenous hydration, nasogastric decompression, and parenteral nutrition if necessary. Ileocolic, colo-colic, or higher colorectal strictures may be managed with endoluminal therapy or stricturoplasty, with resection and anastomosis reserved for refractory cases. In a meta-analysis of 13 studies and 347 patients, endoscopic balloon dilation was technically successful in 86% of cases with a reported major complication rate less than 2% [59]. The same study noted that a short stricture length (≤ 4cm) predicted endoscopic success without the need for future surgery, but up to half of patients will require repeat dilation. Various forms of stents, including self-expanding metal stents, plastic stents, and biodegradable stents have been used to treat stenoses in CD. While small studies provide some evidence for a marginal success rate (60% success with a median follow-up at 17 months), various complications including bowel perforation, distal migration, and incorporation of the stent into the bowel mucosa have also been described [60]. Lower colorectal anastomoses can also be dilated digitally or with serial dilators.

Hemorrhage

Intra- and post-operative bleeding in CD patients can be minor or major and is thought to occur due to inadequate clearance of the mesentery prior to division and/or stapling of the bowel. There may be an increased tendency to bleed due to the inherent friability of the blood vessels, coupled with the inflammatory process that surrounds the vessels in a thick, fatty coat. Minor bleeding from the staple or suture line manifests as passage of blood or dark stool with the patient's first bowel movement. This bleeding is typically self-limited and resolves within 24 hours.

Major bleeding occurs in 0.5-4.2% of patients undergoing anastomosis following all cause colorectal surgery [61, 62]. For CD patients, risk factors for anastomotic hemorrhage include ischemia, NSAIDs, antiplatelet medications, and increased disease activity [63]. The technique of anastomosis (stapled vs. hand-sewn) does not appear to have an effect on the incidence of bleeding [62].

Management of postoperative bleeding in CD patients follows the same principles of a lower gastrointestinal bleed in any surgical patient. Initial measures are aimed at adequate resuscitation with intravenous crystalloid or blood products and correction of underlying coagulopathy. Those that fail conservative management may require surgery, angiography, and/or endoscopy. Early endoscopy can be performed safely, utilizing minimal insufflation to help prevent anastomotic dehiscence and disruption of friable tissue [63]. Persistent bleeding from a low anastomosis may be assessed transanally with a proctoscope and managed with suture ligation. Higher anastomoses need endoscopy, angiography, or re-operation. Angiography is particularly useful to identify and possibly treat the bleeding source either without surgery or before surgery. Intraoperative enteroscopy can also be used, but may be difficult to perform in the presence of many strictures [36].

Major bleeding can also occur intraoperatively if the patient has a very thickened, friable mesentery [64]. The associated diseased bowel loop must be handled and resected with extreme caution, as tearing the mesentery can result in profuse bleeding. It is advisable that patients with thickened mesenteries on pre-operative evaluation undergo open laparotomy in case the surgeon needs to control hemorrhage quickly. In the event of mesenteric tearing or difficult-to-perform vascular control of a thick mesentery, the surgeon should obtain proximal control of the root of the mesentery with large, non-crushing non-traumatizing clamps to minimize further blood loss. Upon release of the clamp, bleeding areas can be controlled with hemostats, suture ligatures, or an energy device [36]. In general, the mesenteric division should occur with clamps and ties rather than relying on energy devices, which may not have the same efficacy in the thickened mesentery of CD.

Recurrence

Post-surgical recurrence is a common complication in CD patients. In fact, without proper medical therapy, ultimately, all patients with CD can be expected to experience disease recurrence. Recurrent disease carries significant economic burden and is associated with lower quality of life, regardless of surgical approach [65].

Recurrence can be identified during endoscopy (i.e., endoscopic recurrence), or by recurrence of symptoms, defined as a clinical recurrence. If the recurrence of symptoms requires surgical intervention, it is termed a surgical recurrence. The most common location for disease recurrence is the anastomosis and neo terminal ileum. Active surveillance is recommended for all patients following resection, even in the absence of clinical recurrence, with ileocolonoscopy starting 6-12 months following resection [66, 67].

Following ileocolic resection (ICR), endoscopic recurrence occurs in approximately 60% of patients within 1-year, manifesting as aphthous and serpiginous ulceration [68]. The severity of endoscopic recurrence is characterized according to the Rutgeerts scoring system, ranging from i0 (least severe) to i4 (most severe) [58]. Endoscopic recurrence predicts both clinical recurrence and the need for future surgery and procedures. Those with more severe endoscopic disease are at even higher risk.

The risk of recurrent clinical disease after a primary operation for CD is approximately 17-55% at 5 years, 32-76% at 10 years, and 72-73% at 20 years [5, 69, 70]. The risk of surgical recurrence is approximately 30% at 5-years, 40% at 10-years, and 55% at 20-years [2]. Repeated surgery for CD is associated with increased postoperative complications, increased incidence of short bowel syndrome, increased risk of ostomy, and increased risk for requiring a future surgery, further emphasizing the importance of preventing recurrence [71].

Modifiable patient factors that can decrease the risk of disease recurrence include smoking cessation, and exclusive enteral nutrition (EEN). Smoking cessation following ICR decreased recurrence by four-fold [72, 73]. EEN has been found to decrease the risk of both clinical and endoscopic recurrence following surgery for CD [74-76]. These beneficial effects may be more significant for those patients who are significantly malnourished or previously identified to be high risk for recurrence. Fecal microbiota transplantation is currently under investigation for inducing remission with promising, although limited, results [77].

Historically, one performed conservative mesenteric resections for CD, preferring to divide the mesentery flush along the bowel. However, multiple investigations hypothesize that the pathognomonic creeping fat and associated hypertrophy of the mesentery may be a primary driving force behind the intestinal pathology in CD [78-80]. Testing this theory, an RCT of 64 patients undergoing ICR for CD found that an extended mesenteric dissection was associated with decreased risk for surgical recurrence when compared to conservative resection [81]. However, the authors note that experience is required to manipulate and excise the friable and thickened mesentery.

The high rate of recurrence after CD surgery has spurred significant research in postoperative medical prophylactic therapy. The mechanisms of action and drug profiles of the various medical therapies available are beyond the scope of this chapter, but it is prudent to discuss the current literature regarding their efficacy in preventing disease recurrence.

Prophylactic corticosteroid therapy does not reduce recurrence rate [82]. On the other hand, a number of investigations suggest that mesalamine [83], nitroimidazole antibiotics (metronidazole, ornidazole) [84, 85], and thiopurines (6-mercaptopurine and azathioprine) are effective in reducing post-operative clinical and endoscopic recurrence [86-89]. However, the utility of these agents should take into consideration the risk of adverse events. Nitroimidazole antibiotics are poorly tolerated, especially with long-term administration (e.g., GI upset, neuropathy) and their beneficial effects do not persist after interruption of therapy. Thiopurines are also associated with multiple adverse effects, including GI upset, pancreatitis, hepatotoxicity, and myelotoxicity, and show similar benefits as mesalamine, a medication typically tolerated well [90, 91].

Biologic therapy is the most effective prophylactic treatment for preventing postoperative recurrence. Multiple studies have demonstrated decreased risk for endoscopic and/or clinical recurrence with infliximab or adalimumab therapy [92-95]. Therefore, the AGA recommends anti-TNF therapy or thiopurines for prophylaxis within 3 months of resection for CD patients, especially for those at higher risk for disease recurrence. Regular endoscopy can guide treatment in these patients, as medications can be initiated or stepped-up for those that have endoscopic evidence of recurrent disease.

Venous Thromboembolism (VTE)

Venous thromboembolic events (VTE), which includes deep vein thrombosis (DVT) and pulmonary embolism (PE), are a major cause of post-operative morbidity for all patients. Patients with inflammatory bowel disease (IBD) are at a two-fold higher risk for VTE compared to the general population, with rates reported to be between 1 – 8% [96], although this is likely to be underreported or underdiagnosed. For post-operative IBD patients, approximately 3% will have a thromboembolic complication within 90 days of discharge [97].

There are currently no American guidelines regarding prescribing VTE prophylaxis to post-operative CD patients after discharge, and there is insufficient data to suggest there is a morbidity or mortality benefit. Additionally, a modeling study demonstrated that extended VTE prophylaxis in CD patients was not cost-effective [98]. Despite this, a 2021 statement from an international group of experts recommended prescribing low-molecular-weight heparin for VTE prophylaxis in high-risk patients with active CD [99]. Additionally, patients should be advised to wear compression stockings and regularly mobilize. Interestingly, the usage of anti-TNF medications can reduce the risk of VTE in CD patients [99].

Short Bowel Syndrome

Short bowel syndrome (SBS) is the number one cause of chronic intestinal failure (CIF) in patients with CD, occurring in approximately 5 – 10% of patients [100, 101]. Additionally, CD is the most common cause of CIF [100]. SBS can occur after a single large resection, or several repeated smaller resections. CIF occurs when the remaining small intestine lacks the surface area and capacity to digest and absorb nutrients. SBS is typically defined as < 200 cm of small intestine; while signs of malabsorption usually occur when < 110-130 cm of small bowel remain with no colon present or <70-90 cm of small bowel remain with an intact colon.

The risk factors for SGS include diagnosis of CD before age 16, early age at first surgery, and penetrating disease phenotype [102, 103]. Septic complications following surgery is the most frequent event subsequently leading to CIF [104]. CD patients that undergo more bowel resections are at increased risk for SBS, as are those that experience a delay in diagnosis [105].

In general, SBS can be treated by optimizing nutritional status and fluid balance by careful coordination with medical physicians, dieticians, and pharmacists. Patients will commonly require parenteral nutrition, while a select few may be candidates for transplant, both of which are associated with additional morbid complications.

General Risk Factors for Complications

Malnutrition has long been known to be a risk factor for multiple post-operative complications including anastomotic leak and surgical site infection. Patients with CD have increased risk of protein-calorie as well as micronutrient malnutrition when compared to other populations of patients undergoing abdominal surgery [106]. Approximately 80% of patients with active CD are malnourished, with about 40% of patients affected even when disease is in remission [107]. Multiple mechanisms can explain the high incidence of malnutrition in CD patients. This includes decreased intake, decreased nutrient absorption (which may be due to alterations of the gut mucosa, decreased gut length, as well as alterations in the gut microbiota affecting absorption), as well as increased energy requirements due to systemic inflammation [108].

Preoperative hypoalbuminemia, a classic marker of malnutrition, is associated with increased risk of infectious complications in CD patients undergoing a bowel resection. Yet, albumin and prealbumin should be interpreted with care as both are also negative acute phase reactants and may represent the inflammatory status of a patient as opposed to nutritional status. Low levels of these markers may be more related to increased vascular permeability secondary to inflammation; as observational studies have noted that patients with anorexia nervosa usually have normal to mildly decreased albumin levels [109].

For these reasons, the European Society for Clinical Nutrition and Metabolism (ESPEN) recommends using body mass index (BMI) and preoperative weight loss to screen for malnutrition, although they admit these would likely underestimate the true incidence of malnutrition in the IBD population [110]. Despite these concerns, preoperative weight loss of greater than 10% has been found to be associated with increased risk for SSIs [111, 112]. Furthermore, while low BMI (<18.5 kg/m^2) has been associated with poor surgical outcomes, obesity (BMI ≥ 30 kg/m^2) has also shown to be associated with increased risk for SSIs [113]. Therefore, while one can see that patients with CD have metabolic disturbances associated with malnutrition, and these alterations predispose this population of patients to infectious complications, it is not always clear exactly how one should accurately identify and quantify this risk.

It is estimated that preoperative anemia is present in up to a third of patients with CD [114, 115]. Anemia is a risk factor for infectious complications in patients undergoing colorectal surgery [116]. Patients with CD likely develop anemia due to a combination of iron deficiency secondary to decreased oral intake, impaired iron absorption, and blood loss due to disease activity, as well as anemia of chronic disease secondary to the disease's inflammatory nature. Preoperative anemia has also been found to predict overall postoperative complications and need for hospital readmission, in patients undergoing bowel resection for CD [117-119]. Due to higher rates of baseline anemia, Crohn's patients may receive blood transfusions at a greater rate than the general population, although this has not been demonstrated in the literature. Perioperative blood transfusion, has also been shown to have immunosuppressive effects and may impair wound healing. However, it is important to note, that the presence of preoperative anemia may simply represent increased disease activity, which also increases risk for postoperative complications [120].

CD is commonly characterized according to disease phenotype as stricturing or penetrating disease. The latter phenotype is associated with the development of fistulous tracts and associated abscesses. CD patients with penetrating disease are more likely to develop postoperative SSIs and intraabdominal abscesses, thought to be due to contamination of the surgical field and the patient's proinflammatory state [117, 118]. Additionally, the presence of an intra-abdominal abscess at time of surgery increases the risk for anastomotic leaks. Specifically, for CD patients with a fistulous tract present at the time of surgery, preoperative anemia, a positive bacterial culture from the fistula tract, and preoperative enteral nutrition for less than 3 months predicted the development of an SSI [117]. The presence of fistula and/or post-operative intra-abdominal sepsis have also been identified as risk factors for early recurrence [121].

Perioperative Infection Control

If an abscess is present prior to surgery, percutaneous drainage has been shown to significantly reduce the occurrence of postoperative IASCs and to reduce hospital length of stay [122]. Percutaneous drainage allows time for medical optimization with parenteral nutrition, bowel rest, and antibiotics, and reduces contamination at the time of surgery to permit anastomosis creation and avoid a stoma. Timing of surgery after percutaneous drainage is variable, with most surgeons recommending a 4-6 week interval to allow for resolution.

Medical optimization helps improve outcomes prior to an elective procedure for CD. This would include correction of anemia, restoration of volume, correction of electrolyte and acid-base disorders, and improvement of nutrition. Preoperative TPN for at least 18 days is recommended for patients with moderate to severe CD to minimize risk of early postoperative complications [123]. Preoperative imaging with either CT or MR enterography may assist in adequate planning and identification of extraluminal complications, which may aid in identification of potential complicating factors to reduce operative duration and infectious risk. However, CT imaging should be ordered with discretion in CD patients, since they may require repeated scans over time leading to increased radiation exposure [124]. Mechanical bowel preparation may decrease rates of infectious complications for ICR, especially for patients with penetrating disease [125], and the addition of oral antibiotics to bowel preparation may further decrease infectious risk over mechanical bowel preparation alone [126]. Regardless, intravenous second-generation cephalosporin or ciprofloxacin plus metronidazole should be given for prophylaxis 30 minutes before surgery and every 3 hours during the procedure.

Perioperative Medical Management

Corticosteroids remain widely prescribed to the CD patient population despite the well-documented concerns with both wound healing and immunosuppression [127]. However, investigations into the effects of chronic steroid use and SSIs remains unclear in the CD patient population. Some studies have found an association between SSI incidence and preoperative steroid use [128, 129], although it is important to note that other studies have not found such an association [130]. Corticosteroids may impair anastomotic healing through multiple mechanisms: they decrease activation and infiltration of inflammatory cells (macrophages and neutrophils) that are critical in the initial phases of wound healing, and they inhibit growth factors, as well as proteins, and collagen synthesis. However, there is no consistent evidence describing the specific dose or duration of steroids that cause anastomotic complications. One study that defined steroid use as 10mg or more of prednisone or equivalent for at least 4 weeks and within two weeks of surgery found an increased risk for anastomotic complications [21, 131]. Despite the lack of specific guidance on steroid dosing, most experts suggest that steroid doses exceeding 20mg a day confer a significant additional risk. If other risk factors are present, surgeons should consider fecal diversion instead of primary anastomosis. Additionally, steroid use also increased the risk of VTE in Crohn's patients, although the mechanism behind this is not well elucidated [99].

Anti-TNFα therapy (Infliximab, Adalimumab) has revolutionized management of CD although the immunomodulatory nature of these medications raises concerns for their infectious risk. However, multiple observational studies have failed to find a connection between anti-TNFα therapy and risk for postoperative SSI [129, 132-134]. A meta-analysis did not demonstrate a difference in incidence of SSI with those that received their last infusion 4-weeks, 8-weeks, or 12-weeks from surgery [135], and another observational study found that infliximab may be protective against SSI for patients with penetrating disease [136]. A large, prospective cohort study found that anti-TNF therapy within 3 months of surgery was associated with increased risk for anastomotic complications [137]. However, a meta-analysis that included 4100 CD patients failed to find a connection between recent biologic use and AL [138]. Increased doses of infliximab are associated with postoperative infection risk, Ustekinumab-treated patients were found to have increased risk of return to the operating room (due to AL or SSI) compared to patients on anti-TNF agents [139]. It is important to note that patients on higher doses of anti-TNF therapy likely have more aggressive disease behavior further confounding the conclusions from these studies [140]. Historically, guidelines have recommended holding immunomodulators in the perioperative period, however more recent guidelines state that immunomodulators can be continued, and furthermore, that surgery should not be delayed due to immunomodulator therapy [141]. The literature regarding the risk of AL with these newer biologics is lacking.

Vedolizumab is a human monoclonal antibody to the $\alpha 4\beta 7$ integrin, blocking leukocyte transmigration to the intestinal mucosa. Despite the theoretical concerns with infectious complications, it continues to gain market share as a second-line treatment option for CD.

Multiple trials have investigated this risk with conflicting results. Perhaps most convincingly, a multicenter, retrospective review demonstrated a 6-fold increased risk for all SSIs as well as a significant increase in superficial SSIs for patients receiving Vedolizumab compared to anti-TNF therapy [142]. However, patients receiving Vedolizumab in this study most likely failed treatment with first-line anti-TNF therapy and may thus represent a subset of patients with more severe disease. Despite this uncertainty, other investigations have also found increased SSI risk for patients on Vedolizumab compared to those on anti-TNF therapy and no biologic therapy [143], although multiple meta-analyses did not detect differences in infectious outcomes for patients on Vedolizumab [144-146].

Procedure Factors

Longer OR time has been demonstrated to increase risk for postoperative SSI in multiple retrospective, observational studies [136, 147-149]. While it is tempting to view OR time as a modifiable variable, in observational studies, prolonged OR time likely correlates with increased surgical complexity, which with CD patients, also likely represents an increased risk of surgical field contamination, which also increases risk for SSIs [148, 150]. Interestingly, patients with CD undergoing colorectal procedures were found to be more likely to have contaminated or dirty wounds when compared to other colorectal surgical populations [6].

Minimally Invasive vs Open Techniques

Compared to open approaches for ICR, laparoscopic procedures have decreased overall rate of postoperative complications, shorter postoperative stay, and decreased pain [151]. A laparoscopic approach for ICR was also associated with improved cosmesis and decreased risk of incisional hernia [152]. However, there does not appear to be differences in rates of clinical recurrence, surgical recurrence, postoperative bowel obstruction, or long-term quality of life for ICR done laparoscopically versus open [152-154]. A retrospective review of the NSQIP dataset for CD patients undergoing ICR found a slight decrease in the incidence of wound infections when utilizing a laparoscopic approach whereas no difference was found in a meta-analysis [155, 156]. While a meta-analysis has found decreased overall postoperative complications with a laparoscopic compared to an open surgical approach, no difference was found in the incidence of postoperative AL (2.7% vs. 2.7%) [153]. In particular, open surgical repair was found to increase the risk of post-operative VTE [99].

In experienced hands, laparoscopy can be performed safely, even for complicated CD, characterized by recurrent disease, abscesses, inflammatory masses, and enteric fistulas. There remains a learning curve for surgeons utilizing laparoscopic technique, as one group found that rates of conversion to a laparotomy decreased with experience [157]. Another compared outcomes of laparoscopic ICR for patients with recurrent disease found that the conversion rate and incidence of enteric fistula did not differ compared to patients undergoing their first procedure, although, as expected, operative times were longer for those with recurrent disease [158].

Low anterior resection and male gender are risk factors for postoperative complications with laparoscopic colorectal procedures. Low rectal pathology is generally considered a risk factor for high-grade complications such as intraoperative bleeding, ureteral injury, and anastomotic complications, most likely due to the challenges of extensive pelvic dissection [159]. Age is not considered a risk factor for complications after laparoscopic surgery; in fact, a laparoscopic approach for colorectal resections is generally considered lower risk than open surgery in older patients [160]. Together, these investigations suggest that patients who present with low rectal pathology, especially male patients, should be approached with an open or modified hybrid approach (such as laparoscopic vessel ligation, splenic flexure mobilization, and open pelvic dissection through a low midline incision). Surgeons should maintain a low threshold for conversion to open in patients with both recurrent flares of CD or with intraabdominal sepsis at initial laparoscopy.

Conversion from laparoscopic to open surgery is associated with higher rates of both minor and major complications [159]. Common reasons for conversion include encountering complex masses, dense adhesion, abscesses, fistulas, or other complications of a prior resection [161]. Studies have placed the conversion rate for CD patients undergoing ICR at about 20%, identifying recurrent disease, thickened mesentery, and large inflammatory mass as factors that predict the need for conversion [157].

To reduce risk of conversion, decrease operative time, and enable tactile feedback, hand-assisted laparoscopic surgery (HALS) is a viable alternative to laparoscopic or laparoscopic-assisted surgery. The HALS technique involves inserting a hand via a Gelport device into the abdomen while using laparoscopic tools with the other hand [162]. HALS has been reported to be safe and feasible in complex Crohn's colitis and to decrease operative times with no increase in postoperative complications [163].

Single-incision laparoscopic surgery (SILS) is another available minimally invasive approach. The single port site is utilized for the entire procedure and can subsequently function as an extraction site [162]. SILS is associated with a similar conversion and complication rates when compared to traditional laparoscopic surgery and is associated with decreased analgesic requirements and shorter length of stay [164, 165].

Robotic approaches have gained popularity for colorectal surgery due to the improved 3-dimensional visualization, tremor reduction, improved articulation, and improved ergonomics compared to conventional laparoscopy [166-168]. However, there remain concerns that the loss of haptic feedback, longer operative times, and increased cost may limit the general use of robotic platforms for colorectal surgery [168-170]. Compared to an open approach, robotic ICR was associated with a shorter hospital stay and a lower 30-day complication rate, but longer operative times in a retrospective, propensity-matched study [171]. However, a retrospective review of NSQIP data comparing laparoscopic to robotic ICR for CD did not find significant differences in postoperative complications, but did again find that robotic surgery was associated with longer operative times [172]. Further investigations are required to assess the advantages and disadvantages of robotic surgery for CD.

Ostomy creation was found to be associated with postoperative SSI in an observational study of CD patients undergoing abdominal surgery [136]. However, patients with penetrating disease are more likely to undergo ostomy creation, either for diversion or to avoid a primary anastomosis, than those with a fibrostenotic phenotype [24]. Furthermore, other studies observed ostomy creation decreased the risk of postoperative infection, thought to be due to the lack of anastomosis or diversion of stool from a new anastomosis.

The need for emergency surgery compared to elective surgery also predicted SSI development in a propensity-matched, retrospective review of the NSQIP database for CD patients [148]. Additionally, both ileostomy creation and emergency surgery were risk factors for the development of VTE [99].

Elevated intraoperative lactate predicts incidence of SSI in a retrospective case-control study of CD patients undergoing bowel resection [135], as does the need for intraoperative or postoperative blood transfusion. Preoperative transfusion carries no increased risk of SSI [173]. Malperfusion and inadequate oxygenation correlate with impaired wound healing and increased infectious risk, but blood transfusions specifically may alter patients' immune function by multiple mechanisms, including alteration of pro- and anti-inflammatory balance and cytokine release from allogenic leukocytes [173].

Conclusion

The main complications of surgery for CD are related to the inherent inflammatory nature of the disease and clinical features of the patient population. They include an increased risk for wound infections, intra-abdominal abscesses, hemorrhage, anastomotic complications, enterocutaneous fistulas, and venous thromboembolic events than the general surgical population. The risk for complications is greater in patients who smoke tobacco, have penetrating disease behavior, malnutrition and weight loss, chronic steroid use, and/or intra-abdominal sepsis at the time of operation. Complications lead to re-operation in about half of patients. Strategies to reduce post-operative complications include cessation of smoking, optimization of preoperative nutrition, preoperative antibiotics and percutaneous drainage of abscesses, limited resection techniques, routine endoscopic follow-up, use of standard VTE prophylaxis, and judicious use of steroid-sparing immunomodulating and biologic agents.

References

[1] Gajendran M, Loganathan P, Catinella AP, Hashash JG. A comprehensive review and update on Crohn's disease. *Dis Mon* 2018;64:20–57.

[2] Bernell O, Lapidus A, Hellers G. Risk Factors for Surgery and Postoperative Recurrence in Crohn's Disease: *Ann Surg* 2000;231:38.

[3] Frolkis AD, Dykeman J, Negrón ME, et al. Risk of Surgery for Inflammatory Bowel Diseases Has Decreased Over Time: A Systematic Review and Meta-analysis of Population-Based Studies. *Gastroenterology* 2013;145:996–1006.

[4] Fornaro R, Caratto E, Caratto M, et al. Post-operative recurrence in Crohn's disease. Critical analysis of potential risk factors. An update. *The Surgeon* 2015;13:330–347.

[5] Yamamoto T. Factors affecting recurrence after surgery for Crohn's disease. *World J Gastroenterol* 2005;11:3971.

[6] Wideroff M, Xing Y, Liao J, Byrn JC. Crohn's Disease but not Diverticulitis Is an Independent Risk Factor for Surgical Site Infections in Colectomy. *J Gastrointest Surg* 2014;18:1817–1823.

[7] Nguyen GC, Elnahas A, Jackson TD. The impact of preoperative steroid use on short-term outcomes following surgery for inflammatory bowel disease. *J Crohns Colitis* 2014;8:1661–1667.

[8] Luglio G, Pellegrini L, Rispo A, et al. Post-operative morbidity in Crohn's disease: what is the impact of patient-, disease- and surgery-related factors? *Int J Colorectal Dis* 2022;37:411–419.

[9] Bossuyt P, Debeuckelaere C, Ferrante M, et al. The operative risk and natural history after the diagnosis of ileal penetrating Crohn's disease. *Eur J Gastroenterol Hepatol* 2018;30:539–545.

[10] Tiberi A, Pesi B, Giudici F, et al. Laparoscopic ileo-colic resection and right hemicolectomy for Crohn's disease and colon cancer: a preliminary comparative study on post-operative outcome. *Updat Surg* 2020;72:821–826.

[11] Tolstrup M-B, Watt SK, Gögenur I. Morbidity and mortality rates after emergency abdominal surgery: an analysis of 4346 patients scheduled for emergency laparotomy or laparoscopy. *Langenbecks Arch Surg* 2017;402:615–623.

[12] Freund MR, Emile SH, Horesh N, et al. Redo ileocolic resection for recurrent Crohn's disease: A review and meta-analysis of surgical outcomes. *Surgery* 2022;172:1614–1621.

[13] Freund MR, Kent I, Horesh N, et al. Redo ileocolic resection in Crohn's disease – does time passed since previous surgery matter? *Colorectal Dis* 2022;24:484–490.

[14] Iesalnieks I, Kilger A, Glaß H, et al. Intraabdominal septic complications following bowel resection for Crohn's disease: detrimental influence on long-term outcome. *Int J Colorectal Dis* 2008;23:1167–1174.

[15] Alves A, Panis Y, Bouhnik Y, et al. Risk Factors for Intra-Abdominal Septic Complications After a First Ileocecal Resection for Crohn's Disease: A Multivariate Analysis in 161 Consecutive Patients. *Dis Colon Rectum* 2007;50:331–336.

[16] Myrelid P, Olaison G, Sjödahl R, et al. Thiopurine Therapy Is Associated with Postoperative Intra-Abdominal Septic Complications in Abdominal Surgery for Crohn's Disease. Dis Colon Rectum 2009;52:1387–1394.

[17] Garner JS, Jarvis WR, Emori TG, et al. CDC definitions for nosocomial infections, 1988. *Am J Infect Control* 1988;16:128–140.

[18] Strobel RM, Leonhardt M, Förster F, et al. The impact of surgical site infection—a cost analysis. *Langenbecks Arch Surg* 2022;407:819–828.

[19] Maeda K, Nagahara H, Shibutani M, et al. A preoperative low nutritional prognostic index correlates with the incidence of incisional surgical site infections after bowel resection in patients with Crohn's disease. *Surg Today* 2015;45:1366–1372.

[20] Bhakta A, Tafen M, Glotzer O, et al. Increased Incidence of Surgical Site Infection in IBD Patients. *Dis Colon Rectum* 2016;59:316–322.

[21] Huang W, Tang Y, Nong L, Sun Y. Risk factors for postoperative intra-abdominal septic complications after surgery in Crohn's disease: A meta-analysis of observational studies. *J Crohns Colitis* 2015;9:293–301.

[22] Yamamoto T, Allan RN, Keighley MRB. Risk factors for intra-abdominal sepsis after surgery in Crohn's disease. *Dis Colon Rectum* 2000;43:1141–1145.

[23] Yamaguchi A, Matsui T, Sakurai T, et al. The clinical characteristics and outcome of intraabdominal abscess in Crohn's disease. *J Gastroenterol* 2004;39:441–448.

[24] Bellolio F, Cohen Z, MacRae HM, et al. Outcomes following surgery for perforating Crohn's disease. *Br J Surg* 2013;100:1344–1348.

[25] Choy PYG, Bissett IP, Docherty JG, et al. Stapled versus handsewn methods for ileocolic anastomoses - Choy, PYG - 2011 | Cochrane Library.

[26] Gutierrez A, Lee H, Sands BE. Outcome of Surgical Versus Percutaneous Drainage of Abdominal and Pelvic Abscesses in Crohn's Disease. *Am J Gastroenterol* 2006;101:2283–2289.

[27] Masoomi H, Carmichael JC, Mills S, et al. Predictive Risk Factors of Early Postoperative Enteric Fistula in Colon and Rectal Surgery. *Am Surg* 2013;79:1058–1063.

[28] Pritts TA, Fischer DR, Fischer JE. Postoperative enterocutaneous fistula. *Surgical Treatment: Evidence-Based and Problem-Oriented*. Zuckschwerdt; 2001.

[29] Evenson AR, Fischer JE. Current management of enterocutaneous fistula. *J Gastrointest Surg* 2006;10:455–464.

[30] Tang Q, Hong Z, Ren H, et al. Nutritional Management of Patients With Enterocutaneous Fistulas: Practice and Progression. *Front Nutr* 2020;7.

[31] Weimann A, Braga M, Carli F, et al. ESPEN guideline: Clinical nutrition in surgery. *Clin Nutr* 2017;36:623–650.

[32] Mitrev N, Huang H, Hannah B, Kariyawasam VC. Review of exclusive enteral therapy in adult Crohn's disease. *BMJ Open Gastroenterol* 2021;8:e000745.

[33] Hu D, Ren J, Wang G, et al. Exclusive Enteral Nutritional Therapy Can Relieve Inflammatory Bowel Stricture in Crohn's Disease. *J Clin Gastroenterol* 2014;48:790.

[34] Matsueda K. Therapeutic efficacy of elemental enteral alimentation in Crohn's disease. | *J Gastroenterol* | EBSCOhost. 2000;35:19. Available at: https://openurl.ebsco.com/contentitem/gcd:18221977?sid=ebsco:plink:crawler&id=ebsco:gcd:18221977. Accessed July 20, 2024.

[35] Yan D, Ren J, Wang G, et al. Predictors of response to enteral nutrition in abdominal enterocutaneous fistula patients with Crohn's disease. *Eur J Clin Nutr* 2014;68:959–963.

[36] Michelassi F, Sultan S. Surgical Treatment of Complex Small Bowel Crohn Disease. *Ann Surg* 2014;260:230–235.

[37] Dodiyi-Manuel A, Wichendu PN. Current concepts in the management of enterocutaneous fistula. *Int Surg J* 2018;5:1981.

[38] Poritz LS, Gagliano GA, McLeod RS, et al. Surgical management of entero and colocutaneous fistulae in Crohn's disease: 17 year's experience. *Int J Colorectal Dis* 2004;19:481–485.

[39] Ren J, Liu S, Wang G, et al. Laparoscopy improves clinical outcome of gastrointestinal fistula caused by Crohn's disease. *J Surg Res* 2016;200:110–116.

[40] Agwunobi AO, Carlson GL, Anderson ID, et al. Mechanisms of intestinal failure in Crohn's disease. *Dis Colon Rectum* 2001;44:1834–1837.

[41] Hyman N, Manchester TL, Osler T, et al. Anastomotic Leaks After Intestinal Anastomosis: It's Later Than You Think. *Ann Surg* 2007;245:254.

[42] Smallwood N, Mutch MG, Fleshman JW. The Failed Anastomosis. In: Steele SR, Maykel JA, Champagne BJ, Orangio GR, eds. *Complexities in Colorectal Surgery: Decision-Making and Management*. New York, NY: Springer; 2014:277–304.

[43] Lim M, Akhtar S, Sasapu K, et al. Clinical and Subclinical Leaks After Low Colorectal Anastomosis: A Clinical and Radiologic Study. *Dis Colon Rectum* 2006;49:1611.

[44] Gouya H, Oudjit A, Leconte M, et al. CT Antegrade Colonography to Assess Proctectomy and Temporary Diverting Ileostomy Complications Before Early Ileostomy Takedown in Patients With Low Rectal Endometriosis. *Am J Roentgenol* 2012;198:98–105.

[45] Anon. Radiological evaluation of colorectal anastomoses | *Int J Colorect Dis*. Available at: https://link.springer.com/article/10.1007/s00384-008-0487-z. Accessed July 16, 2024.

[46] Jeganathan NNA, Koltun WA. Special Considerations of Anastomotic Leaks in Crohn's Disease. *Clin Colon Rectal Surg* 2021;34:412–416.

[47] Choi H-K, Law W-L, Ho JWC. Leakage After Resection and Intraperitoneal Anastomosis for Colorectal Malignancy: Analysis of Risk Factors. *Dis Colon Rectum* 2006;49:1719–1725.

[48] Neary PM, Aiello AC, Stocchi L, et al. High-Risk Ileocolic Anastomoses for Crohn's Disease: When Is Diversion Indicated? *J Crohns Colitis* 2019;13:856–863.

[49] Sánchez-Guillén L, Frasson M, García-Granero Á, et al. Risk factors for leak, complications and mortality after ileocolic anastomosis: comparison of two anastomotic techniques. *Ann R Coll Surg Engl* 2019;101:571–578.

[50] Damen N, Spilsbury K, Levitt M, et al. Anastomotic leaks in colorectal surgery. *ANZ J Surg* 2014;84:763–768.

[51] Sciuto A, Merola G, Palma GDD, et al. Predictive factors for anastomotic leakage after laparoscopic colorectal surgery. *World J Gastroenterol* 2018;24:2247–2260.

[52] Kann BR. Anastomotic Considerations in Crohn's Disease. *Clin Colon Rectal Surg* 2023;36:63–73.

[53] Simillis C, Purkayastha S, Yamamoto T, et al. A Meta-Analysis Comparing Conventional End-to-End Anastomosisvs.Other Anastomotic Configurations After Resection in Crohn's Disease. D*is Colon Rectum* 2007;50:1674.

[54] He X, Chen Z, Huang J, et al. Stapled Side-to-Side Anastomosis Might Be Better Than Handsewn End-to-End Anastomosis in Ileocolic Resection for Crohn's Disease: A Meta-Analysis. *Dig Dis Sci* 2014;59:1544–1551.

[55] Guo Z, Li Y, Zhu W, et al. Comparing Outcomes Between Side-to-Side Anastomosis and Other Anastomotic Configurations After Intestinal Resection for Patients with Crohn's Disease: A Meta-Analysis. *World J Surg* 2013;37:893–901.

[56] Resegotti A, Astegiano M, Farina EC, et al. Side-to-Side Stapled Anastomosis Strongly Reduces Anastomotic Leak Rates in Crohn's Disease Surgery. *Dis Colon Rectum* 2005;48:464–468.

[57] Scarpa M, Ruffolo C, Bertin E, et al. Surgical predictors of recurrence of Crohn's disease after ileocolonic resection. *Int J Colorectal Dis* 2007;22:1061–1069.

[58] Rutgeerts P, Geboes K, Vantrappen G, et al. Predictability of the postoperative course of Crohn's disease. *Gastroenterology* 1990;99:956–963.

[59] Hassan C, Zullo A, De Francesco V, et al. Systematic review: endoscopic dilatation in Crohn's disease. *Aliment Pharmacol Ther* 2007;26:1457–1464.

[60] Alastruey CL, Murcia XA, Comas ME. The role of stents in the treatment of Crohn's disease strictures. *Endosc Int Open* 2016;04:E301–E308.

[61] Martínez-Serrano M-A, Parés D, Pera M, et al. Management of lower gastrointestinal bleeding after colorectal resection and stapled anastomosis. *Tech Coloproctology* 2009;13:49–53.

[62] Neutzling CB, Lustosa SA, Proenca IM, et al. Stapled versus handsewn methods for colorectal anastomosis surgery. *Cochrane Database Syst Rev* 2012.

[63] Shen B. Interventional inflammatory bowel disease: endoscopic therapy of complications of Crohn's disease. *Gastroenterol Rep* 2022;10:goac045.

[64] Person B. Laparoscopic surgery for inflammatory bowel diseases. *Minerva Chir* 2008;63:151–160.

[65] Kiran RP, Nisar PJ, Church JM, Fazio VW. The role of primary surgical procedure in maintaining intestinal continuity for patients with Crohn's colitis. *Ann Surg* 2011;253:1130–1135.

[66] Ble A, Renzulli C, Cenci F, et al. The Relationship Between Endoscopic and Clinical Recurrence in Postoperative Crohn's Disease: A Systematic Review and Meta-analysis. *J Crohns Colitis* 2022;16:490–499.

[67] Cruz PD, Kamm MA, Hamilton AL, et al. Crohn's disease management after intestinal resection: a randomised trial. *Lancet* 2015;385:1406–1417.

[68] Pascua M, Su C, Lewis JD, et al. Meta-analysis: factors predicting post-operative recurrence with placebo therapy in patients with Crohn's disease. *Aliment Pharmacol Ther* 2008;28:545–556.

[69] Bergamaschi R, Haughn C, Reed JFI, Arnaud J-P. Laparoscopic Intracorporeal Ileocolic Resection for Crohn's Disease: Is It Safe? *Dis Colon Rectum* 2009;52:651.

[70] Mirow L, Hauenschild L, Hildebrand P, et al. [Recurrence of Crohn's disease after surgery--causes and risks]. *Zentralbl Chir* 2008;133:182–187.

[71] Colombo F, Frontali A, Baldi C, et al. Repeated surgery for recurrent Crohn's disease: does the outcome keep worsening operation after operation? A comparative study of 1224 consecutive procedures. *Updat Surg* 2022;74:73–80.

[72] Valibouze C, Desreumaux P, Zerbib P. Post-surgical recurrence of Crohn's disease: Situational analysis and future prospects. *J Visc Surg* 2021;158:401–410.

[73] Bolckmans R, Kalman T, Singh S, et al. Does Smoking Cessation Reduce Surgical Recurrence After Primary Ileocolic Resection for Crohn's Disease? *Dis Colon Rectum* 2020;63:200.

[74] Yamamoto T, Nakahigashi M, Umegae S, et al. Impact of long-term enteral nutrition on clinical and endoscopic recurrence after resection for Crohn's disease: a prospective, non-randomized, parallel, controlled study. *Aliment Pharmacol Ther* 2007;25:67–72.

[75] Yamamoto T, Shiraki M, Nakahigashi M, et al. Enteral nutrition to suppress postoperative Crohn's disease recurrence: a five-year prospective cohort study. *Int J Colorectal Dis* 2013;28:335–340.

[76] Esaki M, Matsumoto T, Hizawa K, et al. Preventive effect of nutritional therapy against postoperative recurrence of Crohn disease, with reference to findings determined by intra-operative enteroscopy. *Scand J Gastroenterol* 2005;40:1431–1437.

[77] Fehily SR, Basnayake C, Wright EK, Kamm MA. Fecal microbiota transplantation therapy in Crohn's disease: Systematic review. *J Gastroenterol Hepatol* 2021;36:2672–2686.

[78] Akobeng AK, Zhang D, Gordon M, MacDonald JK. *Oral 5-aminosalicylic acid for maintenance of medically-induced remission in Crohn's disease* - Akobeng, AK - 2016 | Cochrane Library.

[79] Coffey JC, O'Leary DP, Kiernan MG, Faul P. The mesentery in Crohn's disease: friend or foe? *Curr Opin Gastroenterol* 2016;32:267.

[80] Soucy G, Wang HH, Farraye FA, et al. Clinical and pathological analysis of colonic Crohn's disease, including a subgroup with ulcerative colitis-like features. *Mod Pathol* 2012;25:295–307.

[81] Coffey CJ, Kiernan MG, Sahebally SM, et al. Inclusion of the Mesentery in Ileocolic Resection for Crohn's Disease is Associated With Reduced Surgical Recurrence. *J Crohns Colitis* 2018;12:1139–1150.

[82] Gionchetti P, Dignass A, Danese S, et al. 3rd European Evidence-based Consensus on the Diagnosis and Management of Crohn's Disease 2016: Part 2: Surgical Management and Special Situations. *J Crohns Colitis* 2017;11:135–149.

[83] Doherty G, Bennett G, Patil S, et al. *Interventions for prevention of post-operative recurrence of Crohn's disease* - Doherty, G - 2009 | Cochrane Library.

[84] Rutgeerts P, Hiele M, Geboes K, et al. Controlled trial of metronidazole treatment for prevention of crohn's recurrence after ileal resection. *Gastroenterology* 1995;108:1617–1621.

[85] Rutgeerts P, van Assche G, Vermeire S, et al. Ornidazole for prophylaxis of postoperative Crohn's disease recurrence: A randomized, double-blind, placebo-controlled trial. *Gastroenterology* 2005;128:856–861.

[86] D'Haens GR, Vermeire S, Van Assche G, et al. Therapy of Metronidazole With Azathioprine to Prevent Postoperative Recurrence of Crohn's Disease: A Controlled Randomized Trial. *Gastroenterology* 2008;135:1123–1129.

[87] Ardizzone S, Maconi G, Sampietro GM, et al. Azathioprine and mesalamine for prevention of relapse after conservative surgery for Crohn's disease. *Gastroenterology* 2004;127:730–740.

[88] Reinisch W, Angelberger S, Petritsch W, et al. Azathioprine versus mesalazine for prevention of postoperative clinical recurrence in patients with Crohn's disease with endoscopic recurrence: efficacy and safety results of a randomised, double-blind, double-dummy, multicentre trial. *Gut* 2010;59:752–759.

[89] Peyrin-Biroulet L, Deltenre P, Ardizzone S, et al. Azathioprine and 6-Mercaptopurine for the Prevention of Postoperative Recurrence in Crohn's Disease: A Meta-Analysis. *J Am Coll Gastroenterol* 2009;104:2089.

[90] Gordon M, Taylor K, Akobeng AK, Thomas AG. Azathioprine and 6-mercaptopurine for maintenance of surgically-induced remission in Crohn's disease - Gordon, M - 2014 | Cochrane Library.

[91] Chaparro M, Ordás I, Cabré E, et al. Safety of Thiopurine Therapy in Inflammatory Bowel Disease: Long-term Follow-up Study of 3931 Patients. *Inflamm Bowel Dis* 2013;19:1404–1410.

[92] Sorrentino D, Terrosu G, Avellini C, Maiero S. Infliximab With Low-Dose Methotrexate for Prevention of Postsurgical Recurrence of Ileocolonic Crohn Disease. *Arch Intern Med* 2007;167:1804–1807.

[93] Sorrentino D, Paviotti A, Terrosu G, et al. Low-Dose Maintenance Therapy With Infliximab Prevents Postsurgical Recurrence of Crohn's Disease. *Clin Gastroenterol Hepatol* 2010;8:591-599.e1.

[94] Yoshida K, Fukunaga K, Ikeuchi H, et al. Scheduled Infliximab Monotherapy to Prevent Recurrence of Crohn's Disease Following Ileocolic or Ileal Resection: A 3-year Prospective Randomized Open Trial. *Inflamm Bowel Dis* 2012;18:1617–1623.

[95] Papamichael K, Archavlis E, Lariou C, Mantzaris GJ. Adalimumab for the prevention and/or treatment of post-operative recurrence of Crohn's disease: A prospective, two-year, single center, pilot study. *J Crohns Colitis* 2012;6:924–931.

[96] Arvanitakis KD, Arvanitaki AD, Karkos CD, et al. The risk of venous thromboembolic events in patients with inflammatory bowel disease: a systematic review and meta-analysis. *Ann Gastroenterol* 2021;34:680–690.

[97] Brady MT, Patts GJ, Rosen A, et al. Postoperative Venous Thromboembolism in Patients Undergoing Abdominal Surgery for IBD: A Common but Rarely Addressed Problem. *Dis Colon Rectum* 2017;60:61.

[98] 98. Leeds IL, DiBrito SR, Canner JK, et al. Cost-benefit limitations of extended, outpatient venous thromboembolism prophylaxis following surgery for Crohn's disease. *Dis Colon Rectum* 2019;62:1371–1380.

[99] Olivera PA, Zuily S, Kotze PG, et al. International consensus on the prevention of venous and arterial thrombotic events in patients with inflammatory bowel disease. *Nat Rev Gastroenterol Hepatol* 2021;18:857–873.

[100] Aksan A, Farrag K, Blumenstein I, et al. Chronic intestinal failure and short bowel syndrome in Crohn's disease. *World J Gastroenterol* 2021;27:3440–3465.

[101] Thompson JS, Iyer KR, DiBaise JK, et al. Short bowel syndrome and crohn's disease. *J Gastrointest Surg* 2003;7:1069–1072.

[102] Elriz K, Palascak-Juif V, Joly F, et al. Crohn's disease patients with chronic intestinal failure receiving long-term parenteral nutrition: a cross-national adult study. *Aliment Pharmacol Ther* 2011;34:931–940.

[103] Uchino M, Ikeuchi H, Bando T, et al. Risk factors for short bowel syndrome in patients with Crohn's disease. *Surg Today* 2012;42:447–452.

[104] Soop M, Khan H, Nixon E, et al. Causes and Prognosis of Intestinal Failure in Crohn's Disease: An 18-year Experience From a National Centre. *J Crohns Colitis* 2020;14:1558–1564.

[105] Limketkai BN, Parian AM, Shah ND, Colombel J-F. Short Bowel Syndrome and Intestinal Failure in Crohn's Disease. *Inflamm Bowel Dis* 2016;22:1209–1218.

[106] Jabłońska B, Mrowiec S. Nutritional Status and Its Detection in Patients with Inflammatory Bowel Diseases. *Nutrients* 2023;15:1991.

[107] Sokulmez P, Demirbag AE, Arslan P, Disibeyaz S. Effects of enteral nutritional support on malnourished patients with inflammatory bowel disease by subjective global assessment. *Turk J Gastroenterol* 2014;25.

[108] 108Balestrieri P, Ribolsi M, Guarino MPL, et al. Nutritional Aspects in Inflammatory Bowel Diseases. *Nutrients* 2020;12:372.

[109] Nguyen GC, Du L, Chong RY, Jackson TD. Hypoalbuminaemia and Postoperative Outcomes in Inflammatory Bowel Disease: the NSQIP Surgical Cohort. *J Crohns Colitis* 2019;13:1433–1438.

[110] Abd-El-Aziz MA, Hübner M, Demartines N, et al. Simple Clinical Screening Underestimates Malnutrition in Surgical Patients with Inflammatory Bowel Disease—An ACS NSQIP Analysis. *Nutrients* 2022;14:932.

[111] Alavi K, Sturrock PR, Sweeney WB, et al. A Simple Risk Score for Predicting Surgical Site Infections in Inflammatory Bowel Disease. *Dis Colon Rectum* 2010;53:1480–1486.

[112] Aydinli HH, Aytac E, Remzi FH, et al. Factors Associated with Short-Term Morbidity in Patients Undergoing Colon Resection for Crohn's Disease. *J Gastrointest Surg* 2018;22:1434–1441.

[113] McKenna NP, Habermann EB, Zielinski MD, et al. Body mass index: Implications on disease severity and postoperative complications in patients with Crohn's disease undergoing abdominal surgery. *Surgery* 2019;166:703–708.

[114] Reinisch W, Staun M, Bhandari S, Muñoz M. State of the iron: How to diagnose and efficiently treat iron deficiency anemia in inflammatory bowel disease. *J Crohns Colitis* 2013;7:429–440.

[115] Wallaert JB, De Martino RR, Marsicovetere PS, et al. Venous Thromboembolism After Surgery for Inflammatory Bowel Disease: Are There Modifiable Risk Factors? Data from ACS NSQIP. *Dis Colon Rectum* 2012;55:1138–1144.

[116] Liu L, Liu L, Liang L-C, et al. Impact of Preoperative Anemia on Perioperative Outcomes in Patients Undergoing Elective Colorectal Surgery. *Gastroenterol Res Pract* 2018;2018:1–7.

[117] Guo K, Ren J, Li G, et al. Risk factors of surgical site infections in patients with Crohn's disease complicated with gastrointestinal fistula. *Int J Colorectal Dis* 2017;32:635–643.

[118] Hu T, Wu X, Hu J, et al. Incidence and risk factors for incisional surgical site infection in patients with Crohn's disease undergoing bowel resection. *Gastroenterol Rep* 2018;6:189–194.

[119] El-Hussuna A, Iesalnieks I, Horesh N, et al. The effect of pre-operative optimization on post-operative outcome in Crohn's disease resections. *Int J Colorectal Dis* 2017;32:49–56.

[120] Wilson A, Reyes E, Ofman J. Prevalence and outcomes of anemia in inflammatory bowel disease: a systematic review of the literature. *Am J Med* 2004;116:44–49.

[121] Iesalnieks I, Dederichs F, Kilger A, et al. [Postoperative morbidity after bowel resections in patients with Crohn's disease: risk, management strategies, prevention]. *Z Gastroenterol* 2012;50:595–600.

[122] Müller-Wille R, Iesalnieks I, Dornia C, et al. Influence of percutaneous abscess drainage on severe postoperative septic complications in patients with Crohn's disease. *Int J Colorectal Dis* 2011;26:769–774.

[123] Jacobson S. Early postoperative complications in patients with Crohn's disease given and not given preoperative total parenteral nutrition. *Scand J Gastroenterol* 2012;47:170–177.

[124] Swanson G, Behara R, Braun R, Keshavarzian A. Diagnostic Medical Radiation in Inflammatory Bowel Disease: How to Limit Risk and Maximize Benefit. *Inflamm Bowel Dis* 2013;19:2501–2508.

[125] Iesalnieks I, Hoene M, Bittermann T, et al. Mechanical Bowel Preparation (MBP) Prior to Elective Colorectal Resections in Crohn's Disease Patients. *Inflamm Bowel Dis* 2018;24:908–915.

[126] Uchino M, Ikeuchi H, Bando T, et al. Efficacy of Preoperative Oral Antibiotic Prophylaxis for the Prevention of Surgical Site Infections in Patients With Crohn Disease: A Randomized Controlled Trial. *Ann Surg* 2019;269:420–426.

[127] Moghadamyeghaneh Z, Hanna MH, Blondet JJ, et al. Impact of chronic steroid use on outcomes of colorectal surgery. *Am J Surg* 2015;210:1003–1009.

[128] Aberra FN, Lewis JD, Hass D, et al. Corticosteroids and immunomodulators: postoperative infectious complication risk in inflammatory bowel disease patients. *Gastroenterology* 2003;125:320–327.

[129] Lightner AL, McKenna NP, Alsughayer A, et al. Biologics and 30-Day Postoperative Complications After Abdominal Operations for Crohn's Disease: Are There Differences in the Safety Profiles? *Dis Colon Rectum* 2019;62:1352–1362.

[130] Bruewer M, Utech M, Rijcken EJM, et al. Preoperative Steroid Administration: Effect on Morbidity among Patients Undergoing Intestinal Bowel Resection for Crohn's Disease. *World J Surg* 2003;27:1306–1310.

[131] Tzivanakis A, Singh JC, Guy RJ, et al. Influence of Risk Factors on the Safety of Ileocolic Anastomosis in Crohn's Disease Surgery. *Dis Colon Rectum* 2012;55:558–562.

[132] Uchino M, Ikeuchi H, Horio Y, et al. Association between preoperative biologic use and surgical morbidity in patients with Crohn's disease. *Int J Colorectal Dis* 2022;37:999–1010.

[133] Kotze PG, Saab MP, Saab B, et al. Tumor Necrosis Factor Alpha Inhibitors Did Not Influence Postoperative Morbidity After Elective Surgical Resections in Crohn's Disease. *Dig Dis Sci* 2017;62:456–464.

[134] Syed A, Cross RK, Flasar MH. Anti-Tumor Necrosis Factor Therapy Is Associated With Infections after Abdominal Surgery in Crohn's Disease Patients. *Am J Gastroenterol* 2013;108:583–593.

[135] Qiu Y, Zheng Z, Liu G, et al. Effects of preoperative anti-tumour necrosis factor alpha infusion timing on postoperative surgical site infection in inflammatory bowel disease: A systematic review and meta-analysis. *United Eur Gastroenterol J* 2019;7:1198–1214.

[136] Uchino M, Ikeuchi H, Matsuoka H, et al. Risk Factors for Surgical Site Infection and Association With Infliximab Administration During Surgery for Crohn's Disease. *Dis Colon Rectum* 2013;56:1156–1165.

[137] Brouquet A, Maggiori L, Zerbib P, et al. Anti-TNF Therapy Is Associated With an Increased Risk of Postoperative Morbidity After Surgery for Ileocolonic Crohn Disease: Results of a Prospective Nationwide Cohort. *Ann Surg* 2018;267:221–228.

[138] Waterland P, Athanasiou T, Patel H. Post-operative abdominal complications in Crohn's disease in the biological era: Systematic review and meta-analysis. *World J Gastrointest Surg* 2016;8:274.

[139] Lightner AL, McKenna NP, Tse CS, et al. Postoperative Outcomes in Ustekinumab-Treated Patients Undergoing Abdominal Operations for Crohn's Disease. *J Crohns Colitis* 2018;12:402–407.

[140] Lau C, Dubinsky M, Melmed G, et al. The Impact of Preoperative Serum Anti-TNFα Therapy Levels on Early Postoperative Outcomes in Inflammatory Bowel Disease Surgery. *Ann Surg* 2015;261:487–496.

[141] Lightner AL, Vogel JD, Carmichael JC, et al. The American Society of Colon and Rectal Surgeons Clinical Practice Guidelines for the Surgical Management of Crohn's Disease. *Dis Colon Rectum* 2020;63:1028–1052.

[142] Lightner AL, McKenna NP, Tse CS, et al. Postoperative outcomes in vedolizumab-treated Crohn's disease patients undergoing major abdominal operations. *Aliment Pharmacol Ther* 2018;47:573–580.

[143] Lightner AL, Raffals LE, Mathis KL, et al. Postoperative Outcomes in Vedolizumab-Treated Patients Undergoing Abdominal Operations for Inflammatory Bowel Disease. *J Crohns Colitis* 2017;11:185–190.

[144] Law CCY, Narula A, Lightner AL, et al. Systematic Review and Meta-Analysis: Preoperative Vedolizumab Treatment and Postoperative Complications in Patients with Inflammatory Bowel Disease. *J Crohns Colitis* 2018;12:538–545.

[145] Moosvi Z, Duong JT, Bechtold ML, Nguyen DL. Systematic Review and Meta-Analysis: Preoperative Vedolizumab and Postoperative Complications in Patients with IBD. *South Med J* 2021;114:98–105.

[146] Yung DE, Horesh N, Lightner AL, et al. Systematic Review and Meta-analysis: Vedolizumab and Postoperative Complications in Inflammatory Bowel Disease. *Inflamm Bowel Dis* 2018;24:2327–2338.

[147] Liu S, Miao J, Wang G, et al. Risk factors for postoperative surgical site infections in patients with Crohn's disease receiving definitive bowel resection. *Sci Rep* 2017;7:9828.

[148] Wilson MZ, Connelly TM, Hollenbeak CS, Messaris E. Organ space infection following ileocolectomy for Crohn's disease: a National Surgical Quality Improvement Project study. *Am J Surg* 2014;208:749–755.

[149] Ikeshima R, Mizushima T, Takahashi H, et al. The efficacy of active drainage for preventing postoperative organ/space surgical site infections in patients with Crohn's disease. *Surg Today* 2018;48:25–32.

[150] Culver DH, Horan TC, Gaynes RP, et al. Surgical wound infection rates by wound class, operative procedure, and patient risk index. *Am J Med* 1991;91:S152–S157.

[151] Pak SJ, Kim YI, Yoon YS, et al. Short-term and long-term outcomes of laparoscopic vs open ileocolic resection in patients with Crohn's disease: Propensity-score matching analysis. *World J Gastroenterol.* 2021;27:7159–7172.

[152] Eshuis EJ, Slors JFM, Stokkers PCF, et al. Long-term outcomes following laparoscopically assisted versus open ileocolic resection for Crohn's disease. *Br J Surg* 2010;97:563–568.

[153] Patel SV, Patel SV, Ramagopalan SV, Ott MC. Laparoscopic surgery for Crohn's disease: a meta-analysis of perioperative complications and long term outcomes compared with open surgery. *BMC Surg* 2013;13:14.

[154] Bellinger J, Munoz-Bongrand N, Pariente B, et al. Endoscopic and clinical recurrences after laparoscopic or open ileocolic resection in Crohn's disease. *J Laparoendosc Adv Surg Tech A* 2014;24:617–622.

[155] Tilney HS, Constantinides VA, Heriot AG, et al. Comparison of laparoscopic and open ileocecal resection for Crohn's disease: a metaanalysis. *Surg Endosc* 2006;20:1036–1044.

[156] Lee Y, Fleming FJ, Deeb AP., et al. A laparoscopic approach reduces short-term complications and length of stay following ileocolic resection in Crohn's disease: an analysis of outcomes from the NSQIP database. *Colorectal Dis* 2012;14:572–577.

[157] Mege D, Michelassi F. Laparoscopy in Crohn Disease: Learning Curve and Current Practice. *Ann Surg* 2020;271:317.

[158] Hasegawa H, Watanabe M, Nishibori H, et al. Laparoscopic surgery for recurrent Crohn's disease. *Br J Surg* 2003;90:970–973.

[159] Asa Z, Greenberg R, Ghinea R, et al. Grading of complications and risk factor evaluation in laparoscopic colorectal surgery. *Surg Endosc* 2013;27:3748–3753.

[160] Person B, Cera SM, Sands DR, et al. Do elderly patients benefit from laparoscopic colorectal surgery? *Surg Endosc* 2008;22:401–405.

[161] Evans J, Poritz L, MacRae H. Influence of Experience on Laparoscopic Ileocolic Resection for Crohn's Disease. *Dis Colon Rectum* 2002;45:1595.

[162] Liu W, Zhou W. Minimally invasive surgery in Crohn's disease: state-of-the-art review. *Front Surg* 2023;10.

[163] Nakajima K, Nezu R, Hirota M, Nishida T. The role of hand-assisted laparoscopic surgery in subtotal and total colectomy for Crohn's colitis. *Surg Endosc* 2010;24:2713–2717.

[164] Celentano V, Pellino G, Rottoli M, et al. Single-incision laparoscopic surgery (SILS) for the treatment of ileocolonic Crohn's disease: a propensity score–matched analysis. *Int J Colorectal Dis* 2021;36:605–608.

[165] Carvello M, de Groof EJ, de Buck van Overstraeten A, et al. Single port laparoscopic ileocaecal resection for Crohn's disease: a multicentre comparison with multi-port laparoscopy. *Colorectal Dis* 2018;20:53–58.

[166] Lanfranco AR, Castellanos AE, Desai JP, Meyers WC. Robotic Surgery: A Current Perspective. *Ann Surg* 2004;239:14.

[167] Rockall TA, Darzi A. Robot-assisted laparoscopic colorectal surgery. *Surg Clin* 2003;83:1463–1468.

[168] Trinh BB, Jackson NR, Hauch AT, et al. Robotic Versus Laparoscopic Colorectal Surgery. *JSLS* 2014;18:e2014.00187.

[169] Lim DR, Min BS, Kim MS, et al. Robotic versus laparoscopic anterior resection of sigmoid colon cancer: comparative study of long-term oncologic outcomes. *Surg Endosc* 2013;27:1379–1385.

[170] Bertani E, Chiappa A, Biffi R, et al. Assessing appropriateness for elective colorectal cancer surgery: clinical, oncological, and quality-of-life short-term outcomes employing different treatment approaches. *Int J Colorectal Dis* 2011;26:1317–1327.

[171] Raskin ER, Gorrepati ML, Mehendale S, Gaertner WB. Robotic-assisted ileocolic resection for Crohn's disease: outcomes from an early national experience. *J Robot Surg* 2019;13:429–434.

[172] Hota S, Parascandola S, Smith S, et al. Robotic and laparoscopic surgical techniques in patients with Crohn's disease. *Surg Endosc* 2021;35:4602–4608.

[173] Lan N, Stocchi L, Li Y, Shen B. Perioperative blood transfusion is associated with post-operative infectious complications in patients with Crohn's disease. *Gastroenterol Rep* 2018;6:114–121.

Chapter 14

Short Bowel Syndrome

Nicole J. Kus[1], MD
Lindsay Kohan[2]
and Stephen M. Kavic[2,*], MD, MSHPE
[1]University of Maryland Medical Center, Baltimore, Maryland, USA
[2]University of Maryland School of Medicine, Baltimore, Maryland, USA

Abstract

The small bowel plays an essential role in the absorption of nutrients, vitamins, and water. The length of the small bowel in an adult ranges between 275 to 850 cm. Short gut syndrome (SBS) can occur when there is an average of less than 200 cm of remaining small bowel. SBS may occur for various reasons, with extensive surgical resection or congenital intestinal diseases as the two top causes. The most common pathologies linked with SBS in adults are Crohn's disease, post-operative complications, mesenteric ischemia, and radiation enteritis. The cardinal symptoms of SBS are diarrhea and steatorrhea leading to global malabsorption and the subsequent complications. SBS can be managed medically and surgically, but both play an important role in treating this devastating disease. Therapy of SBS ultimately depends on the degree of small bowel losses and the resulting functional disturbances but can be individualized based on the underlying cause. The goal of surgical management of SBS is to increase absorption by either slowing the gastrointestinal transit or increasing the absorptive surface area of the bowel. In this chapter, we will introduce short bowel syndrome and delve into the treatment of this disease, highlighting the importance of both medical and surgical management. We will conclude this chapter by discussing the complications that may arise from SBS and the life expectancy patients with this disease face.

Keywords: short bowel syndrome, intestinal failure, Bianchi, STEP, small bowel transplantation

Introduction

The normal length of small bowel varies based on age. In neonates, small bowel is estimated to have a mean length of 270 cm, while in infants an average of 350 cm is documented[1]. Small bowel length in adults, on the other hand, ranges from 275 to 850 cm. The small bowel is

---

* Corresponding Author's Email: skavic@som.umaryland.edu

In: Surgery for Crohn's Disease. Second Edition
Editors: Stephen M. Kavic, Rebecca Brown and Kerri Lopez
ISBN: 979-8-89530-676-5

primarily responsible for the absorption of nutrients, with the absorption of most nutrients occurring within the first 100 cm of the jejunum [1]. Absorption in the small bowel varies based on the segment, as demonstrated in Figure 14.1.

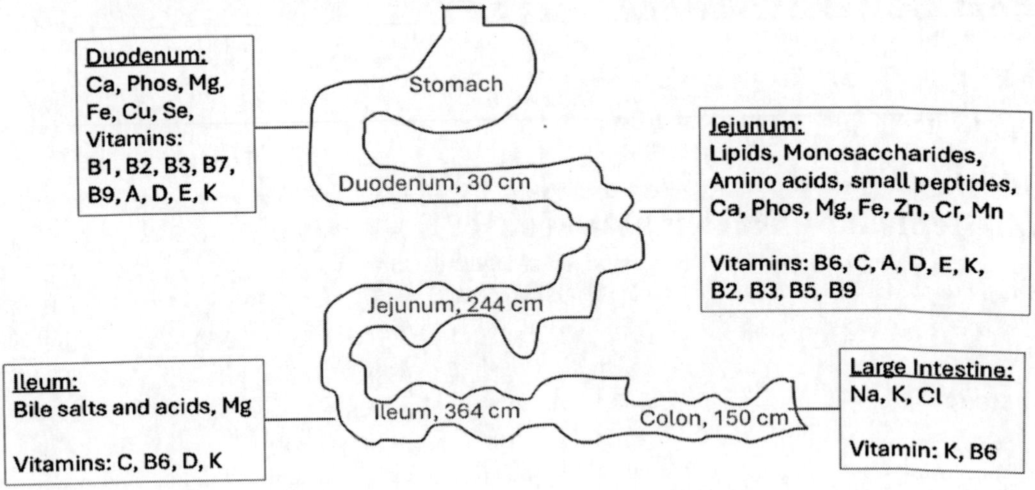

Figure 14.1. Absorptive properties of the small bowel and large intestine.

Short bowel syndrome (SBS) is a form of intestinal failure that compromises nutrient, fluid, electrolyte, and vitamin absorption. It may occur in adults when insufficient small bowel is present for normal function. By consensus definition, this occurs when less than 180-200 cm of small bowel remains, leading to the need for additional nutritional and fluid supplementation [2]. In children, short bowel syndrome occurs in children when less than 25% of small bowel remains that is expected for the gestational age is present [2].

There are varying etiologies of SBS, with extensive surgical resection or congenital intestinal diseases listed as the top two causes. The most common pathologies which can lead to SBS in adults are Crohn's disease, post-operative complications, mesenteric ischemia, and radiation enteritis [2]. In children, the most common pathologies include volvulus, intestinal malformations, and necrotizing enterocolitis [2]. SBS has an estimated prevalence of 3-4 per million individuals, affecting 15% of patients with intestinal resection, 75% of which had massive resection and 25% of which had multiple resections [3, 4].

Patients with SBS exhibit global malabsorption due to the decreased absorptive capacity and disrupted gastrointestinal (GI) regulation [5]. The cardinal symptoms of SBS are diarrhea and steatorrhea. The symptoms of SBS lead to dehydration secondary to diarrhea, malabsorption of macro- and micro- nutrients, failure to thrive, weight loss, and ultimate malnutrition [6, 7].

The severity of the symptoms patients may experience are related to the portions of small bowel that are missing. For instance, resection of the duodenum can lead to malabsorption of iron, folate and calcium, whereas resection of the jejunum can lead to massive fluid loss. Patients who have had their duodenum or terminal ileum removed are found to have more severe symptoms.

Intestinal insufficiency may result and depends on the severity of the malabsorption and the degree of resection based on the type of SBS. The degree of functional insufficiency has been classified into three types: 1) acute, short term, and self-limited, 2) acute and prolonged, requiring parenteral nutrition (PN) over weeks to months, and 3) chronic, requiring PN over months to years. SBS symptoms may be mitigated by the presence of colon and ileocecal valve, as this improves the patient's prognosis [8].

Type 1 SBS is a patient who has a terminal enterostomy, type 2 is a patient who has a jejuno-colonic anastomosis, and type 3 is a patient with a jejuno-ileal anastomosis, with the entire colon and ileocecal valve in continuity [8]. Patients with SBS may develop intestinal insufficiency depending on the different anatomical type when the remaining bowel is <115 cm, <60cm, and <35 cm, for type 1, type 2, and type 3 respectively [9].

Patients with SBS can be treated through medical or surgical management. Most patients will require nutritional supplementation, often through the form of total parenteral nutrition (TPN). TPN remains the standard of care with patients who have developed severe intestinal insufficiency [8]. Patients that are eligible may undergo surgical procedures which focus on lengthening the native small bowel, or reducing motility. As a last resort, small bowel may be replaced through transplantation. Ultimately, the care of patients with SBS is complex and requires a multidisciplinary approach of physicians, dieticians, and nurses to provide nutritional support, rehabilitation, and improvement in life quality [10].

Crohn's Disease and SBS

Crohn's is a common disease encountered among western Europe and Northern America, with a prevalence of 100-300 per 100,000 people [11]. It is typically managed with medications including immunosuppressants, but severe or refractory Crohn's disease may require surgical resection. Within 10 years of the initial diagnosis, over 50% of patients will undergo intestinal resection and fully a third may undergo a repeat intestinal resection within 5 years. Patients with Crohn's disease are at a high risk of developing SBS and consequently malnutrition due to the chronic inflammatory mucosal damage and diminished functional short bowel length [10]. While SBS may be defined as occurring when less than 200 cm of combined jejunum-ileum exist following small bowel resection, patients with Crohn's disease may have more than 200 cm but still experience symptoms as the remaining bowel is often diseased [7]. Irrespective of length, these patients are managed like standard SBS patients. It is focused on optimizing nutritional status and fluid balance while obtaining appropriate weight gain or maintenance [12].

Patients with Crohn's disease are more likely to develop chronic intestinal failure (CIF), a complication of reduced gastrointestinal function which requires IV supplementation to maintain health and growth as there is enteral absorption of micronutrients, electrolytes, and water [12]. According to the European Society for Clinical Nutrition and Metabolism, CIF is characterized by an anatomical, clinical, functional, or pathophysiological cause. CIF in Crohn's disease is most commonly due to SBS, and 60% of Crohn's patients with CIF will be permanently dependent on parenteral nutrition [12]. Disease location affects the severity of Crohn's disease and the development of CIF, with ileocolonic involvement carrying the greatest risk of CIF and parental nutrition dependance. Penetrating Crohn's disease is more commonly involved in patients who are dependent on parenteral nutrition and is associated with a longer length of bowel resection in contrast to perianal Crohn's disease which is associated with more frequent bowel resections. Corticosteroid use for acute Crohn's flares also increases the risk of

CIF due to more intestinal resections from steroid-induced post-operative complications and an earlier onset of CIF [10]. Overall, due to the inflammatory changes causing impaired nutrition absorption, especially with ileocolonic involvement, and the intestinal resections and risk for reresections, Crohn's disease poses a significant risk of developing SBS.

Medical Management of SBS

The small intestine can adapt to less extensive resections by increasing the absorptive surface area to improve digestive and absorptive functions. These adaptations can further be aided by the administration of factors which promote enterocyte and colonocyte proliferation [13]. While intestinal adaptation may improve absorption, secondary dilation can prevent effective peristalsis [14]. Thus, dilated bowel has poor motility, poor absorption, and is a prime environment for bacterial overgrowth [14].

Successful management of SBS is dependent on timing. There are three phases of treatment: the acute phase, the adaptation phase, and the maintenance phase. The acute phase occurs within the first 4 weeks. The primary goal of the acute phase is to stabilize the patient. These patients require aggressive rehydration, broad spectrum antibiotic coverage as they are at risk of sepsis, and proton pump inhibitors to reduce gastric secretion [7]. This is followed by the adaptation phase which occurs within the first 1-2 years and focuses on inducing maximal adaptation by gradually increasing nutrient exposure to the remaining small bowel. The final phase, referred to as the maintenance phase, occurs once maximal nutrition has been reached and focuses on maintaining the current state of the patient. Therapy of SBS ultimately depends on the degree of small bowel losses and on the resulting functional disturbances. Therapy can also be individualized as it depends on the underlying cause of pathophysiology. In patients with Crohn's disease, optimal treatment of underlying disease to avoid further reduction.

Medications for SBS focus on slowing gut transit or treating the complications associated with SBS (Table 14.1). These may include loperamide, H2 blockers, proton pump inhibitors (PPI), and cholestyramine. H2 blockers and PPIs reduce gastric fluid secretions and fluid losses during the first 6 months [15]. Anti-motility agents are then required after 6 months to further reduce fluid losses, through medications like loperamide or diphenoxylate [15]. If these are ineffective, uses of codeine or tincture of opium may be necessary [15]. Octreotide is only used when the fluid losses exceed 3 liters, as it may impair post resection intestinal adaptation and increase the risk of cholelithiasis [15]. If necessary to treat bacterial overgrowth, treatment includes antibiotic therapy with oral antibiotics like metronidazole or tetracyclines [15].

Table 14.1. Medical management of Short Bowel Syndrome

Purpose	Medications
Slow gut transit	Loperamide Diphenoxylate Codeine Tincture of opium
Decrease gastric secretions	H2 Blockers PPI
Minimize bacterial overgrowth	Metronidazole Tetracyclines
Mitigate large fluid losses	Consider octreotide when losses are > 3L

The chronic intestinal failure of SBS leads to the requirement of nutritional supplementation, often in the form of TPN. The risk of parenteral nutrition dependence in patients with SBS is associated with location and type of resection. Patients with SBS and <30 to 35 cm jejunoileal anastomoses, <60 to 65 cm jejuno-colonic anastomoses, or <100 to 115 cm end jejunostomy will require parenteral nutrition [10].

Surgical Management of SBS

When deficient in overall length, the intestine undergoes adaptation to improve peristalsis and nutrient absorption. However, this process may actually be maladaptive, as the bowel often becomes dilated and inefficient at both absorption and motility. For this reason, surgeons have attempted to design methods that may mitigate these changes.

The goal of surgical management of SBS is to increase nutrient and water absorption by slowing GI transit or increasing the absorptive surface area of the bowel. Since the 19th century, surgeons have developed a variety of methods to enhance the length of small bowel in SBS. Techniques have ranged from constructing valves within the small bowel or providing electrical retrograde small bowel stimulation to lengthening procedures and providing interposition grafts of antiperistaltic small bowel segments or colon. These surgical procedures will be described in the following paragraphs.

One of the first surgical techniques was developed by Adrian Bianchi, considered a pioneer in intestinal lengthening surgery. In a paper published in 1980, Bianchi described a method to creating two segments of bowel that were anastomosed in an isoperistaltic fashion. In this technique, blunt division of the peritoneum of the small bowel mesentery is carried out to create two distinct halves which may supply the bowel [16]. The small bowel is then divided longitudinally along the mesenteric and antimesenteric walls and each half is tubularized to create two vascularized loops of bowel with half of the original diameter. These are then anastomosed in an end-to-end isoperistaltic fashion. This technique is now referred to as the Bianchi or the Longitudinal Intestinal Lengthening and Tapering (LILT) [16]. Unfortunately, the LILT procedure may be prohibitive in patients which only have the remaining duodenum and colon as the procedure depends on adequate mesentery [16].

To combat these prohibitions, the Kimura technique was developed. The Kimura technique, also known as the isolated bowel segment or Iowa model, is a staged approach for isoperistaltic bowel elongation. In this approach, the dilated segment of small bowel undergoes a seromyotomy to expose the mucosa of the bowel [16, 17]. This mucosa is then fixed to a "donor" organ, such as the liver or abdominal wall. An interval duration of 8-10 weeks then occurs in which collaterals are formed to the fixed mucosa. Patients then return to the OR where the dilated, but now dually perfused intestine, is split longitudinally and subsequently re-anastomosed in an end-to-end isoperistaltic manner.

In 2003, another procedure was developed for lengthening the small bowel, the serial transverse enteroplasty procedure (STEP) [16]. STEP uses a stapler to elongate the dilated bowel. The stapler is applied in alternating directions, both perpendicular to the long axis of the intestine, parallel to the direction of the blood supply. These staple lines are 2 cm apart from each other and leave 2 cm of the bowel uncut. This uncut bowel creates a zigzag common channel. STEP is now one of the most commonly performed bowel lengthening procedures, alongside LILT [16].

Table 14.2. Surgical techniques for Short Bowel Syndrome

	Main Concept	Benefits	Complications
LILT (Bianchi)	Mesenteric leaflets are split and used as dual blood supply to the newly formed halves of dilated bowel	Isoperistaltic	Ischemia of hemiloop and strictures; unable to perform in patients with only duodenum and colon. Cannot be repeated.
Kimura (Iowa)	Coaptation induces collateral formation to the dilated bowel, allowing for surgical lengthening	Can be performed on bowel with restrictions with other procedures; isoperistaltic	Failure of appropriate collateral development; multiple operations are required.
STEP	Transverse staple firings parallel to the blood supply allow for increased length of the dilated bowel	Less anatomic limitations; can be performed on duodenum and proximal jejunum; can be repeated	Disrupts muscle fibers; can lead to staple line ulcers, bacterial overgrowth, or re-dilation of bowel

Unfortunately, as STEP gained more popularity, complications from this procedure came to fruition with one of the most common being re-dilation of the bowel after this procedure [16]. Systematic reviews comparing STEP and LILT demonstrate similar increase in intestinal length and successful weaning from parenteral nutrition [18]. Bleeding and re-dilation were found to occur more frequently with step, but these postoperative complications, along with stricture and leakage, were not significantly different between the two procedures [18]. However, data from this systemic review found advantages of STEP, namely that it was able to be performed in the duodenum and proximal jejunum, where LILT was not possible, and that STEP was able to be repeated.

Bianchi himself recognized that intestinal lengthening surgeries should be coupled with maximal medical therapies as the primary management of SBS [14]. He stressed the importance of individualized and multidisciplinary management of these patients [14]. The benefits and complications of each described surgical procedure are summarized in Table 14.2.

Intestinal transplantation is often reserved for those who are unable to receive surgical correction or have failed medical management for SBS. It is proposed to patients as a last resort for those who are dependent on PN or whose condition becomes life-threatening as a result of a severe complication of PN, such as ongoing liver failure, thrombosis, or frequent severe dehydration [8].

Ultimately, SBS is the most common indication for small bowel transplantation [10]. Intestinal transplantation may involve the small intestine itself, the liver and the intestine, or multiple organs (liver, pancreas, stomach) [8]. Isolated small bowel transplantation has a 5-year survival of 56.3%, while combined transplantations have a survival of 25% [19].

Complications of SBS and Life Expectancy

Patients with SBS are at risk for various complications. These include intestinal failure associated liver disease, gallstone development, chronic renal failure, electrolyte imbalances, vitamin deficiencies, and metabolic bone disease [2].

Complications of fluid and nutrient malabsorption and deficiencies put patients at risk of metabolic derangements and malnutrition. Patients with SBS should take in 1.5 to 2 times greater oral intake throughout the day than prior to when they were diagnosed with SBS. The exception to this is patients with SBS and proximal jejunostomies as these patients might be net "secretors," meaning that their fecal and fluid losses increase as their enteral intake increases [20].

The nutritional deficiencies of SBS depend on the section of bowel that was resected or is non-functional. For example, resection of the terminal ileum may cause deficiencies in vitamin B12, bile acids, and the fat-soluble vitamins A, D, E, K [21]. Other nutritional deficiencies include iron, selenium, zinc, and copper. D-lactic acidosis can occur related to gut microbiota fermentation of unabsorbed simple carbohydrates and other nutrients [4].

Reduced absorption or reduced binding of intestinal calcium in SBS can lead to hypocalcemia, necessitating repletion of calcium, magnesium, and vitamin D [4]. Metabolic bone disease can occur in these patients characterized as either osteomalacia or osteoporosis. It is associated with decreased vitamin C, E, K levels, although vitamin D levels are reduced in all patients with SBS. It can occur in almost 85% of patients with SBS on parenteral nutrition [20].

Nephrolithiasis is also a common complication of SBS. Hyperoxaluria may occur in patients with SBS due to reduced intestinal calcium levels causing increased reabsorption of free oxalate in the colon. Patients with SBS are thus at risk of forming calcium oxalate stones in the ureter and renal pelvis. Prevention includes a diet low in oxalate, a diet high in citrate to compete with calcium for oxalate in the urine, and bile salt replacement to increase fat absorption and decrease calcium saponification in the gut [20].

Intestinal failure-associated liver disease is another dreaded complication. It is thought to occur due to increased intestinal permeability, altered circulation of bile acids, and alterations in the gut microbiota. The liver disease may progress to end-stage liver disease requiring a liver transplant, with or without a concurrent small bowel transplant [21]. Although parenteral nutrition supplementation is key in the management of SBS, it has inherent risks. Central venous access is required for TPN and thus carries a risk of catheter-related bloodstream infections, including fungal infections which are difficult to treat.

Patients with SBS have been shown to have reduced long-term survival. A 2013 review documented a survival probability of 94% at one year, 70% at 5 years, and 52% at 10 years [22]. Home-based parenteral nutrition is a well-known factor for increased mortality and has been associated with an increased likelihood of death than enteral nutrition [22]. Survival of patients with SBS dependent on parenteral nutrition demonstrated a survival probability of 87%, 67-80%, and 60% at 1, 3, and 5 years, respectively [23]. For patients with intestinal transplants, patient survival rates between 1998 and 2002 were shown to be 77% and 49% at 1 and 5 years, respectively, with a graft survival rate of 66% and 34% at 1 and 5 years, respectively [24].

Overall mortality of SBS is difficult to assess but can vary with underlying conditions. Age greater than 55 is associated with a three times higher mortality, active neoplasia with a 23 times higher mortality, radiation enteritis with a four times higher mortality, and systemic sclerosis with a six times higher mortality [20].

The quality of life for patients with SBS may be poor due to symptomatology and complications. Patients often face poor sleep due to frequent nighttime awakenings, changes in their appetite, and reduced physical strength due to diarrhea, steatorrhea, bloating, dehydration, weight loss, and abdominal cramping [25]. Additionally, there is a significant economic burden on these patients related to out-of-pocket costs, non-reimbursed co-payments, and costs related to TPN [20]. Overall, it is important to discuss the impact of SBS on the quality and quantity of life with the patient and their loved ones.

Conclusion

Short bowel syndrome is a rare disease that occurs when an adult patient has < 200 cm of remaining small bowel. It most often occurs because of extensive resection or an underlying disease pathology, such as Crohn's disease. SBS can lead to the development of intestinal failure and patients may become dependent on parenteral nutrition. Surgical techniques have been developed to improve gastrointestinal motility and ideally absorption, but these are not without risks. While SBS may be the leading cause of intestinal transplantation, transplantation is a last resort option for patients. In the end, the treatment of SBS is individualized and requires a multidisciplinary team. Most often, it requires maximal medical therapy with surgical supplementation.

Recommended Readings

1. Greig CJ, Oh PS, Gross ER, Cowles RA. Retracing our STEPs: Four decades of progress in intestinal lengthening procedures for short bowel syndrome. *Am J Surg*. 2019 Apr;217 (4):772-782. doi: 10.1016/j.amjsurg.2018.11.025. Epub 2018 Nov 27. PMID: 30514435.
2. Abu-Elmagd, K., Costa, G. (2019). Intestinal Lengthening and Transplantation Surgery: Candidacy, Logistics, and Techniques. In: Oniscu, G. C., Forsythe, J. L. R., Pomfret, E. A. (eds) *Transplantation Surgery*. Springer Surgery Atlas Series. Springer, Berlin, Heidelberg. https://doi.org/10.1007/978-3-540-73796-4_23

References

[1] Bardwell C, El Demellawy D, Oltean I, Murphy M, Agarwal A, Hamid JS, Reddy D, Barrowman N, de Nanassy J, Nasr A. Establishing normal ranges for fetal and neonatal small and large intestinal lengths: results from a prospective postmortem study. *World J Pediatr Surg*. 2022 May 16;5(3):e000397. doi: 10.1136/wjps-2021-000397. PMID: 36475045; PMCID: PMC9717316.

[2] Guillen B, Atherton NS. Short Bowel Syndrome. [Updated 2023 Jul 17]. In: StatPearls [Internet]. Treasure Island (FL): StatPearls Publishing; 2024 Jan-. Available from: https://www.ncbi.nlm.nih.gov/books/NBK536935/.

[3] Lakkasani S, Seth D, Khokhar I, Touza M, Dacosta TJ. Concise review on short bowel syndrome: Etiology, pathophysiology, and management. *World J Clin Cases*. 2022 Nov 6;10(31):11273-11282. doi: 10.12998/wjcc.v10.i31.11273. PMID: 36387822; PMCID: PMC9649563.

[4] Thompson JS, Iyer KR, DiBaise JK et al. Short bowel syndrome and Crohn's disease. *J Gastrointest Surg* 7, 1069–1072 (2003). https://doi.org/10.1016/j.gassur.2003.08.007.

[5] Keller J, Panter H, Layer P. Management of the short bowel syndrome after extensive small bowel resection, *Best Prac Res Clin Gastroenterol*. 2004;18(5):977-992, https://doi.org/10.1016/j.bpg.2004.05.002.

[6] Vanderhoof JA, Langnas AN. Short-bowel syndrome in children and adults. *Gastroenterology*. 1997 Nov;113(5):1767-78.

[7] Robinson MK, Wilmore DW. Short bowel syndrome. In: Holzheimer RG, Mannick JA, editors. Surgical Treatment: Evidence-Based and Problem-Oriented. Munich: Zuckschwerdt; 2001. Available from: https://www.ncbi.nlm.nih.gov/books/NBK6974/

[8] Pironi L, Arends J, Bozzetti F, Cuerda C, Gillanders L, Jeppesen PB, Joly F, Kelly D, Lal S, Staun M, Szczepanek K, Van Gossum A, Wanten G, Schneider SM Home Artificial Nutrition & Chronic

Intestinal Failure Special Interest Group of ESPEN. ESPEN guidelines on chronic intestinal failure in adults. *Clin Nutr*. 2016;35:247–307.

[9] Carbonnel F, Cosnes J, Chevret S, et al. The role of anatomic factors in nutritional autonomy after extensive small bowel resection. *J Parenter Enteral Nutr* 1996;20(4):275—80.

[10] Limketkai BN, Parian AM, Shah ND, Colombel JF. Short Bowel Syndrome and Intestinal Failure in Crohn's Disease. *Inflamm Bowel Dis*. 2016 May;22(5):1209-18. doi: 10.1097/MIB.0000000000000698. PMID: 26818425.

[11] MedlinePlus [Internet]. Bethesda (MD): National Library of Medicine (US). Crohn's disease; [updated 2022 Jan 3; reviewed 2024 Jun 30. Available from: https://medlineplus.gov/genetics/condition/crohns-disease/#frequency.

[12] Aksan A, Farrag K, Blumenstein I, Schröder O, Dignass AU, Stein J. Chronic intestinal failure and short bowel syndrome in Crohn's disease. *World J Gastroenterol*. 2021 Jun 28;27(24):3440-3465. doi: 10.3748/wjg.v27.i24.3440. PMID: 34239262; PMCID: PMC8240052.

[13] Mayeur C, Gillard L, Le Beyec J, Bado A, Joly F, Thomas M. Extensive Intestinal Resection Triggers Behavioral Adaptation, Intestinal Remodeling and Microbiota Transition in Short Bowel Syndrome. *Microorganisms*. 2016 Mar 8;4(1):16. doi: 10.3390/microorganisms4010016. PMID: 27681910; PMCID: PMC5029521.

[14] Greig CJ, Oh PS, Gross ER, Cowles RA. Retracing our STEPs: Four decades of progress in intestinal lengthening procedures for short bowel syndrome. *Am J Surg*. 2019 Apr;217(4):772-782. doi:10.1016/j.amjsurg.2018.11.025. Epub 2018 Nov 27. PMID: 30514435.

[15] American Gastroenterological Association. American Gastroenterological Association medical position statement: short bowel syndrome and intestinal transplantation. *Gastroenterology*. 2003 Apr;124(4):1105-10. doi: 10.1053/gast.2003.50139. PMID: 12671903.

[16] Abu-Elmagd, K., Costa, G. (2019). Intestinal Lengthening and Transplantation Surgery: Candidacy, Logistics, and Techniques. In: Oniscu, G.C., Forsythe, J.L.R., Pomfret, E.A. (eds) Transplantation Surgery. Springer Surgery Atlas Series. Springer, Berlin, Heidelberg. https://doi.org/10.1007/978-3-540-73796-4_23.

[17] Kimura K, Soper RT. A new bowel elongation technique for the short-bowel syndrome using the isolated bowel segment Iowa models. *J Pediatr Surg*. 1993 Jun;28(6):792-4. doi: 10.1016/0022-3468(93)90328-i. PMID: 8331504.

[18] Frongia G, Kessler M, Weih S, et al. Comparison of LILT and STEP procedures in children with short bowel syndrome – a systematic review of the literature. *J Pediatr Surg*. 2013 Aug;48(8):1794e1805. PubMed PMID: 23932625. Epub 2013/08/13. Eng.

[19] Elsabbagh AM, Hawksworth J, Khan KM, Kaufman SS, Yazigi NA, Kroemer A, Smith C, Fishbein TM, Matsumoto CS. Long-term survival in visceral transplant recipients in the new era: A single-center experience. *Am J Transplant*. 2019 Jul;19(7):2077-2091. doi: 10.1111/ajt.15269. Epub 2019 Mar 26. PMID: 30672105; PMCID: PMC6591067.

[20] Carroll, R.E., Benedetti, E., Schowalter, J.P. et al. Management and Complications of Short Bowel Syndrome: an Updated Review. *Curr Gastroenterol Rep* 18, 40 (2016). https://doi.org/10.1007/s11894-016-0511-3

[21] Massironi S, Cavalcoli F, Rausa E, Invernizzi P, Braga M, Vecchi M. Understanding short bowel syndrome: Current status and future perspectives. *Dig Liv Dis*. 2020;52(3):253-261, https://doi.org/10.1016/j.dld.2019.11.013.

[22] Wrinkler M, Tappenden K. Epidemiology, survival, costs, and quality of life in adults with short bowel syndrome. *Nutr Clin Prac*. 2023 Apr 28;38(1):S17-S26. https://doi.org/10.1002/ncp.10964.

[23] Noelting J, Gramlich L, Whittaker S, Armstrong D, Marliss E, Jurewitsch B, Raman M, Duerksen D, Stevenson D, Lou W, Saha S, Allard J. Survival of patients with short-bowel syndrome on home parenteral nutrition: a prospective cohort study. *J Parent Ent Mutr*. 2021;45(5):1083-1088. https://doi.org/10.1002/jpen.1984.

[24] DeLegge, M., Alsolaiman, M.M., Barbour, E. et al. Short Bowel Syndrome: Parenteral Nutrition Versus Intestinal Transplantation. Where Are We Today?. *Dig Dis Sci* 52, 876–892 (2007). https://doi.org/10.1007/s10620-006-9416-6.

[25] Chen Y, Yan M, Chen H, Sheng Y, Wang Z, Wu B. A Systematic Review of Quality of Life in Patients with Short Bowel Syndrome and Their Caregivers. *Patient Prefer Adherence*. 2024 Jun 13;18:1217-1230. doi: 10.2147/PPA.S443026. PMID: 38895637; PMCID: PMC11182759.

Chapter 15

Surveillance and Follow Up

Seema Patil*, **MD**
University of Maryland School of Medicine, Baltimore, Maryland, USA

Abstract

The complex, chronic, and systemic nature of Crohn's disease warrants a unified approach by a multidisciplinary team of providers. Special clinical situations such as complex perianal disease and perioperative medical treatment require collaboration between medical and surgical providers, as well as nurses, radiologists, dietitians, and specialty consultants. The long-term postoperative care of the Crohn's disease patient is focused on preventing future need for surgery. The onset of histologic recurrence occurs within days of surgery, and is eventually followed by endoscopic and clinical recurrence. Risk stratifying patients for recurrence, instituting prophylactic therapy, and regularly surveying for recurrence can improve outcomes.

Role of the Multidisciplinary Team

Caring for the patient with Crohn's Disease (CD) in the perioperative period and beyond requires a multidisciplinary approach. The multidisciplinary team should include the surgeon, gastroenterologist, nurse educator, dietitian, pathologist, and radiologist. Each team member possesses skills that are vital to the optimal care of patients with IBD.

The partnership between the IBD surgeon and gastroenterologist offers the patient multiple perspectives on their care. Cooperation between these two providers can optimize preoperative planning, perioperative management, patient education and informed consent, postoperative recovery, and prophylaxis against recurrent disease. Special situations exist in which this partnership is particularly important, such as complex perianal disease. In a 2012 study, clinical healing rates in patients treated with both infliximab and surgical intervention were higher than in those who were treated with surgery alone (71% vs 36%, $p = 0.001$) [1]. Compared to patients receiving infliximab alone, patients with complex perianal disease who had an exam under anesthesia prior to infliximab infusions had a better initial response (100% vs.82.6%,$p = 0.014$), lower recurrence rate (44% vs. 79%, $p = 0.001$), and longer time to recurrence (13.5 months vs. 3.6 months, $p = 0.0001$) [2]. A recent systematic review of existing literature comparing combined medical and surgical therapy to each strategy alone concluded additional benefit in

* Corresponding Author's Email: spatil@som.umaryland.edu

In: Surgery for Crohn's Disease. Second Edition
Editors: Stephen M. Kavic, Rebecca Brown and Kerri Lopez
ISBN: 979-8-89530-676-5

complete healing of perianal fistulae is gained with the combined approach [3]. Cooperation between the surgeon and the gastroenterologist can lead to improved outcomes in this setting.

The risk for postoperative complications in the setting of anti-TNF-alpha therapy is an evolving area of IBD patient care that requires continued collaboration of surgeons and gastroenterologists. Several studies have not detected an increased risk of postoperative complications with preoperative anti-TNF use. For example, a retrospective study of patients at the Mayo Clinic who underwent an abdominal surgery for CD found no difference in complication rates with preoperative use of corticosteroids, immunosuppressant medications, or infliximab [4]. Additional studies focused on preoperative infliximab echoed this finding, including a large retrospective cohort study, which did not find an increased rate of postoperative complications in patients on infliximab. However, an overwhelming majority of patients underwent elective, not emergency, surgery, and the overall number of surgeries was lower than expected [5].

On the other hand, some studies have detected significant differences in the rate of complications. In a retrospective cohort study, preoperative infliximab use was associated with increased risk for 30-day sepsis (OR 2.62, 95% CI 1.12-6.13) and intraabdominal abscess (OR 5.78, 95% CI 1.69-19.7) [6]. A separate study found that CD patients receiving infliximab within 8 weeks of an abdominal surgery were at increased of postoperative infectious (OR 2.43, 95% CI 1.18-5.03) and surgical site (1.96, 95% CI 1.02-3.77) complications [7]. Although further investigation in a prospective fashion will be required for clarification of this issue, it illustrates the interconnected nature of medical and surgical treatments of CD patients in the perioperative period.

The nurse can also play an important role in the care of the IBD patient, particularly in the areas of patient advocacy and education. As advocates, nurses help connect patients to resources that can assist them with the physical, financial, and emotional needs that may arise due to their disease. Frequent communication with CD patients is a vital part of their care.

A recent study by Ramos-Rivers analyzed telephone activity between patients and nurse coordinators in a busy tertiary care IBD practice. The subgroup of patients who generated a particularly high volume of telephone calls had increased rates of ED visits and hospital admissions in the ensuing 12 months [8]. These encounters represent an important opportunity for nurses to triage symptoms, offer education, direct appropriate resource utilization, reinforce provider recommendations, and lend an empathetic ear. A nurse specialized in stoma management can also be a tremendous resource and support to the patient and family after stoma creation [9]. As a liaison between patients and providers, the nurse is a crucial component of the multidisciplinary team.

Malnutrition is frequently seen in CD patients (see Chapter 4). The proportion of outpatients with CD experiencing weight loss has been found to be 20% to 40%, and even higher numbers (approaching 80%) are seen in hospitalized patients with CD [10]. Malnutrition has been found to be a significant risk factor for postoperative complications and for mortality in hospitalized IBD patients [11].

A Swedish study compared the outcomes of malnourished CD patients who received preoperative TPN to historical controls who did not receive TPN. Patients were on TPN for a mean of 46 days. Patients in the TPN group had statistically significant increases in body weight, BMI, and serum albumin. A significantly higher rate of early postoperative complications was seen in the control cohort compared to the TPN cohort (28% vs 0%, $p < 0.05$) [12].

Preoperative TPN and bowel rest can also be useful in the setting of penetrating phenotype CD. In a retrospective cohort study from France, 78 patients with penetrating ileal CD characterized by intraabdominal abscess and/or fistulizing disease underwent ileocecal resection. The inflammatory process in patients with intraabdominal abscess was found to be diminished after 2 weeks of bowel rest [13].

Finally, surgical intervention in patients with CD can put them at risk for nutritional deficiencies. Most commonly, terminal ileal resection can lead to B12 deficiency. Multiple small bowel resections can lead to malabsorption of multiple micronutrients, including B vitamins, fat-soluble vitamins, iron, and zinc. Clinical manifestations of these deficiencies include anemia, osteoporosis, hypercoagulability, and poor wound healing [14].

Stomates may require significant dietary modification to manage their output. In a nutrition survey, 82% of IBD patients reported problems with food and nutrition, and 63% perceived food and nutrition as "important" or "extremely important." On the other hand, fewer than half of patients had consulted with a dietitian [15]. Approaching these issues with the assistance of a dietician can result in more frequent screening, intensive management, and patient education.

Psychiatric comorbidities can have a significant negative impact on the course of disease, outcome of treatments, and quality of life [22]. As psychiatric disorders can often go unrecognized in CD, screening at regular intervals is recommended [23]. A patient-focused strategy, in which options of pharmacological, psychological, or combined therapies are offered, is preferred. While pharmacological therapy for depression or anxiety in CD patients is often initiated by primary care or even gastroenterology providers, there is evidence that patients are more likely to receive an adequate trial of medication with the involvement of a specialized mental health provider [24]. Establishing a consulting relationship with a mental health provider can help to facilitate the referral process [25].

Chronic diseases are often associated with increased rates of depression and anxiety, and CD is no exception. A large nested case-control study in the UK compared rates of depression and anxiety in the IBD population to those of controls. The rates of both depression and anxiety were 5 times higher in CD patients than in controls [16]. A large population-based Canadian study showed IBD patients are more than twice as likely as the general population to be diagnosed with major depression in their lifetime (OR 2.20; 95% CI 1.64-2.95) [17]. Levels of anxiety and depression have also been found to be higher in IBD patients when compared to patients with irritable bowel syndrome and colon cancer [18]. In addition, corticosteroids, a common therapeutic agent, have been associated with psychiatric side effects including depressive symptoms and mania [19, 20]. Psychiatric symptoms can also worsen in the time surrounding a surgical intervention [21].

The value of working with radiologists and pathologists with specialized training in or experience with inflammatory bowel disease can also improve care. Preoperative imaging is essential for recommendation of surgical intervention as well as operative planning. It can also offer benefit over endoscopy in some situations, particularly with impassable strictures, small bowel involvement, and extraluminal complications [26]. An experienced pathologist can also significantly influence preoperative planning and postoperative prognosis. In addition, the management of extraintestinal manifestations of CD may require the involvement of a rheumatologist, dermatologist, ophthalmologist, and infectious disease provider.

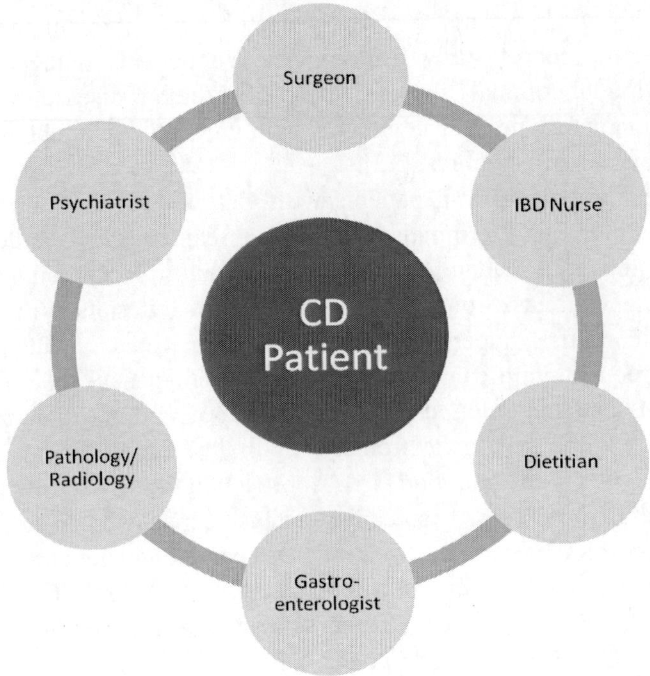

Figure 15.1. The multidisciplinary IBD team.

The multidisciplinary team can offer the CD patient a comprehensive, multifaceted treatment and monitoring plan (see Figure 15.1). Maintaining good communication between team members is essential. Regular multidisciplinary conferences to discuss complex aspects of care and invite new ideas and approaches can further improve provider relationships and lead to the development of a unified plan. Multidisciplinary clinics give the patient the opportunity to consult with multiple team providers in one visit and can build confidence in the collective approach being taken towards their care. In addition, these clinics can expedite multidisciplinary decisions regarding the care of these patients.

Postoperative Recurrence

Surgical intervention on complications of CD and medically-refractory disease can induce remission and significantly improve quality of life, but the clock for recurrence of CD starts soon after the patient leaves the operating room. Histologic recurrence in the neoterminal ileum after terminal ileal resection has been shown to occur as early as 1 week after surgery [27]. Endoscopic recurrence in the neoterminal ileum has been seen in 73% of patients within 1 year of surgery, and 85% within 3 years. Only 20% and 34% of these patients had symptomatic recurrence, respectively [28].

Exposure to the fecal stream appears to be a prerequisite for recurrence, as diversion by loop ileostomy above ileocolonic anastomoses has been shown to prevent recurrent lesions in the neoterminal ileum at 6 months. Endoscopic recurrence developed in these patients within 6 months of ileostomy closure [29]. For the 25% of the CD population with isolated colonic disease who undergo total colectomy and end ileostomy, ileal recurrence rates are lower. In one retrospective study, the 10-year cumulative probability of surgical recurrence in the ileum after total colectomy and ileostomy was 18%, vs. 34% after subtotal colectomy with ileorectal anastomosis (p = 0.03) [30].

Smoking tobacco products can have a dramatic impact on the course of CD. A meta-analysis from 2008 included 16 studies comparing outcomes of CD patients according to smoking status. Smokers are twice as likely to have postoperative clinical recurrence (OR 2.07; 95% CI 1.25-3.44) than nonsmokers. They also have more than a twofold risk of surgical recurrence at 10 years (OR 2.56; 95% CI 1.79-3.67) [31].

Multiple additional risk factors for recurrence have been identified. Perianal disease has been shown in multiple studies to increase risk of postoperative recurrence. In an Italian referral center cohort, only perianal disease was found to significantly increase the risk of clinical recurrence (HR 16.9; 95% CI 7.6-37.7) [32]. A history of prior intestinal resection appears to correlate with increased likelihood of recurrence after surgery. Studies from both Sweden and the UK revealed more frequent recurrence in those who had undergone a previous operation for CD [33, 34]. The length of small bowel resected may also have an impact on recurrence. A resection of more than 50 cm of small bowel was associated with an increased risk of recurrence in a Swedish population-based cohort (RR 1.4; 95% CI 1.0-1.8) [35]. Another study found increased risk of endoscopic recurrence with resections greater than 20 cm [36].

Other clinical factors have been proposed as risk factors for increased postoperative recurrence, but studies have been conflicting. Inconsistent data exist regarding disease behavior and risk for postoperative recurrence. In a 2008 meta-analysis including 13 studies from referral centers, penetrating phenotype was associated with a higher rate of surgical recurrence (HR 1.50; 95% CI 1.16-1.93), but there was significant heterogeneity among studies [37]. However, in a population-based study from the Mayo Clinic, risk of endoscopic recurrence in penetrating CD was found to be lower than that in inflammatory disease [38].

There is also great variation in conclusions regarding recurrence risk and disease location. In a Swedish population-based study, ileal and ileocolonic disease location was associated with a clinical recurrence rate of about 30% at 5 years after surgery, 50% at 10 years, and 55-60% at 15 years. Recurrence rates in isolated colonic disease were lower in comparison: 20% at 5 years and 35% at 10 years [33]. A population-based study from the Mayo Clinic, however, found no difference in risk of recurrence by disease location [39].

Histologic characteristics have also been evaluated for possible influence on recurrence rates. The existence of myenteric plexitis at the margins of the resection specimen was found to be associated with higher rates of endoscopic and clinical recurrence in one study [40]; however, it was not found to significantly impact rates in another study [41]. A meta-analysis including 6 studies found a decreased rate of surgical recurrence with the laparoscopic approach (OR 0.51; 95% CI 0.28-0.93), but possible confounding factors include patient selection for this approach as well as use of maintenance medical therapy [42]. A retrospective cohort study has found side-to-side ileocolonic anastomoses have a lower surgical recurrence rate than stapled end-to-side anastomoses [43]. Various studies are in disagreement about the influence of genetic and biochemical factors on recurrence rates [44, 45, 46].

Based on these risk factors, gastroenterologists can consider instituting postoperative medical therapy in an effort to prevent the onset of recurrence. The efficacy of available therapies to stave off recurrence is variable. Aminosalicylates have shown a modest benefit in this setting. In a recent met-analysis including randomized placebo-controlled trials, mesalamine did reduce postoperative recurrence at a 12 month or longer follow up (RR 0.6;

95% CI 0.37-0.88). However, mesalamine did not prevent endoscopic recurrence (RR 0.67; 95% CI 0.39-1.08) [47]. Nitroimidazole antibiotics (metronidazole, ornidazole) have been shown to significantly reduce both endoscopic and clinical recurrence in two placebo-controlled trials [48, 49]. Budesonide is ineffective in preventing both clinical (RR 0.93; 95% CI 0.40-1.84) and endoscopic (RR 0.86; 95% CI 0.61-1.22) [47]. Thiopurines also decrease postoperative recurrence of symptoms and endoscopic disease. The combination of thiopurine and nitroimidazole antibiotics has been proposed as another therapeutic options, but the aforementioned meta-analysis did not show a benefit of combination therapy over either thiopurine monotherapy (RR 0.54; 95% CI 0.12-1.59) or antibiotic monotherapy (RR 0.43; 95% CI 0.10-1.19) [47].

Anti-TNF therapy has been shown to hold significant promise in prophylaxis against recurrence. The first randomized placebo-controlled trial examining this issue was a pilot study of 24 patients. The 11 patients who received infliximab had a significantly lower rate of recurrence than the placebo-treated group (9.1% vs. 84.6%, p = 0.0006) [50]. A long-term extension of this study followed patients out to at least 5 years. The adjusted rate ratio for being in endoscopic remission while on infliximab was 13.47 when compared to no infliximab (95% CI 3.52-61.53) [51]. A subsequent study comparing infliximab to azathioprine for postoperative prophylaxis found superiority in prevention of histologic recurrence (18% vs. 80%, p = 0.008), but not in endoscopic or clinical recurrence [52]. In one study, adalimumab has been shown to reduce the rate of endoscopic recurrence when compared to azathioprine and mesalamine [53]. Anti-TNF monotherapy was the most effective postoperative prophylaxis when compared with other therapies in the aforementioned meta-analysis (endoscopic relapse RR 0.005-0.04; clinical relapse 0.02-0.20) [47].

Although anti-TNF therapy is most effective in preventing postoperative recurrence, universally treating all patients is not practical from a risk or cost perspective. Stratifying patients based on known risk factors for postoperative recurrence is the most reasonable approach. Higher risk patients are those with tobacco use, penetrating phenotype disease, prior history of resections, and short time from diagnosis to first resection. Lower risk patients are nonsmokers who are status post their first resection for short segment fibrostenotic disease [54]. Therapy should be initiated within 4 weeks of the surgery. Endoscopic surveillance should be performed 6 to 12 months after surgery, and endoscopic recurrence should prompt optimization of therapy.

Endoscopic Surveillance

Endoscopic recurrence precedes clinical and surgical recurrence, so endoscopic surveillance holds great prognostic value. Ileocolonoscopy is the gold standard for surveying for postoperative recurrence of CD. It also offers the provider an opportunity for intervention to change disease course. In 1990, Rutgeerts et al. described a detailed endoscopic scoring system for postoperative surveillance (see Figure 15.2). The absence of recurrent endoscopic lesions is scored as i0. Mild recurrence of ≤5 aphthous ulcers in the neoterminal ileum is scored as i1. Moderate recurrence, or i2 recurrence, includes >5 aphthous lesions with normal intervening mucosa, skip areas of larger lesions, or lesions confined to the anastomosis. Diffuse aphthous ileitis with diffusely inflamed mucosa is scored as i3. Diffuse inflammation with larger ulcers, nodules, and/or stenosis is scored as i4. Both i3 and i4 represent severe recurrence [28]. The Rutgeerts score on surveillance ileocolonoscopy 6 to 12 months after ileocolonic resection can predict outcomes. Severe recurrent disease at 1 year, Rutgeerts i3 or i4, is associated with a greater than 50% risk of clinical recurrence within 1 to 3 years [55].

Endoscopic Score	Endoscopic findings
i0	No lesions
i1	£5 aphthous lesions
i2	>5 aphthous lesions with normal mucosa between the lesions, or skip areas of larger lesions, or lesions confined to the ileocolonic anastomosis
i3	Diffuse aphthous ileitis with diffusely inflamed mucosa
i4	Diffuse inflammation with already larger ulcers, nodules, and/or narrowing

Figure 15.2. Rutgeerts score (adapted from Rutgeerts et al. Gastroenterology 1990).

While ileocolonoscopy is the gold standard for postoperative surveillance, it is an invasive and expensive test. Non-invasive methods that can act as surrogate markers for recurrence are being investigated. In a small prospective study, 13 patients were followed for 1 year after surgery. Fecal lactoferrin and calprotectin were checked serially throughout the study period. The levels of both markers normalized within 2 months of surgery. They rose with the development of clinical symptoms and with any postoperative complications. However, in a second cross-sectional cohort in the study, fecal lactoferrin and calprotectin levels did not differ between patients with and without evidence of endoscopic recurrence [56]. This finding is contradictory to a previous study which compared fecal calprotectin to endoscopic activity of CD, although not in the postoperative setting. A fecal calprotectin concentration ≥200 mcg/g had a 70% sensitivity, 94% specificity, 94% positive predictive value (PPV), and 61% negative predictive value (NPV) in predicting endoscopically active disease. A fecal lactoferrin concentration ≥10 mcg/g had a sensitivity, specificity, PPV, and NPV of 66%, 92%, 94%, and 59%. [57]. These markers may be valuable adjunctive tools, but do not appear appropriate surrogates at this time.

After laboratory markers, radiography exams follow as potential non-invasive tests to consider. MR enteroclysis has been put forth as a contender in a 2008 study from Austria. An MR score was developed to parallel the Rutgeerts scoring system, based on image quality, contrast enhancement, and mural and extramural bowel-wall changes. Comparing MR and Rutgeerts score, the mean observer agreement for the total score rating was 77.8% (kappa 0.67). When comparing only “high grade” (Rutgeerts score >i2) and “low grade” (Rutgeerts score <i2) scores, the mean observer agreement for the overall score improved to a rating of 95% (kappa 0.84) [58].

Small intestine contrast ultrasonography (SICUS) is also gaining popularity as a non-invasive tool with which active CD can be detected and measured. The utility of this method in the setting of postoperative surveillance has not been established. Findings representative of active CD on SICUS include increased bowel wall thickness (BWT), small bowel dilation, small bowel stricture, fistulae, mesenteric adipose tissue alteration and/or masses, and abscesses. In a prospective study from Italy, 72 CD patients who had undergone ileocolonic resection were evaluated with both ileocolonoscopy and SICUS 6 months later. Using ileocolonoscopy as the gold standard, the sensitivity and specificity of SICUS to detect endoscopic recurrence were 92.5% and 20% specificity, respectively, with an accuracy of

87.5%. The BWT correlated well with the Rutgeerts score [59]. SICUS holds potential as a non-invasive surveillance method, but further testing and extensive training of operators would be required beforehand.

Wireless capsule endoscopy (WCE) has also been proposed as a less invasive method of endoscopic surveillance. In a 2006 prospective trial, 32 patients who were status post ileocolonic resection underwent WCE and ileocolonoscopy within 6 months of surgery. WCE was inferior to ileocolonoscopy in detecting recurrence in the neoterminal ileum, with a sensitivity of 62% vs. 90% ($p < 0.05$). WCE did find lesions outside of the scope of ileocolonoscopy, but the clinical significance of those lesions is unclear [60]. A subsequent study found excellent correlation between ileocolonoscopy, WCE, and SICUS, with the exception that 5 of 22 patients could not undergo WCE due to stricturing disease (61). Further investigation is required before WCE can perform as a tool for postoperative surveillance.

Patients should undergo endoscopic surveillance 6 to 12 months after surgery. The Rutgeerts score can allow providers to make decisions on need for optimization of medical management and risk stratify patients for surgical intervention in the future. Further research is needed to determine if non-invasive methods can be used to provide prognostic information regarding postoperative recurrence.

References

[1] El-Gazaaz G, Hull T, Church JM. Biological immunomodulators improve the healing rate in surgically treated perianal Crohn's fistulas. *Colorectal Dis* 2012; 14: 1217-23.

[2] Regueiro M, Mardini H. Treatment of perianal fistulizing Crohn's disease with infliximab alone or as an adjunct to exam under anesthesia with seton placement. *Inflamm Bowel Dis* 2003; 9: 98-103.

[3] Yassin NA, Askari A, Warusavitarne J, et al. Systematic review: the combined surgical and medical treatment of fistulising perianal Crohn's disease. *Aliment Pharmacol Ther* 2014; 40: 741-49.

[4] Colombel JF, Loftus EV Jr, Tremaine WJ, et al. Early postoperative complications are not increased in patients with Crohn's disease treated perioperatively with infliximab or immunosuppressive therapy. *Am J Gastroenterol* 2004; 99: 878-83.

[5] Kunitake H, Hodin R, Shellito PC, et al. Perioperative treatment with infliximab in patients with Crohn's disease and ulcerative colitis is not associated with an increased rate of postoperative complications. *J Gastrointest Surg* 2008; 12: 1730-37.

[6] Appau KA, Fazio VW, Shen B, et al. Use of infliximab within 3 months of ileocolonic resection is associated with adverse postoperative outcomes in Crohn's patients. *J Gastrointest Surg* 2008; 12: 1738-44.

[7] Syed A, Cross RK, Flasar MH. Anti-tumor necrosis factor therapy is associated with infections after abdominal surgery in Crohn's disease patients. *Am J Gastroenterol* 2013; 108: 583-93.

[8] Ramos-Rivers C, Regueiro M, Vargas EJ, et al. Association between telephone activity and features of inflammatory bowel disease. *Clin Gastroenterol Hep* 2014; 12: 986-94.

[9] Lee DT, Choi KC, Chan CW, et al. The impact on patient health and service outcomes of introducing nurse consultants: a historically matched controlled study. *BMC Health Serv Res* 2013 Oct; 23: 431.

[10] Hartman C, Eliakim R, Shamir R. Nutritional status and nutritional therapy in inflammatory bowel disease. *World J Gastroenterol* 2009; 15: 2570-78.

[11] Nguyen GC, Munsell M, Harris ML. Nationwide prevalence and prognostic significance of clinically diagnosable protein-calorie malnutrition in hospitalized inflammatory bowel disease patients. *Inflamm Bowel Dis* 2008; 14: 1105-11.

[12] Jacobson S. Early postoperative complications in patients with Crohn's disease given and not given preoperative total parenteral nutrition. *Scand J Gastroenterol* 2012; 47: 170-77.

[13] Zerbib P, Koriche D, Truant S, et al. Pre-operative management is associated with low rate of post-operative morbidity in penetrating Crohn's disease. *Aliment Pharmacol Ther* 2010; 32: 459-465.
[14] Hwang C, Ross V, Mahadevan U. Micronutrient deficiencies in inflammatory bowel disease: from A to zinc. *Inflamm Bowel Dis* 2012; 18: 1961-81.
[15] Prince A, Whelan K, Moosa A, et al. Nutritional problems in inflammatory bowel disease: the patient perspective. *J Crohn's Colitis* 2011; 5: 443-50.
[16] Kurina LM, Goldacre MJ, Yeates D, et al. Depression and anxiety in people with inflammatory bowel disease. *J Epidemiol Community Health* 2001; 55: 716-20.
[17] Walker JR, Ediger JP, Graff LA, et al. The Manitoba IBD cohort study: a population-based study of the prevalence of lifetime and 12- month anxiety and mood disorders. *Am J Gastroenterol* 2008 Aug; 103(8): 1989-97.
[18] Kovacs Z, Kovacs F. Depressive and anxiety symptom, dysfunctional attitudes, and social aspects in irritable bowel syndrome and inflammatory bowel disease. *Int J Psychiatry Med* 2007; 37: 245-55.
[19] Yang Y, Lichtenstein GR. Corticosteroids in Crohn's disease. *Am J Gastroenterol* 2002; 97: 803-23.
[20] Cross RK, Lapshin O, Finkelstein J. Patient subjective assessment of drug side effects in inflammatory bowel disease. *J Clin Gastroenterol* 2008; 42: 244-51.
[21] Nahon S, Lahmek P, Durance C, et al. Risk factors of anxiety and depression in inflammatory bowel disease. *Inflamm Bowel Dis* 2012; 18: 2086-91.
[22] Maunder RG. Evidence that stress contributes to inflammatory bowel disease: evaluation, synthesis, and future directions. *Inflamm Bowel Dis* 2005; 11: 600-8.
[23] Caprilli R, Gassull MA, Escher JC, eta l. European evidence based consensus on the diagnosis and management of Crohn's disease: special situations. *Gut* 2006; 55 (suppl 1): 36-58.
[24] Wang PS, Lane M, Olfson M, et al. Twelve-month use of mental health services in the United States: results from the national co-morbidity survey replication. *Arch Gen Psychiatry* 2005; 62: 629-40.
[25] Graff LA, Walker JR, Bernstein CN. Depression and anxiety in inflammatory bowel disease: a review of comorbidity and management. *Inflamm Bowel Dis* 2009; 15: 1105-18.
[26] Panes J, Bouhnik Y, Reinisch W, et al. Imaging techniques for assessment of inflammatory bowel disease: joint ECCO and ESAGAR evidence-based consensus guidelines. *J Crohns Colitis* 2013; 7: 556-85.
[27] D'Haens GR, Geboes K, Peeters M, et al. Early lesions of recurrent Crohn's disease caused by infusion of intestinal contents in excluded ileum. *Gastroenterology* 1998; 114: 262-7.
[28] Rutgeerts P, Geboes K, Vantrappen G, et al. Predictability of the postoperative course of Crohn's disease. *Gastroenterology* 1990; 99: 956-63.
[29] Rutgeerts P, Geboes K, Peeters M, et al. Effect of faecal stream diversion on recurrence of Crohn's disease in the neoterminal ileum. *Lancet* 1991; 338: 771-4.
[30] Yamamoto T, Keighley MR. Fate of the rectum and ileal recurrences after total colectomy for Crohn's disease. *World J Surg* 2000; 24: 125-9.
[31] Reese GE, Nanidis T, Borysiewicz C, et al. The effect of smoking after surgery for Crohn's disease: a meta-analysis of observational studies. *In J Colorectal Dis* 2008; 23: 1213-21.
[32] Parente F, Sampietro GM, Molteni M, et al. Behaviour of the bowel wall during the first year after surgery is a strong predictor of symptomatic recurrence of Crohn's disease: a prospective study. *Aliment Pharmacol Ther* 2004; 20: 959-68.
[33] Hellers G. Crohn's disease in Stockholm County 1955-1974. A study of epidemiology, results of surgical treatment and long-term prognosis. *Acta Chir Scand Suppl* 1079; 490: 1-84.
[34] Ng SC, Lied GA, Arebi N, et al. Clinical and surgical recurrence of Crohn's disease after ileocolonic resection in a specialist unit. *Eur J Gastroenterol Hepatol* 2009. 21: 551-7.
[35] Bernell O, Lapidus A, Hellers G. Risk factors for surgery and recurrence in 907 patients with primary ileocaecal Crohn's disease. *Br J Surg* 2000; 87: 1697-1701.
[36] Welsch T, Hinz U, Loffler T, et al. Early re-laparotomy for post-operative complications is a significant risk factor for recurrence after ileocaecal resection for Crohn's disease. *Int J Colorectal Dis* 2007; 22: 1043-9.

[37] Simillis C, Yamamoto T, Reese GE, et al. A meta-analysis comparing incidence of recurrence and indication for reoperation after surgery for perforating versus nonperforating Crohn's disease. *Am J Gastroenterol* 2008; 103: 196-205.

[38] Peyrin-Biroulet L, Loftus EV, Zinsmeister A, et al. Postoperative recurrence of Crohn's disease in a population-based cohort. (abstracts 1183). *Dig Dis Week New Orleans* 2010; 138: S198-9.

[39] Agrez MV, Valente RM, Pierce W, et al. Surgical history of Crohn's disease in a well-defined population. *Mayo Clin Proc* 1982; 57: 747-52.

[40] Sokol H, Polin V, Lavergne-Slove A, et al. Plexitis as a predictive factory of early postoperative clinical recurrence in Crohn's disease. Gut 2009; 58: 1218-25.

[41] Ng SC, Lied GA, Kamm MA, et al. Predictive value and clinical significance of myenteric plexitis in Crohn's disease. *Inflamm Bowel Dis* 2009; 15: 1499-507.

[42] Rosman AS, Melis M, Fichera A. Metaanalysis of trials comparing laparoscopic and open surgery for Crohn's disease. *Surg Endosc* 2005; 19: 1549-55.

[43] Scarpa M, Ruffolo C, Bertin E, et al. Surgical predictors of recurrence of Crohn's disease after ileocolonic resection. *Int J Colorectal Dis* 2007; 11: 1061-9.

[44] Buning C, Genschel J, Buhner S, et al. Mutations in the NOD2/CARD15 gene in Crohn's disease are associated with ileocecal resection and are a risk factor for reoperation. *Aliment Pharmacol Ther* 2004; 19: 1073-8.

[45] Maconi G, Colombo E, Sampietro GM, et al. CARD15 gene variants and risk of reoperation in Crohn's disease patients. *Am J Gastroenterol* 2009; 104: 2483-91.

[46] Caprilli R, Corrao G, Taddei G, et al. Prognostic factors for postoperative recurrence of Crohn's disease. Gruppo Italiano per lo Studio del Colon e del Retto (GISC). *Dis Colon Rectum* 1996; 39: 335-41.

[47] Singh S, Garg SK, Pardi DS, et al. Comparative efficacy of pharmacologic interventions in preventing relapse of Crohn's disease after surgery: a systematic review and network meta-analysis. *Gastroenterology* 2015; 148: 64-76.

[48] Rutgeerts P, Hiele M, Geboes K, et al. Controlled trial of metronidazole treatment for prevention of Crohn's recurrence after ileal resection. *Gastroenterology* 1995; 108: 1617-21.

[49] Rutgeerts P, Van Assche G, Vermeire S, et al. Ornidazole for prophylaxis of postoperative Crohn's disease recurrence: a randomized, double-blind, placebo-controlled trial. *Gastroenterology* 2005; 128: 856-61.

[50] Regueiro M, Schraut W, Baidoo L, et al. Infliximab recurrence prevents Crohn's disease recurrence after ileal resection. *Gastroenterology* 2009; 136: 441-50.

[51] Regueiro M, Kip KE, Baidoo L, et al. Postoperative therapy with infliximab prevents long-term Crohn's disease recurrence. *Clin Gastroenterol Hepatol* 2014; 12: 1494-502.

[52] Armuzzi A, Felice C, Papa A, et al. Prevention of postoperative recurrence with azathioprine or infliximab in patients with Crohn's disease: an open-label pilot study. *J Crohns Colitis* 2013; 7: e623-9.

[53] Savarino E, Bodini G, Dulbecco P, et al. Adalimumab is more effective than azathioprine and mesalamine at preventing postoperative recurrence of Crohn's disease: a randomized controlled trial. *Am J Gastroenterol* 2013; 108: 1731-42.

[54] Swoger J, Regueiro M. Preventive therapy in postoperative Crohn's disease. *Curr Opin Gastroenterol* 2010; 26: 337-43.

[55] Pallone F, Boirivant M, Stazi M, et al. Analysis of clinical course of postoperative recurrence in Crohn's disease of distal ileum. *Dig Dis Sci* 1992; 37: 215-19.

[56] Lamb CA, Mohiuddin MK, Gicquel J, et al. Faecal calprotectin or lactoferrin can identify postoperative recurrence in Crohn's disease. *Br J Surg* 2009; 96: 663-74.

[57] Sipponen T, Savilhati E, Kohlo KL, et al. Crohn's disease activity index assessed by fecal calprotectin and lactoferrin: correlation with Crohn's disease activity index and endoscopic findings. *Inflamm Bowel* Dis 2008; 14: 40-6.

[58] Sailer J, Peloschek P, Reinisch W, et al. Anastomotic recurrence of Crohn's disease after ileocolonic resection: comparison of MR enteroclysis with endoscopy. *Eur Radiol* 2008); 18: 2512-21.

[59] Calabrese E, Petruzziello C, Onali S, et al. Severity of postoperative recurrence in Crohn's disease: correlation between endoscopic and sonographic findings. *Inflamm Bowel Dis* 2009; 15: 1635-42.

[60] Bourreille A, Jarry M, D'Halluin PN, et al. Wireless capsule endoscopy versus ileocolonoscopy for the diagnosis of postoperative recurrence of Crohn's disease: a prospective study. *Gut* 2006; 55: 978-83.
[61] Biancone L, Calabrese E, Petruzziello C, et al. Wireless capsule endoscopy and small intestine contrast ultrasonography in recurrence of Crohn's disease. *Inflamm Bowel Dis* 2007. 13: 1256-65.

Index

F

G

H

I

J

L